Patient Z

STEFAN FRANZEN

Fulton Books, Inc.
Meadville, PA

Published by Fulton Books 2021

ISBN 978-1-64952-033-3 (paperback)
ISBN 978-1-64952-035-7 (hardcover)
ISBN 978-1-64952-034-0 (digital)

Printed in the United States of America

CONTENTS

⤳

LIST OF FIGURES

LIST OF ABBREVIATIONS

AMA: American Medical Association
APS: American Pain Society
AAPM: American Association for Pain Medicine
BPI: brief pain inventory
CARA: Comprehensive Addiction and Recovery Act
CDC: Centers for Disease Control and Prevention
CNCP: chronic noncancer pain
COT: chronic opioid treatment
DEA: Drug Enforcement Administration
DHHS: Department of Health and Human Services
DOJ: Department of Justice
DOR: delta-opioid receptor
FDA: Food and Drug Administration
KOR: kappa-opioid receptor
MAT: medication-assisted treatment
MEDD: morphine equivalent daily dose
MOR: mu-opioid receptor
MRI: magnetic resonance imaging
NAC: nucleus accumbens
NCQA: National Committee for Quality Assurance
NIH: National Institutes of Health
NSAID: nonsteroidal anti-inflammatory drug
OIH: Opioid-induced hyperalgesia
OUD: opioid use disorder
PCP: primary care physician
PET: positron emission tomography

PROP: Physicians for Responsible Opioid Prescribing
RCT: randomized controlled trial
SAMHSA: Substance Abuse and Mental Health Services Administration
SN: substantia nigra
TNF: tumor necrosis factor
VTA: ventral tegmental area
WHO: World Health Organization
WHYMPI: West Haven-Yale Multidimensional Pain Inventory

INTRODUCTION

⟨⟨⟩⟩

Patient Z did not start out as a pain patient. He was athletic and very healthy up to the age of forty-two. Then his life began to change. He never thought that he would take an opioid in his life. But when his health failed him, he had pain that could only be controlled by opioid medications. Years after that, when a pain clinic began the process of limiting his medication to the point where he could no longer function, he came to understand that the *prescription opioid crisis* is the most recent chapter in the history of mistreatment of pain patients in the United States.

The government caused the opioid crisis by literally declaring a *war on prescription drugs*. The Drug Enforcement Agency's (DEA's) *war on drugs* was a bad idea, and it failed more completely than any government program in the history of the United States. The *war on prescription drugs* that was born in 2004 to justify the continued existence of the DEA was an even more absurd idea. Now, the full power of the federal government was being turned against the people of the United States, not all the people, but against those who were most vulnerable and least able to fight back. People with chronic pain became the victims of the public outrage over the advertising and sale of opioid drugs on a massive scale. The DEA was the agency that authorized the manufacture and sale of opioids with ever greater production quotas. During this same period, the DEA declined to investigate the diversion of prescription drugs for illicit use by major opioid manufacturers and pharmacies. The DEA turned a blind eye while blatant criminals ran pill mills in Florida, California, and elsewhere for over a decade. Instead, the agency focused its resources on investigation and prosecution of small pain clinics including the few doctors who were treating people in extreme pain. Despite the evident massive diversion, policy failures at the highest level, and history of failed drug enforcement policy, the current drug problem has been blamed on doctors' overprescribing and the intrinsic addictive nature of pain patients. This was the reality that Patient Z came to understand merely because he needed pain medication.

Addiction is a word so difficult to utter that most doctors cannot talk about it openly with their patients. Yet the fear of addiction explains why pain patients are treated so badly. Many in the medical community are worried that pain patients who take opioids will become addicted or even that they already are addicted. We must solve the problem of the treatment of pain together with that of addiction. But how do we do this in a punitive society where the DEA sees opioid medication as an illegal narcotic and prosecutes doctors and patients alike for any perceived transgression? This is a multifaceted problem that requires knowledge of the scientific, legal, medical, historical, and political aspects of pain medicine to establish the basis for patients' rights. The undertreatment of pain is embedded in the fabric of how medicine is practiced in a patchwork of different offices with specialists who do not communicate with one another. The doctors who want to rise to the challenge to treat severe pain can easily find themselves without support, facing the Department of Justice (DOJ) in a distorted legal system where pain medication is classified as a dangerous narcotic. There are doctors who would like to help patients like Patient Z, but they feel that matters are out of their hands. There is not likely to be major change until the citizens of the United States realize that the denial of pain management care is an attack on patients' rights and that what happened to Patient Z could happen to anyone.

Since the government has set down explicit and implicit rules for opioid prescribing that have the force of law, doctors write in hushed tones in medical journals decrying the fact that they no longer have real autonomy to make medical decisions in the field of pain medicine. However, some doctors have begun to speak out on behalf of pain patients and medical community's responsibility.[1-3] While the petitions, letters, and policy analyses may receive a formal response from the government agency, they are being ignored by most of the pain clinics.[1] Unfortunately, today patients are left to fend for themselves by a medical system that is divided. The DEA looms in the background as a silent enforcer of a medical policy that applies to the entire population. The current policy on opioid prescribing in government agencies is based on the conclusion that "evidence is insufficient to determine the effectiveness" of long-term pain relief by opioids.[4] All prior studies were excluded from the final systematic review based on a new criterion that a valid study required a one-year observation period. This criterion is at variance with the Food and Drug Administration (FDA) protocols that always stipulate a twelve-week period of observation. To unilaterally redefine the terms of valid studies so that one can exclude all prior data is an unscientific and clearly biased procedure. Any policy based on such a procedure ignores the needs of the majority of patients since no effort has been made to examine their disease or the nature of their pain. Ironically, this approach is the opposite of personalized medicine, which is supposed to be the new trend in modern treatment. More seriously, ignoring the needs of individual patients by applying a universal standard makes this a problem in medical ethics.[5] Clearly the group of doctors, which has managed to impose its judgment on clinical practice guidelines should justify their decisive action. One justification of their stance would be to prove that opioids are not effective for long-term, persistent pain. If this could be proven, then doctors would be justified to arbitrarily limit treatment. To this end, the members of this advocacy group have reanalyzed existing studies using meta-analyses and evidence reviews after changing the basis of evaluation. Over a period of years, their conclusions became progressively less favorable to treatment of persistent pain with opioids.[4,6–10] That case would be greatly strengthened if it could further be shown that pain patients are prone to addiction. This is a second argument made by the advocacy coalition, not using studies, but commentary and analysis.[11,12] The academic publications were financially beneficial to some of the members of the advocacy coalition, because they serve as highly paid expert witnesses in the court cases against the opioid manufacturers.

Taking opioids, even large doses, does not indicate addiction. Addiction is characterized by behavior, and it has a textbook definition that involves self-destructive behavior as one of the most important aspects.[13] A *pain patient*, "a person who is genuinely in pain," *seeks drugs* in the same way that someone with a headache seeks aspirin in the medicine cabinet. The desire to alleviate pain is the opposite of a self-destructive tendency. Some pain patients need opioid medication, quite literally for their survival. Others may need opioid pain medicine to go to work. These are not destructive behaviors. The clinical data and neurophysiological evidence explain how and why a very small percentage of pain patients succumb to addiction. The vast majority follow their prescriptions. In reality, it should not matter. No one should have to live in pain. Until American society begins to treat addiction as a medical condition, a disease instead of a crime, pain patients will be suspected of addiction and will be treated as badly as addicts. To be in pain and be doubted to the point of being a social outcast is all too common a fate for a pain patient in the United States.[14]

Pain patients have faced a stigma throughout modern times. Chronic pain has been renamed intractable pain and is often referred to as persistent pain today to destigmatize pain patients. In the neurobiology and psychology literature, there is also a distinction made between chronic pain—which had its origin in a physical lesion that heals with time but leaves an intact neural pain circuit—and persistent pain, which continues because of an ongoing medical condition, an incurable disease, or an injury that does not heal. Not everyone makes the distinction between chronic and persistent pain, which leads to some confusion in the literature.[15–20]

The American Pain Society embraced a new concept in the treatment of chronic and persistent pain in the late 1990s that I will call the *compassionate care movement*.[21,22] Based on the success of opioid prescribing for cancer patients since the 1960s,[23–25] by the 1980s, clinical observations were underway to extend the treatment to sickle cell disease.[26–28] Clinicians did not downplay either the side effects or the potential for addiction in making these medical advances, but they recognized that opioids frequently are the only viable option for pain relief. When opioid prescribing was proposed for other types of pain in 1996, mistakes were made by the medical community, but also at every level of the government. The movement was hijacked. Because of the diversion of opioids for illicit use, corporate dishonesty, and aggressive marketing, the compassionate care movement led to a rise in opioid addiction; and the set of events led to a resurgence of heroin use and new use of fentanyl. The professional pain societies should have insisted on mandatory education for prescribing doctors. The overdose rate increased, primarily because of diversion of opioid drugs for sale on the black market during the years 2000–2010. The overprescribing narrative in the media, medical journals, and political speeches ignores the strong evidence that corporate greed and government corruption hijacked the compassionate care movement, permitting blatantly criminal diversion on a large scale. Instead, doctors and patients have received the blame for opioid addiction and overdoses. While doctors also made mistakes during this time, those who did were, perhaps naively, following both the prevailing medical guidelines and the aggressive marketing of Purdue Pharmaceuticals (Purdue Pharma), a small but well-positioned opioid manufacturer, which played a major role in subverting the medical focus of the compassionate care movement. The recent criminal conviction of Purdue Pharma for paying kickbacks to doctors to increase opioid prescribing constitutes diversion. The diversion through pill mills involved criminal distribution by people who had a doctor's license but did not have the minimum pretense of treating patients. Kickbacks are more insidious because they occurred wherever doctors were susceptible to the enticements, not just in criminal enterprises. These various forms of diversion were the major cause of crisis. Today, doctors receive the majority of the blame even though there is strong evidence of failures in regulation and enforcement at every level. Every stakeholder involved made mistakes, but assigning blame only to one party misses important aspects of systemic failure. While pharmaceutical companies are held to account in the courtroom, the press focuses on families who accuse doctors in cases of opioid deaths. The media most often fails to mention that millions of people receive pain medication through legitimate channels and many of them need it for their survival. The prosecuting law firms have no interests in patient's rights. They will make the most money by focusing the public rage against the pharmaceutical companies and doctors. It is in their interest to portray pain patients as addicts because it furthers the narrative that nothing good can come from opioid medication. The law firms are using their large profits to lobby Congress to preserve tough attitudes toward prescribing. Rather than simply prosecuting Purdue Pharma and a few other companies, their goal is to prosecute every opioid manufacturer, pharmacy, and professional organization. That maximizes their profit. They want to line up public and political support for tough prescribing guidelines to strengthen the legal case. It is irrelevant to them if vilifying opioids harms pain patients.

Appropriate policies would prevent opioid manufacturers from exercising influence on medical decisions, provide training for physicians, and combine pain management with opioid-use counseling. Doctors should be empowered to meet patients' needs with resources for pain and addiction services alike. However, these ideas have not been given serious consideration. Instead, the approach by the advocacy coalition has been to advocate for a universal limit on opioid dose and even limits on how long a patient may receive treatment. For someone who has incurable cancer, sickle cell disease, or an inflammatory arthritis, what sense does it make to limit the prescribing of pain medication to ninety days total? That would only make it available for terminal patients. Many pain patients in the United States who lack a terminal diagnosis receive substandard care. Nonetheless, the United States is also attempting to export their language and thinking to international bodies such as the International Association for the Study of Pain (IASP).[29] While some countries are receptive, most are rightfully resistant to follow the lead of a country with the highest addiction, overdose, and incarceration rates in the world, combined with a pain management crisis caused overly restrictive regulation.

The backlash against the *compassionate care movement* in the United States extended beyond the pharmaceutical companies, pharmacies, and doctors to eliminate any remnant of support for pain patients. For example, the American Pain Society (APS) no longer exists. The APS filed for bankruptcy in a lawsuit in 2019, despite the fact that it was merely a nonprofit organization to help doctors organize conferences to professional standards and patient relations, much like the American Medical Association (AMA). Many professional organizations went bankrupt in the series of lawsuits that followed the lawsuits against every opioid manufacturer, major pharmacy, or any organization in any way connected with the purveyance of medication to pain patients.[30–34] The advocacy coalition views any funding received from pharmaceutical companies (even for conferences or medical school education) as evidence of corrupt intent. The advocacy coalition strains credulity when they suggest that pain patients too have been corrupted by the pharmaceutical companies. While the media communicates allegations against pharmaceutical companies, pharmacies, and doctors, the DEA receives much less attention.[35] There is no call to scrutinize the agency despite its significant role in the crisis. It was supposed to be fighting a war on prescription drugs, however flawed that concept is, but instead the United States experienced the greatest escalation in prescription-drug abuse in American history. In fact, much or most of the abuse was a result of diversion of opioid drugs, which was exactly what the DEA was supposed to be controlling since its inception in 1970. Yet legitimate prescribing has been blamed. Using language focused on *war* creates enemies, rather than looking at people seeking medication as some of our society's most vulnerable people who are most often deserving of compassion.

The DEA has little incentive to concern itself with the consequences of its policies for pain patients, despite its mandate to ensure that opioids are available for medicinal use. While the agency pays lip service to the needs of Americans in pain, agency actions most often run counter to any expressed commitment to ensure that medications reach those who need them. Throughout the compassionate care movement, agency actions were harmful to many pain patients with the greatest need. Many of the doctors who prescribed to patients with serious diseases had their offices shut down by the DEA. Today most pain patients must go to a pain clinic that is beholden to the DEA in a more direct way than any medical clinic or doctor's office ever has been before. The less the pain clinics know concerning the actual limit that would trigger an investigation, the more fearful they are of overstepping the line. When the National Commission on Quality Assurance (NCQA) posted an opioid dose as a quality standard on their official website, pain clinics interpreted that as a hard limit, a maximum dose that applies to all patients. Determining the appropriate opioid dose for patients with extreme pain is difficult and there is some risk, but it should be a medical decision. For that reason, the control that the DEA exerts might not have been possible without the help of a group of doctors whose interests as the same advocacy coalition that is working with lawyers suing the pharmaceutical companies. Chapter 4 describes the advocacy coalition called Physicians for Responsible Opioid Prescribing (PROP).

Media coverage of the opioid crisis has been focused on drug overdoses, the lawsuits against pharmaceutical companies, and scandalous cases of medical malpractice or malfeasance, rather than the plight of pain patients. There are a few stories of pain patients, but journalists frame the problem in a way that encourages outrage over the criminal nature of the companies such as Purdue Pharma and the pharmacies that sold opioids without explaining the context and need for opioids in medicine. The point that most doctors with legitimate patients have prescribed in a responsible manner is not news and so it is not mentioned in the articles. Many people have suffered because of the generalizations that have been applied to prescribing as a whole. To make it appear that all the problems arose mainly because of legitimate prescriptions is misleading and harmful to hundreds of thousands of people who rely on long-term opioids. The news accounts convey the incorrect idea that addiction is inevitable and perhaps the only expected outcome of opioid prescribing.[35-37]

It is important to explain why there is a different reaction to opioids between people in persistent pain and the rest of the population. In chapter 3, I will take the reader through the medical and neurobiological evidence that explains how a person in severe pain is physiologically different from a person without pain, a pain-naive person. Persistent pain activates the natural opioid system in the body, which also induces a high level of stress. Natural opioids activate the opioid receptors in both the spine and many parts of the brain of a pain patient. An opioid medication will further the signaling in these pathways that we can call a *pain circuit*. In a pain-naive person there is no pain circuit and no opioid receptors in the spine that accompany the response to ongoing pain signaling. Instead, opioids migrate directly to the pleasure center of the brain of a pain-naive person. Experiments based on neurophysiology, chemistry, and brain imaging provide evidence for the hypothesis that pain patients have muted response to opioids in their brain's pleasure center because the pain circuit dominates their consciousness.

In chapter 4, I show how the leaders of PROP ignored the preponderance of the evidence and argued that pain patients are highly likely to become addicts. Using their influence in government agencies, PROP intentionally changed acceptance criteria in order to invalidate all prior studies. This permitted a few influential doctors to claim that there are no studies that support efficacy of long-term opioid therapy. Irrespective of their motivations, medical professionals must base their judgments on evidence, clinical and observational studies, often summarized using two types of publication; meta-analysis and evidence review. In chapter 5, meta-analysis is described as a powerful tool, which summarizes the information in the medical literature for convenience of researchers and doctors.

Chapter 6 describes how the leaders of PROP systematically changed the conclusions regarding efficacy of opioid therapy in a series of meta-analyses and evidence reviews over the seventeen years from 2003 to 2020. The ethical implications are staggering, since this academic fraud also forms the basis for expert witness testimony against pharmaceutical companies by certain members of the advocacy coalition. Recent meta-analyses conducted in Canada[38],[39] and Germany[40–47] arrived at different conclusions based on the same basic data. Given the real-world consequences for millions of patients, this is anything but an academic issue. When a group imposes its idea of appropriate treatment with arbitrary limits on the entire medical community, it is doing what religious zealots do when they impose their belief system on others. In chapter 6 and the appendix, we examine the evidence that has served as the foundation for medical advocacy to limit opioid prescribing.

Today pain clinics are acutely aware of the regulatory climate and want to make sure that they never cross the line defined by the DEA. In chapter 7, I will discuss how pain clinics behave in a system where the DEA does not publish the limit for opioid prescriptions, but every clinic understands what the limit is based on other government agency publications.[48] The clinics know what is permissible based on state regulations, Center for Disease Control and Prevention (CDC) guidelines, and the NCQA quality standard. The implementation of these policies has been devastating since the authors of the new CDC guidelines in 2016 misunderstood the causes of the overdose problem and ignored the medical need of pain patients. Patient Z's experience with this type of pain clinic is documented in chapter 8.

Chapter 9 presents data from the CDC showing an exponential growth in overdose deaths over the past forty years. The claim that prescription drugs caused a drug crisis ignores the major drug crisis that has existed for as long as any of us have been alive. In chapter 10, I discuss how companies and government agencies subverted the movement to try to treat persistent pain. The consequence of their interference with a medical movement led a backlash that is manifest today in the increase in patient death from the health consequences of tapering (reducing the dose) of very sick patients, suicide, and patients who turn to street drugs in desperation.[49] In chapter 11, I address the myth that the overdose crisis is driven by prescription drugs. While prescription drugs did play a role for a few years and we should learn from that unfortunate experience, the overdose fatalities have primarily been from heroin and fentanyl for nearly a decade.[50] Historically, heroin addiction has been a significant problem. The reason that heroin addiction rates went down during the 1980s was caused by the rise of cocaine, not because of a reduction in overall drug use. Blaming prescription drugs and the pain patients need for relief for the illegal drug problem is unethical.

In chapter 12, I discuss the fact that there is a paucity of alternatives to opioid therapy for persistent pain. The notion that pain patients are clinging to their medication and refusing the alternatives is a false narrative. Electrostimulation and nerve blocks are among the only possible alternatives, and these are not feasible for most types of severe pain. Chapter 13 discusses the consequences of untreated pain, which can be as harmful as any of the side effects of opioids. Indeed, pain can kill a person, although it is not recognized as a cause of death. Chapter 14 is dedicated to the topic of opioid-induced hyperalgesia, a heightened sensitivity to pain observed in some patients who have received strong opioids like remifentanil prior to surgery and in recovering heroin addicts. While this type of hypersensitivity is observed in lab rats, there is no conclusive evidence that it is an important phenomenon in humans. Nonetheless, it has become a buzzword in pain clinics because doctors see it as a justification for reducing the dose.

Patient Z was unfamiliar with the way our society treats people who live in persistent pain when his journey through pain clinics began. He now knows that medical ethics support a patient-based approach to long-term pain medication given the scientific uncertainties.[5] Yet today more than any time in the past thirty years, academic medical professionals are making the argument that pain patients are likely to develop dependence and opioid use disorder.[10,51,52] These arguments are constructed on ethical quicksand because they are generalizations for an entire patient population based on woefully incomplete data. In formulating a response to zealots, science, clinical studies, history, and patient experience, each has a role to play in explaining the unique situation of a person in pain in our society today. Patient Z is not an addict, yet Patient Z needs pain medication to walk or even to stand. Is this dependence? How do the experts characterize a person whose body has been racked with pain to the point where he can no longer work and barely is able to walk? As the medical establishment inexorably takes what little comfort he has in life away from him, Patient Z has resolved to speak out. Many have spoken out before him, and it seems futile, but this is the only way that Patient Z can find any meaning in what has happened to him.

Patient Z's disease is inflammatory, debilitating, and incurable. Patient Z's pain is representative of the extreme type of pain that patients experience in a number of rare diseases. Although the diseases are rare, the total patient population in the United States is in the millions (parentheses indicate millions of patients in the US where data are readily available). These diseases include ankylosing spondylitis (0.7), reactive arthritis, rheumatoid arthritis (1.3), psoriatic arthritis (0.3), adhesive arachnoiditis, Ehlers-Danlos syndrome, lupus erythematosus (1.5), multiple sclerosis (0.4), Crohn's disease (0.7), muscular dystrophy (0.25), Parkinson's disease (0.06), uveitis (0.11), Sjogren's disease, Lou Gehrig's disease, fibromyalgia, and many others. Other extremely painful conditions include burns, and wounds of various kinds whether from the battlefield, industrial accident, or car crash. Any of these conditions could be as painful as cancer or sickle cell anemia—two painful conditions that have received authorization for opioid treatment, even at high doses. The point of listing diseases is not to rank them on a pain scale, but merely to say that each of the above conditions has the potential to be so painful that a person would rather die than continue in the state of pain. It is also obvious that I cannot list every single disease, so I mean for the list to include any painful condition in solidarity with those patients who are suffering. Each of the diseases has various forms, some mild, others serious. I am not claiming that five million people have such severe pain that they need high-dose opioids. However, an estimate of patients on high-dose opioids in Vermont can be extrapolated to approximately 360,000 in the United States as a whole.[53] Patient Z's pain is excruciating, and his experience is representative for this group of persistent-pain patients.

It is important to relate some of the personal experiences of patients like Patient Z as they confront the changes in policy and attitude toward pain patients. The news media are focused on the loss of life because of overdoses and the lawsuits against the pharmaceutical companies. There are far fewer stories about the plight of pain patients. The media should distinguish between prescription drug overdoses, which are a small fraction of the total, and illicit or street drug overdoses, which are the vast majority. But they seldom make this distinction. The fact that we seldom hear different points of view is not because the media are biased, but on this topic they appear ill-informed. Pain is a difficult topic and one that is poorly understood. Even some doctors, particularly younger ones, have been exposed to the viewpoint that nothing good can come from opioids. A half century ago opioids were universally respected as important medicines, while they certainly were always feared for their addictive power. The attitudes today are closer to the thought process doctors had in the 1920s, when opioids had recently been criminalized. At that time, pain patients received less sympathy or understanding because of the poor understanding of the causes of pain. By the way, in the nineteenth century when morphine was legal, it was widely used for pain, especially for end-of-life pain regardless of the origin. Today, we know more about pain, its symptoms, and we also have a lot of experience with what can go wrong with prescribing. Is it not better to take that knowledge and try to meet the needs of each individual in the best way we can, rather than implementing rules that apply to everyone uniformly?

We must distinguish between different origins of pain. There are tens of millions of people with low back pain and osteoarthritis without complications. Many of these people need some type of pain medication, but the literature informs us that a significant number became overmedicated during the decade 2000 to 2010, when prescribing was not controlled. The advocacy coalition to limit prescribing, known as PROP, appears to have this patient group in mind in their publications. PROP's journal articles ignore other more serious types of pain, and therefore, advocate for hard limits for all patients, regardless of the severity of pain. If they do not mean to do this, then surely, they must know that this is how their guidelines are being implemented in practice. The leadership of PROP should be aware that there are millions of people like Patient Z for whom opioid medications provide the only alternative to a life of misery. Patient Z's pain is not a transient discomfort that he can just push through. Patients like Z have pain that will never stop and will probably continue to worsen as their disease progresses. I find it hard to believe that any medical professional given the facts of a patient with ankylosing spondylitis would hesitate to treat that a severe case of that disease with opioid pain medication. Only in the event that a definitive study showed that the pain medication has no efficacy would they pause and think that perhaps it is not a good idea to treat the patient. The zealots have sown doubt in the medical community by attacking conclusions that have been in the medical literature for more than thirty-five years. Without a scientific foundation, they have created a narrative that opioids have no efficacy for treatment of chronic pain. This book does not advocate for opioids or any other specific treatment. Rather, the goal is to present evidence that the medical community as a whole has been prevented from exercising its collective best judgment because of corruption, political interference, and bias in the media. The circumstances that lead so many patients to difficulty are most often not because of their behavior or their disease, but rather are a result of advocacy by PROP and biased media coverage that features overdose cases and largely ignores pain management as an issue. Patient Z's experience gives us insight into how these various factors affect patients' clinical treatments.

CHAPTER 1

~⚡~

Patient Z Could Be Any One of Us

Sometimes life deals you a blow. Imagine you got very sick, so sick that you eventually could not walk and every move you made became painful. Then imagine your doctor, Dr. C, understood what you were experiencing, could see the decline in health, and believed you when you said how painful it was. Your doctor prescribed pain-killers, morphine and oxycodone, opioid drugs that you had only heard about in the media and regarded as dangerous. Your doctor explained that you should take these drugs to prevent the pain from getting out of control. At first, you were hesitant. It was not something that you ever thought you would need. But the pain really had become excruciating. So you took the drugs, and the pain became manageable. You discovered that at least you could fight back. Your life was not over. Then, a few years later, without any explanation, your doctor told you that you were required to see a pain specialist. The pain specialist was supposed to be the expert who would take over from the primary care physician (PCP). Your doctor only said that the expert would help you navigate from that point forward. However, you discovered that the pain specialist was not the ally in the fight against pain, which you had in your PCP. You did not realize what was really going on because your PCP was under too much legal pressure to explain to you that he was under investigation. He had no choice. He could not speak to you freely since you were part of an investigation. You did not know it yet, but you had become Patient Z.

Patients X and Z had the same primary care physician, Dr. C. Dr. C did not know Patient X well and had taken on the patient as favor to a friend who was retiring from his practice. Dr. C did not prescribe opioids very often. However, he had prescribed opioids to both Patients X and Z. Rather quickly Dr. C felt compelled to terminate care for Patient X for noncompliance. Soon thereafter, Patient X died of a heroin overdose. There were no prescription drugs involved in Patient X's death. Nonetheless, Patient X's family requested that the state medical board investigate Dr. C. The medical board is duty-bound to look into such a matter. The medical board needed more patient data from Dr. C to determine whether there was a pattern of improper prescribing. That is why they used Patient Z's file. They did so without his knowledge. The designations X and Z were assigned to the patients in the state medical board investigation. Dr. C had known Patient Z for nearly twenty years and had observed his disease progression. It was unclear why Patient Z should be part of the investigation, except for one salient point. Up to the point of the incidents described here, Patient Z lacked a diagnosis. A patient who lacked a diagnosis but received a prescription for a high dose of opioids drew suspicion. In fact, the ground was shifting under everyone's feet during this time. Patient Z was adversely affected by the fact that Dr. C had to answer to allegations, stop writing prescriptions, and refer him to a pain clinic. That was the beginning of Patient Z's odyssey. At first when very disturbing things happened, Patient Z was shocked and felt lonely. Being in pain and feeling helpless about it is one of the worst feelings a person can have. Slowly Patient Z found his way. I hope his story will help other patients who have similar diseases and confront similar adversity from a world of academics, government bureaucrats, legislators, law enforcement officials, and yes, even some doctors who simply have never contemplated the idea that people can live in persistent pain. Many of the diseases listed above take years or decades to mature. The people who have them could be productive members of society, have jobs or a family life, but they cannot do those things if they live in severe persistent pain.

None of us will ever know much about Patient X, Dr. C's other patient. But we can deduce that Patient X had a major impact on Patient Z's life. Patient X was now a statistic since Patient X died of a heroin overdose. Without his consent, Patient Z became part of the investigation into Dr. C's prescriptions of pain medication. Dr. C did what good doctors do. He listened. He believed what the patient told him, and he tried to do his best to treat the disease, which included alleviating pain. The fact that Patient X died of a heroin overdose, not of a prescription-drug overdose, should have been enough to separate the fates of Patients X and Z, but it was not. Patient Z was affected, not because of any fault of Dr. C, but simply because the dose given to Patient Z was high enough to warrant scrutiny. Patient Z knew that the medication was necessary. He had experienced pain strong enough to take over his consciousness, and opioid medication gave him relief. He did not yet realize that he had become a victim of the turmoil in the medical community that mirrored the reaction of the broader society to the opioid crisis.

CHAPTER 2

⸙

Patient Z's Painful Path to a Diagnosis

It took much too long for Patient Z to receive a diagnosis. The sheer number of different experts he was forced to consult was beyond reason. Health care was fragmented in different offices each with its own specialty, and he had to start over with each one.[54] Sadly, few specialists gave him any helpful information, and many of his visits were in vain. There was no evidence that the doctors communicated with one another more than to send the results of a test to the next office. Even office-to-office communication frequently failed; so that Patient Z had to get involved to ensure that his records were complete for the new specialist. The exhausting process of chasing after records took a toll on the patient. He would wait for months for the appointment and then have forty minutes in a new-patient visit to bring the new physician up to date by explaining his medical history. Explanation was invariably necessary because the specialist usually did not have time to read a file as long as Patient Z's. By the time of his diagnosis, the file was 180 pages of handwritten notes and bloodwork, as well as many compact discs (CDs) of images of magnetic resonance images (MRIs) and x-rays. Patient Z began to realize with each new, disappointing experience that there was no overview of the process. His primary care doctor was engaged and tried to help, but it was beyond his job description to organize the disparate information from the specialists who each had their own viewpoint. Dr. C was often disappointed and frustrated with test results and analysis he received from the specialists as well. Often the diagnoses of the symptoms made no sense. It was illogical to explain swelling in one leg by vasculitis in one vein when both legs were swollen. Clearly, the diagnosis would have to be that there was vasculitis in two veins, one in each leg. When Patient Z pointed this out to the specialist, he dismissed the swelling in the second leg as having a different cause.

Specialists often ignored Patient Z's questions or information and then would make a pronouncement about what was wrong, repeating what he already told them, as though they had some great insight.

"We need to determine the source of your back pain," the specialist expounded.

"For a couple of years now my greatest pain has been between the lumbar L5 and S1," Patient Z answered.

"Well, we'll see once the test is done."

Off Patient Z went for a test where they pushed an electrode into his back and cranked up the voltage to *simulate his pain*.

"Is this what your pain is like?" the doctor called out from across the room as Patient Z lay facedown on the bed, nauseous with agonizing pain.

"No," he said, "that is not the pain I normally feel."

"All right, let's try another position then, shall we?" the specialist said cheerfully, as Patient Z felt as though he were going to pass out.

Although nothing was learned on that afternoon, it gave Patient Z another setback. He took nearly a week to recover from the lingering throbbing in his back. On the next visit, a month later, the doctor told Patient Z with some fanfare that he had determined that his pain was located between L5 and S1. It would be pointless for Patient Z to explain to the doctor that he had tried to tell him that to begin with.

Over time, Patient Z's file was full of so many incorrect diagnoses and illogical statements that it would have taken a significant effort to determine whether there was any information of value. Perhaps some doctors assumed that the patient did not know what is in the file, so there would be no point in discussing it. Unfortunately, a medical file has no cover page or annotation to explain the main points of the disease. In all the medical visits, some treatments had marginal benefit. The well-known hormone prednisone alleviated some of the swelling and helped to calm flares to an extent. But prednisone is dangerous, and the fact that it helped was useful mainly as an indication that Patient Z had an inflammatory disease. Cortisone injections given by orthopedic surgeons over the years also had some benefit. Cortisone is also risky, and doctors typically limit cortisone injections to one every three months.

Patient Z did not overreact and did not have a trace of catastrophizing of his pain. Patient Z was empathetic and always had thought about pain and suffering of others when he was young and healthy. Suffering from a debilitating pain might make a person retreat into depression, but Patient Z approached the pain as a scientist might approach it. He documented the pain and the medications he took in endless notes. Although not a great long-term record keeper, he kept a careful record of what he took, what worked, and what did not work. He always had the relevant information at his fingertips. Before the illness he had a near-perfect memory. It was still above average even with the pain. But he was constantly questioning his memory now that pain had invaded his consciousness.

Data Collection Quantifying Patient Perceptions of Pain

Asking patients to estimate their pain should not be a substitute for a medical examination that tests for effects of high blood pressure, hormonal imbalance, and lack of sleep, which are objective measures of the ravages of pain.[55-59] Although used mostly in research, some elaborate pain questionnaires have been developed. The West Haven-Yale Multi-dimensional Pain Inventory (WHYMPI) is a psychometric method for obtaining a clinically relevant assessment of a patient's pain.[58] The inventory has three parts and twelve scales to estimate the impact of pain on the patients' lives. It includes the responses of others to the patients' communications of pain, and it also asks the extent to which patients participate in common daily activities. This method is validated for use in behavioral and psychophysiological assessment strategies.[59] It is deemed appropriate for its wide-ranging set of criteria that help a clinician to get a holistic perspective on a patient's pain. The McGill pain questionnaire has received wider acceptance.[60] However, many pain clinics do not even do a routine medical exam of the patient and they are unlikely to take the time to implement a fifty-two-question inventory. In the current climate when the goal is to administer opioids with minimum potential risk for the clinic, documenting the patient perceptions of pain may raise more questions than it answers. A large WHYMPI study of lupus, jawbone (temporomandibular) disorder, and chronic lower-back pain patients concluded that those with the autoimmune disease lupus had higher pain levels and greater activity interference. Of lupus patients, 88% could be classified as (1) dysfunctional, 14%; (2) interpersonally distressed, 28%; or (3) adapting, 46%.[61] These conclusions of the multidimensional pain inventory profiles for lupus patients are validated, based on external measures. Given the context of such a study, the obvious interpretation is that at least half of the patients in the study have poorly managed pain.

As Patient Z felt his pain increase, he wondered how bad it could get. He also thought about other diseases and wondered how much pain they caused and what medications they used. This is not the type of thing that you normally think about until you are in pain yourself. Cancer is widely understood to be a painful disease. For many years, it has been accepted that cancer patients at the end of life should have their pain alleviated by opioids.[62–65] For many cancer patients, the greatest pain comes at the last stage of the cancer. Later, pain experts concluded that cancer patients who are not in hospice should have access to opioid painkillers as well when their pain is sufficiently great.[66] The pain of sickle cell disease has also been recognized as serious enough that it requires opioid therapy.[28,67] However, many African American patients struggle to get adequate access to healthcare.[26,68,69] Obtaining pain medicine is particularly challenging. Moreover, there is a gap in the pain literature when it comes to autoimmune and degenerative diseases. They are less common than cancer, and they kill more slowly, but they can be as painful.

Cancer pain has been estimated using the Brief Pain Inventory (BPI). The BPI application to cancer patients is global. It has been translated into twelve languages from Greek to Chinese.[70] It consists of four questions on an eleven-point scale with a diagram of the body asking the patient to identify where the pain is located and then how much pain the patient has experienced at the worst point, at the best point, on average, and at the time of the inventory. It asks how effective medication is from 0% to 100%. Finally, it asks how much the pain interferes with general activity, mood, walking, normal activities, sleep, and socializing, each on an eleven-point scale. Although there are hundreds of publications on the BPI applied to cancer, there are only a handful in which it has been validated for noncancer pain.[70,71] There is even less study of autoimmune and other debilitating diseases, but responses from such patients tend to place their pain consistently in the higher range of the pain intensity, while cancer patients tend to show much more variation.[72] The mortality of cancer is thought to be the reason that society has permitted use of opioids for cancer pain.[17] Despite the similarity of pain levels, patients with rare debilitating diseases from cerebral palsy to psoriatic arthritis could live for decades, in some cases; it appears that society scrutinizes their statements about pain with more skepticism.

The Eleven-Point Pain Scale—All Earthly Pain on a Scale from 0 to 10

Patient Z is not the only patient who has questioned the validity of the eleven-point pain scale that physicians are required to use every time they see a patient in an office visit. Of course, an eleven-point scale is hardly subtle since the response from 0 to 10 could cover everything—from stubbing your toe to being burned alive.

"How would you rate your pain today on a scale from 1 to 10?" the nurse asks.

What is 10? Patient Z thinks to himself. *Losing a limb? Having a third-degree burn over most of your body? How am I to rate three rup-*

tured discs, bone-on-bone pain in the hip, and raging inflammation in my pelvis? Is that a 4? A 5?

If only Patient Z had understood the nature of the game from the beginning. After many years, a nurse told him that "if you say seven, they will give you oxycodone." That is the undisclosed threshold value, at least, for that institution. But Patient Z took the question seriously. Should Patient Z report his pain while sitting or while walking? If only Patient Z knew how much importance the doctors would associate to that eleven-point scale from the beginning. As time progressed, the nurses in the pain clinic would pull out his file and look at the numbers. If the recent numbers were higher than average, they would argue his dose needed to be reduced because he was suffering from pain hypersensitivity (hyperalgesia). If the numbers were on the low side, they argued that he was quite comfortable and so the dose could easily be lowered. No one was too worried about Patient Z since he had never reported a 7 or higher. The numbers could not vary by too much since the whole scale from no pain to the most excruciating pain was all in ten steps. Once, Patient Z rated his pain as 5.5. The pain specialist wrote down 5. Decimal places are not permitted on the pain scale.

Why isn't the pain scale logarithmic? We estimate earthquakes on a logarithmic scale, called the Richter scale, for a reason. Earthquakes can be large by factors of ten, one hundred, or one thousand, so a linear scale does not capture the proper range. Likewise, the severity of pain can cover such a range of different responses that linear comparisons break down. Yet the doctors ask for a response on a linear scale. There are many different kinds of pain. And finally, when pain is serious enough, a person cannot even answer the question. Pain does not follow the rules of rational thought. The metric is so unclear that it is practically meaningless, yet the nurse records the number and the doctor reads it on each visit. By objectifying the pain, the pain clinic staff can more easily dismiss it as not being too great. None of this changes the fact that Patient Z's rating of 5 means that he still has three ruptured discs, bone-on-bone pain in the hip, and raging inflammation in his pelvis. It also means he is not walking. If Patient Z takes a step, he should report his pain as an 8 based on my observation. Like many persistent-pain patients, Patient Z has been sick for many years, and the current state of his pain is the cumulative effect of years of damage and a gradual increase in the severity of his immune response.

Without a diagnosis, it is very difficult to find a physician who will take a claim of persistent pain seriously, unless that physician is a PCP who has a long relationship with the patient and corresponding trust in the patient. One possible theoretical concern has been raised by Melzack's neuromatrix theory[73] that a cluster of neural pathways in the brain contains the recorded memory of pain that can emerge later without an actual impulse. To what extent can a patient be replaying old memories of pain through associations? Because of addiction, doctors are skeptical of a patient's claim to be in pain if they lack a somatic or physical cause of the pain. This issue is crucial to patients who lack a diagnosis. This is not a problem with Melzack's theory, but rather with how clinicians view pain in a society where addiction is considered to be a major problem and opioid use can quickly cross the border from legal to illegal, even when the opioids are prescribed by a doctor. Melzack's theory can explain phenomena such as phantom limb syndrome that affects many soldiers who have lost limbs. Their brain still processes pain signals from limbs, and they are just as real to the patient as if the limb were still there. As Melzack points out, prior to the theory, such pains have been thought to be "imagined" by some doctors, and patients were sent to psychiatrists. Melzack's theory suggests that some alternative therapies may help, but he believed in the use of opioids when other modalities have failed. Melzack's gate theory has led to the concept of electrical stimulation of nerves using implanted devices. This is also a means of controlling pain today, but it is not widely used. Melzack has also pointed out that physical therapy and even acupuncture may help with the phantom limb problem. Finding a doctor who understands these issues may require a long search.

There are many physical symptoms of pain that these clinics could use to quantify a patient's pain.[74] Identifying pain biomarkers or other quantifiable indicators could be used to justify treatment. Medical assays for pain today can include micro-RNA, cytokines, and blood chemistry, including metabolomics profiles.[75,76] For many years it has been possible to detect pain by a physical examination of the patient, measuring blood pressure and adrenocorticotropin levels although doctors seldom use this information.[77] One can also observe tissue damage, swelling, and signs of restricted mobility. X-rays provide information on joint damage, and magnetic resonance imaging (MRI) has a range of applications particularly when contrast agents are used.[19,78–81] Trained clinicians know that inflammation most often does not show up in an image, and inferences about pain based on imaging are not necessarily accurate. For a patient with cancer, the progression of tumors and the location and type of tumors in different tissues will determine the level of pain. One has to take into account the patient's history to understand the pain.

The Subjectivity of Pain

It is a maxim of scientific investigation that no scientist, no observer of nature can be truly objective. The lack of objectivity requires each person who submits a scientific report for publication to demonstrate through extensive control experiments that he or she has thought of as many possible points of view and tested them using control experiments. One should skeptically challenge both the theory and experimental observations from as many different angles as possible. Once a publication is submitted, the reviewers of a submitted paper provide another layer of checking, intended to eliminate subjective interpretations of data. Despite all these levels of control, mistakes, incorrect analyses, and even falsifications are published quite frequently. There are strong scientific disagreements grounded in subjective viewpoints published in reputable journals. While these statements are true of all data-based science from physics to medicine, studies of therapeutic outcomes are subject to greater potential bias compared to studies of physical phenomena. Among the therapeutic outcomes, there is no area more subjective than the nature and intensity of pain. Although there are some pain biomarkers, we have no way to render pain objectively through experimental testing.

Perhaps the most direct view of chronic pain is obtained by research on whole brain imaging using MRI and positron emission tomography (PET).[82] Starting in the 1990s, the technique has been applied first to acute pain, which is more systematic in correlation between anatomical location of the stimulus and the section of the brain where changes are observed. However, the more interesting application for our purpose is to chronic pain. While there are a few common features to all kinds of chronic pain, the "pain matrix" is relatively delocalized over various locations in the brain, including the limbic (emotional) and frontal cortex (rational) regions. The intensity of spontaneous pelvic pain is correlated with the density of gray matter within certain regions of the right brain.[83] Other changes include a decrease in the volume of the learning and memory center of the brain in chronic back pain (CBP), complex regional pain syndrome (CRPS), and osteoarthritis patients (OA).[84] Dopamine levels are modulated in both a phasic (burst) and tonic (constant) mode.[85] The phasic mode is needed for learning.[86,87] Changes in dopamine levels induced by pain are associated with learning how to avoid pain. Microinjection experiments using antagonists and measurements of dopamine flux in the brains of mice using electrochemistry reveal that the reward center (nucleus accumbens) is also a center of learning behavior that will prevent or stop pain.[88] The role of the reward center of the brain in chronic pain has been shown by applying high-temperature pain stimuli to patients with chronic back pain while imaging their brains. The acute pain stimuli cause relief of the chronic back pain observed by changes in the reward center.[78] These methods are expensive, and it will be some time before they are routinely available for use to diagnose pain.[80]

Pain clinics do not use measurement science to diagnose pain, despite the fact there are other much less expensive physiological indicators than whole brain MRI that could be used to detect whether a person is in pain. Perhaps pain professionals should consult with dentists. Dentists will note the signs of grinding of teeth. An astute dentist will suspect that a patient is in pain based on the shape of the molars after the grinding motion that occurs in reaction to systemic pain. Or perhaps the pain specialist should consult an ophthalmologist to learn whether the arteries in the retina are showing signs of strain or even bursting because of the elevated blood pressure that accompanies persistent pain. X-rays and routine MRI can reveal damage to joints that are likely to indicate a source of pain, but the lack of a direct correlation between the imaging and reported pain is a commonly known problem. High blood pressure and abnormal stress hormone levels provide two objective measurements that can give an objective indication that a patient is in pain.[89–93] The stress response is very unhealthy if it is prolonged.

Relying on patient reports and experiences is anecdotal. Yet the entire field of pain management and all the published studies are built on data that consist of subjective reports of patient pain, if only in the report of a number on the pain scale. Not only is pain subjective, but the effects of opioid analgesics are also subjective. The doctors who judge the patient's responses are subjective. The judgment that a pain patient is addicted is also subjective. At this point someone with training in psychiatry might point out that we should use the definition of *addiction* in the *Diagnostic and Statistical Manual of Mental Disorder* (*DSM*).[13] Part of the definition is that "an addicted person is self-destructive"—the person is taking the drug despite the harm that it is doing to them. A pain patient needs the "drug" because it is the only medicine that relieves the pain and permits that person to function as a normal person. Yet many people today from the fields of medicine to law enforcement argue that high-dose opioids are harmful regardless of what the patient thinks or even what the effect on function is. People will argue that we must save the patients from the harms of opioids and that they do not realize themselves how much they are suffering because of opioid medications. However, if we examine some of the well-known cases of people in extreme pain who had very high doses of opioids, such as Sean Greenwood or Richard Paey, discussed in chapter 10, we can see that they were rational, loving members of families and had a reasonable quality life, despite the pain, as long as they had the high-dose opioids that made their pain tolerable. In many known cases, when the DEA closed down a clinic and denied such persistent-pain patients access to the opioids, those patients died or committed suicide. We will never know if those patients were on a self-destructive path since the process designed to save them killed them instead.

The doctors and nurses in the pain clinic never doubted Patient Z's reports of his pain. His function was also improved by taking opioids. Specifically, he could walk, at least a few steps, and he could take care of daily needs by himself. When the pain is too intense, a person cannot even manage to carry out those basic functions. Nonetheless, the pain specialists explained that they had to follow clinic policy, and that meant to bring Patient Z down to the level that the clinic had set, regardless of his disease history or what kind of pain it caused him. There are a million Patient Zs in America today. One concern that is used to justify these tapers is that patients are becoming addicted to their medications. Someone fears that a patient is experiencing a "high" when they take their medication. Patient Z will tell you that a pain patient who uses the drugs as prescribed experiences nothing like that high that they are projecting onto him. He feels pain relief. Many other patients have made the same observation.[94] The science of pain tells us that pain patients have a different physiology compared to healthy people. Moreover, their psychological focus is on their pain and pain relief.

Patient Z Obtains a Diagnosis from the National Institutes of Health

Patient Z's x-rays, MRIs, ultrasounds, and blood chemistry had excessive signs of degeneration, inflammation, and pain. For years as Patient Z shuffled from one specialist to another, no one except his PCP mentioned the possibility that Patient Z may have been suffering from ankylosing spondylitis. But Dr. C could not be sure and he was not a specialist, so he refrained from pushing the diagnosis. He did what the AMA tells PCPs to do and let the specialists do their work. The lead physician in rheumatology at a major university hospital pronounced that Patient Z had a classic case of osteoarthritis and that there was no evidence of inflammation. Patient Z provided the diagnosing doctor with a compact disc (CD) from the internal camera of the microsurgery on his back two years prior. He placed the CD on the desk and said, "The surgeon told me he could see extensive and severe inflammation in my back. The microsurgery footage is on this disc."

Dr. J replied, "I don't need to see that. I know what's wrong with you. You have osteoarthritis, and there is no cure. You just have to learn to live with the discomfort."

By that time, Patient Z was already taking opioids. Patient Z will never know whether Dr. J was referring to his reliance on opioids. After all, if his disease were osteoarthritis, many doctors would say that the pain was bearable and a person should not need opioids. At that time, Patient Z did not understand what effects drugs could have on different types of pain. The pain of inflammatory arthritis and similar autoimmune diseases are ameliorated by modern antibody drugs that block immune system signaling. Opioids can relieve some of that pain, but opioids are most effective for inflammatory pain in combination with one of the antibody drugs or equivalent anti-inflammatory treatments. For years, the specialists, including Dr. J, would not provide Patient Z any of the antibody drugs, which are the modern treatment for autoimmune diseases such as ankylosing spondylitis. The doctors did provide steroids and some drugs that have been used for more than fifty years to treat rheumatoid arthritis. Steroids, such as prednisone and cortisone, were once regarded as miracle drugs for the way they relieve the inflammatory pain of autoimmune diseases. But steroids are dangerous.[95] Their serious side effects include increases in cholesterol and blood sugar to the point where it can cause diabetes.[96,97] Steroids can cause bones to weaken. One simply cannot use them for very long or very often. Studies have concluded that steroids trade one serious problem for another that may be even more serious. Despite this fact, prednisone is still used, because the swelling and other symptoms of ankylosing spondylitis can be so serious in the near term that there is no choice. Patient Z knew that he could not take the steroidal drugs over the long term. It was not logical that Patient Z was given drugs for an inflammatory arthritis only to have the doctor deny that his disease was an inflammatory autoimmune disease.

Two years later, once Patient Z had his diagnosis, a different doctor concluded that a biologic drug was necessary. In the interim, by sheer luck, Patient Z became part of a study at the National Institutes of Health (NIH) in Bethesda, Maryland, one year after the misdiagnosis by Dr. J. The study involved clinical observation at the NIH as part of a large study on the diagnosis of ankylosing spondylitis. Apparently, there are different presentations of ankylosing spondylitis, and Patient Z's presentation was not a textbook case. Most patients present their first pain and disability in the pelvis as well as irritation in their eyes.[98] Patient Z had back pain for years, and many doctors had simply viewed him as a low-back-pain patient. Approximately 3% of ankylosing spondylitis patients presents their first symptoms in the lumbar.[98] In fact, some patients have a mild presentation of the disease such that it is not recognized until much later in life.[99] Patient Z's disease was at the other end of the pain-and-disability spectrum. During two days on the NIH campus, several physicians ran tests, interviewed him, and compared their notes to attempt to determine Patient Z's diagnosis.

The lead investigator, Dr. K, was frank about the fact that his interest was in the epidemiology of ankylosing spondylitis. Dr. K had suspected Patient Z had ankylosing spondylitis just from the symptoms he learned about over the phone in conversations leading up to the invitation. The NIH did not see patients, but they provided medical services to make a diagnosis as part of a study. Patient Z was added to the observational study. The tests and medical discussions were free of charge, and the patient may receive a diagnosis with the understanding that the doctors at the NIH were only interested in understanding the larger context of a disease. Dr. K was sympathetic and had a good bedside manner, but he also had a job to do. He was trying to understand how to diagnose the disease in the population as a whole. Given how Patient Z had suffered from incorrect diagnoses for many years, he was more than happy to participate in any learning process that helped Dr. K understand his condition. If his participation could help other patients, it gave him a sense of purpose. It also helped to know that he was not alone. During the two-day visit, the team of doctors confirmed a diagnosis of ankylosing spondylitis, an aggressive incurable autoimmune disease. However, any diagnosis was better than feeling your life fall apart with a reason or a name to call it.[100,101] Ankylosing spondylitis has an incidence of approximately 0.2% of the population, meaning it afflicts two people per thousand. With a diagnosis in hand, Patient Z was able to obtain the biologic drug that Dr. J had previously refused to prescribe. After some time, the biologic drug began to work. It reduced the inflammation and reduced his pain level. But he still had some inflammation and extensive damage to his back and neck, as well as many joints, knees, hips, shoulders, and tendons. Still, when you feel pain in so many places, any significant reduction in pain provides a wave of relief.

The treatment of autoimmune diseases has some relationship to the treatment of cancer. Some of the same medicines are used. One strategy is to use poisons that are toxic to rapidly growing cells. In cancer, these chemotherapy agents cause the tumor cells to die faster than the rest of the body. However, hair and the stomach lining also have rapidly growing cells, so patients taking chemotherapy often lose their hair and feel nauseous. The immune system also experiences cell division when it is preparing for an attack. Moderately toxic drugs like methotrexate stop cell division and growth. Methotrexate is used against cancer but also used at lower dose to fight autoimmune diseases.

The new class of antibody drugs is designed to intercept certain immune system messengers in the blood stream and block immune attack on a patient's own tissues. Messengers known as cytokines are released by the body's T cells (a special aggressive type of immune cell) during the immune response. The most common biologic drugs are human antibodies that intercept certain cytokines or immune messenger proteins during the attack on tissues. A recent editorial in the premier British medical journal, *Lancet*, refers to these drugs as a renaissance for treatment of ankylosing spondylitis.[102] Antibody drugs can have serious side effects in some patients, but when they work, they can be the most effective at slowing the disease progression. As long as the diagnosis involves an autoimmune disease, the treatment will likely involve similar steps involving prednisone, methotrexate (a chemotherapy drug), and eventually one of the antibody drugs.[103–105] Antibody drugs are expensive. They cost tens of thousands of dollars annually.[106] At maximum dose antibody drugs can exceed $100,000 a year. We cannot ignore that each of the drugs has a risk, and a small percentage of patients have serious side effects. But the reason Patient Z was denied treatment with these more effective drugs for more than a year was because he was misdiagnosed. Early diagnosis and treatment are usually important, and ankylosing spondylitis is no exception.[107]

Doctors deserve respect for having assimilated a great deal of knowledge, and the good doctors merit true gratitude when they analytically put the pieces of an illness together, almost like a detective solving a crime. When diagnosing a disease, doctors often need to look for clues, go over old ground just to make sure that nothing was missed. Just like a detective, they need to think about what question might not have been asked. Dr. K did this. It really was a bit like watching a movie to see him go through the notes to confirm that another clue fit. Like a detective in a film, he did not let on who the suspect was until he had the proof. Having witnessed this process of diagnosis, Patient Z expressed extreme admiration for the doctor who got it right. Health care would be greatly enhanced simply by the doctor and patient spending more time talking in the doctor's office, particularly for the diagnosis of severe disease. But time is money, and the trend is to shorten the time spent with the doctor as much as possible.

Ironically, the era of information has made us more isolated than ever. Despite the fact that doctors and nurses carry the patients' entire file and all data on a small laptop, so all information is potentially at their fingertips, the modern doctor's office visit is often spent largely verifying information or reporting the vital signs. For a healthy person this is of little consequence. But once a person begins to suffer symptoms of some kind of disease, lack of communication becomes more frustrating for the patient. Indeed, all patients would all like to know that their symptoms have a diagnosis and, hopefully, that there is treatment available for the ailment. Even if the diagnosis is bad, patients would rather know what they are facing. Pain is highest on the list of symptoms that cause frustration for patients. Pain is also the primary reason that patients decide to go see a doctor.

Patient Z Confronts the Reality of Persistent Pain

The process used by doctors to arrive at a diagnosis and manner in which they proceed to analyze the treatment options are crucial to the determination whether the patient will be eligible for expensive new-generation medications, such as biologic drugs and opioid painkillers. For all rheumatologic conditions, the quality of a patient's life depends heavily on these two treatment options. The antibody drugs can alleviate a certain kind of systemic pain, the pain of inflammation. They can also slow the disease progression and prolong a patient's life span as well as the functional life of joints and tissues. However, joint damage and systemic problems of swelling bring on a pain that is not relieved by the antibody drugs. American medicine most often separates the decision to treat with antibody drugs from the decision to treat with opioid pain management. In the case of ankylosing spondylitis, the former is determined by a rheumatologist, and the latter by a pain specialist. In theory, these two doctors should have close cooperation, but this rarely occurs. In practice, the modern pain clinic is a thinly disguised opioid dispensary with a legal mandate to restrict the prescription amounts regardless of the severity of the pain a patient feels. This is one more example of fragmentation of care, but it is specifically because of the attitudes and fears that accompany prescribing opioids.[108]

Because the inflammatory condition presented in his back, the first doctors Patient Z saw treated him for back pain because of lumbago, then a slipped disc and finally a ruptured disc in his back. For years, doctors could only see him as a patient with low-back pain. In the world of pain management, back pain is one of the common reasons for an opioid prescription and therefore perhaps one of the most suspect. Patient Z never asked for opioids. He never considered the idea of taking opioids on a regular basis. He rejected the idea as something he would never do. However, Dr. C realized that Patient Z had more than simple back pain. He had several ruptured discs and joint pain in his pelvis and hips that went unrecognized for many years as a part of the same illness. Those events were the beginning of a disease that is frightful in the way it destroys the discs in the spine, but also the hips, neck, and finally various organs in the end stage. The disease can cause internal pressure because of extreme swelling. Although it is commonly accepted that cancer can be extremely painful,[24] there is much less awareness of the pain of inflammation despite the fact that millions of Americans suffer from inflammation of various kinds. Ankylosing spondylitis is known for being a particularly painful condition. Depending on the specifics of the case, these diseases can be more painful than cancer.

How can one evaluate how painful the disease is? Patient Z's x-rays and magnetic resonance images (MRIs) showed disease progression. The spine and all his joints had completely lost the cushioning from discs and cartilage. One must also bear in mind that inflammatory diseases sometimes show little change on radiography despite disease progression. Even in Patient Z's case, the changes were subtle and had caused doctors to call the disease "stable." Some doctors suggested that Patient Z's pain was under control. These pronouncements showed a profound misunderstanding of the nature of inflammatory pain and the progression of ankylosing spondylitis. Anyone who watched Patient Z walk could tell he was in great pain. It took him thirty seconds to stand up from a chair. He did so by pushing with one hand off the chair and holding on to a cane with the other hand. He was not stable on his feet, because he had to adjust to the agonizing pain of standing. He made involuntary sounds and winced as he approached a hunched standing position. Yet the staff of the pain clinic never did a physical examination to observe his physical disability or pain in movement. They would come into the consultation room after Patient Z was seated. While seated he appeared to be a healthy man with good skin and no outward signs of disease. That view was completely deceptive. Patient Z's spine had partially fused and his joints were destroyed. Doctors had recommended knee, hip, and shoulder replacements. But his level of inflammation was so high that most surgeons would not even consider operating. He had one knee replacement done, but the pain was greater after the operation.

Comparing Persistent Nonmalignant Pain to Cancer Pain

Epidemiology is important for understanding the implications of a diagnosis. It is best to take a holistic view of in the incidence of disease since we are discovering new variants of existing diseases. Fifty years ago, many of the inflammatory forms of arthritis were not known as separate diseases. Many of them were known as rheumatoid arthritis or lupus. Today, there are many diseases that have similarity to these, but differ in details. Obviously, a rare disease is harder to characterize because the patient population is smaller. The kind of pain and severity of the symptoms in ankylosing spondylitis are common to a patient population of nearly seven hundred thousand people, with variations in symptoms that include lymphedema and arthritis in joints. All the inflammatory autoimmune diseases can be painful, but ankylosing spondylitis is known to be especially painful because of the extent of degeneration in the back. Taken together, inflammatory forms of arthritis are a significant reason for loss of quality of life and pain for more than four million people.[109,110] Adding one million patients who have other rare degenerative diseases, we estimate that five million patients suffer from either autoimmune or degenerative diseases. To put this number in perspective, we can compare that the approximately two million new cases of cancer per year in the United States. Today many of these cancers are treatable. Great progress has been made with some cancers, and others are still terminal diseases. Despite the progress, more than seven hundred thousand people die of cancer annually. The cumulative impact of cancer is greater on the population, but if we look at the steady state population of people living with an incurable disease, a deteriorating quality of life, and moderate to severe pain, then autoimmune and rare genetic diseases account for a greater number of pain patients than cancer patients.

The medical community has long acknowledged that palliative care (terminal or end-of-life care) should include pain medication at a dose that gives comfort to cancer patients.[24] At first, the duration was up to six months, the typical term of a hospice, but not for any longer-term care. As cancer treatment has evolved and more cancer patients survive, there are also patients who suffer cancer pain but are not near death. Cancer also has a large component of inflammatory pain.[854] The mortality of cancer is greater than that of autoimmune diseases, but the types of pain have more similarities than is commonly understood. Pressure from tumors and pressure from swelling in autoimmune responses can be similar. Inflammatory pain is a matter of degree, and it is systemic and aggressive in many autoimmune diseases, just as it is in cancer. There is a policy initiative to make it acceptable to prescribe opioids for nonterminal cancer and even serious noncancer diagnoses in a palliative care setting, depending on the severity of the disease progression. Patient Z's pain intensity rivals some end-stage cancers, but the disease progression is slow. Ankylosing spondylitis can be so painful that a patient cannot walk or carry out normal daily activities because of pain. Although federal laws, such as the CARA law of 2016 discussed in chapter 3, state that palliative care should be expanded to include many types of serious conditions, in practice, most of the providers are still working in the older model of cancer end-of-life care. Even when accepted into palliative care, nonterminal patients still face hurdles to having their pain treated. The climate is so restrictive that even palliative care professionals must proceed with great deference to the limits placed by current policy. To be sure, uncontrolled escalation of opioid treatment is not a solution to pain management. Doctors and nurses should practice opioid rotation more routinely to keep doses as low as reasonable. However, it is not acceptable that patients should live in constant, debilitating pain, which is the current reality for far too many pain patients. Much of the pain literature discusses titrating the dose to the pain, which means increasing the dose until the pain is tolerable. The subjectivity of pain leaves the meaning of tolerable open to interpretation.

Patient Z Accepts Opioid Therapy

One striking observation of the NIH diagnosis is how many different ways the diagnosis described Patient Z's condition as "painful." Joint damage is clearly painful because of the mechanical aspects—the loss of cushioning; and the spurs, tears, and other physical degradation in the back that can be observed in x-rays and MRIs. A patient with an inflammatory arthritis or a rheumatologic condition has occasional spikes in immune-system activity known as flares. The pain of inflammatory flares may be worse than joint or bone pain, and yet it does not show up on an image. Dr. C recognized that despite his inability to prescribe the drugs to fight inflammation, he could treat Patient Z's pain. When Patient Z's pain began to become intolerable, Patient Z was initially reluctant to take any kind of painkiller beyond over-the-counter analgesics such as ibuprofen or acetaminophen. The idea of taking any type of opioid was so foreign to him that all he could think of was the social stigma and the risk of addiction or other bad side effects he had heard about. These risks were what he had heard of through word of mouth and information on the internet and the news. However, his pain was becoming overwhelming. His legs would swell, and the pressure caused extreme discomfort. Patient Z was having great difficulty sleeping and increasing difficulty in walking, both of which are known to accompany the progression of inflammatory spine diseases.[111] His lack of sleep was so serious that he was at risk of falling or burning himself. He could fall asleep in the shower or while holding a hot cup of coffee because he had missed so many nights of sleep because of the pain. He finally relented and began taking the drugs that Dr. C prescribed. He began to feel some relief. He was able to walk again, enjoy a movie, and sleep through the night. His mood improved dramatically. What would have happened if Patient Z had gone to a modern pain clinic with the same circumstance, no diagnosis, and a set of extremely painful but seemingly unrelated conditions in his back, hips, and legs? The lack of a diagnosis alone would have made it difficult for him to get long-term treatment. Current regulations would limit his dose to far lower than what he has had for the past decade.

Although Patient Z lacked a diagnosis, Dr. C gradually increased the opioid dose while having monthly conversations with Patient Z about his pain. Dr. C ended up prescribing a relatively high dose of opioid painkillers because he recognized that Patient Z had a severe illness. Perhaps treatments could alleviate some of the inflammation and joint replacements might help Patient Z to walk again. But he was in great pain. He knew Patient Z very well, and he had confidence that he would take the drugs as prescribed. Dr. C started treating Patient Z with tramadol. Tramadol is approximately ten times weaker than morphine. For years tramadol was considered nonaddictive and had a class V designation. However, because of observed behavior patterns of users, and lobbying by an advocacy coalition, tramadol was reclassified as a class IV drug, making it a controlled substance.[112] Dr. C added morphine and then added oxycodone to his pain treatment plan because he could see that he still felt significant pain on tramadol. Gradually he increased his dose to 420 morphine milligram equivalents daily dose (MEDD), which was in the range of doses given to intractable pain patients with severe pain for many years. Twenty years ago, the borderline from a moderate to a high dose was considered to be 200 MEDD.[113,114] Some cancer patients receive more than 1000 MEDD.[855] The point is not to advocate for higher doses but to observe that patients have gotten pain relief from higher doses when warranted by their condition. These doses should not be discounted from the outset, as they would be today, but rather, we need a rational and personalized plan to treat pain.

Anyone who observed Patient Z's condition would have agreed that he was in extreme pain. His response to the opioid medications was good. The dose made him functional again despite having raging inflammation and systemic pain. Patient Z briefly went through a phase where he had the stereotypical grogginess or lack of mental acuity that many people believe is associated with opioid use. Although, it was never clear to him if he was just sleepy, and for the first time in many years, he felt comfortable enough to sleep. After a short adjustment that lasted a few weeks, he adapted. Once he had adjusted to the dose, no one who spoke with him would have known that he was taking opioids. On the contrary, without the opioids he was often not able to articulate well or to focus on even simple tasks because of lack of sleep or sheer pain. With opioid medication, he had begun to act like his normal self again because he could sleep and had some level of comfort.

Inflammation is one of the hallmarks of autoimmune diseases. In the case of ankylosing spondylitis, inflammation causes degradation of joints and connective tissue; and, in some patients, the swelling can be more extreme than a sprained ankle and may be because of a similar physical reaction to damage caused by the autoimmune attack. Unlike a sprained ankle, the swelling never subsides unless medication can control the immune response. Sometimes the swelling gets so severe that the skin splits open and wounds can form. Only the most uncompassionate doctor could examine Patient Z and fail to conclude that he must be in serious pain. However, those wounds and the oozing and festering were all inside the bandages on his arms and legs that were not visible as he sat in the office. He wore a long-sleeved shirt and long light trousers so that he looked relatively normal as he sat in the doctor's office. Appearances were deceiving in his case, and perhaps that was to his detriment. Ankylosing spondylitis is both painful and debilitating, which leads many patients to depression and suicidal thoughts.[115] A pain patient may be considered fortunate when some of the symptoms are obvious upon examination. The deformation of the back, extreme swelling, and discoloration of the legs were obvious if a doctor simply conducted a cursory physical examination. Of course, Dr. C had examined Patient Z many times over the years. Dr. C saw the changes, and that is why he concluded that Patient Z must be in great pain. But not all doctors took the time to examine Patient Z or understand the sources of the pain he felt.

One could contrast Dr. C's caring attitude with that of any of the pain clinics. Years later, after Patient Z had been forced to leave Dr. C's care, he had moved from one pain clinic to another because a shortage of rheumatologists forced him to change doctors three times. The pain clinics were separate but usually associated with the rheumatologists' offices. Patient Z did not receive a physical examination in a pain clinic until he had reached his third pain clinic. By that time, he needed help going to the doctor. Since I accompanied Patient Z, I went to the pain clinic and saw how they treated Patient Z. On one visit when the nurse made a comment about how Patient Z's pain seemed to have diminished and suggested they could further reduce the opioid dose, I pointed out to her that she had never seen him walk or seen the wounds on his arms and legs.

The nurse looked surprised. "Does he have wounds?"

"Yes," I replied, "he has had them for as long as he has been coming to this pain clinic. I believe it is more than eighteen months."

The nurse asked, "Don't they heal?"

"Usually they do not heal because his skin is also damaged and he is immune-compromised," I responded. "He has had several operations to obtain skin grafts or special cell preparations to help the healing process. However, new wounds form because the swelling continues, the skin expands, and blisters form. It happens constantly."

Patient Z was silent. He was stoic as usual.

The nurse looked taken aback. She had known Patient Z for eighteen months, and it appeared she had no idea that he was actually very ill. When she began to examine his legs and arms, she appeared very distressed. At least, after this experience, she treated Patient Z with greater respect. However, rules were rules. The clinic still was determined to proceed with the taper.

Understanding and Misunderstanding Opioid Therapy for Inflammatory Arthritis

People who knew Patient Z were extremely surprised when they learned he was taking high-dose opioids. It was clear from the comments that the stereotype is that opioids would cause a person to have lower mental ability and become passivated and perhaps incoherent. But Patient Z was mentally as sharp as ever as long as he was able to sleep. Since the increase in his dose was gradual, he had never had any sign of respiratory suppression or confusion. He had nausea from the pain, but the opioids relieved the nausea. Before he began taking opioids, he was sometimes in such pain that he would not lift his feet properly and he would fall. He did experience constipation, but once he found a proper laxative and began eating fruits and vegetables as a large part of his diet, that problem vanished. His blood pressure came down because of the pain relief. Patient Z had always been grateful to Dr. C for understanding what he needed during that particularly stressful period when he lacked a diagnosis. Patient Z said repeatedly that without those painkillers his life may well have ended there. He had no treatment, no diagnosis, and his day-to-day life was unbearably painful. No one seemed to know what to do to give him any kind of relief from any of the awful things that were happening to him. Dr. C was one of the few people in the medical community who gave Patient Z hope.

Although opioid treatment for severe noncancer persistent pain is still at an early stage, there is precedent in the medical literature for treatment of ankylosing spondylitis with opioids, such as morphine, oxycodone, or a fentanyl patch.[116,117] As is often the case, not all studies found efficacy,[118] but the majority did. Studies of treatments of rheumatoid arthritis using nonsteroidal anti-inflammatory drugs (NSAIDs), such as diclofenac, which is not an opioid, found threefold increased morbidity because of heart failure.[119] NSAIDs sometimes have efficacy that rivals opioids, but they are ineffective for severe pain. Many authors in recent years have focused on the side effects of opioids, such as nausea, constipation, tolerance, and addiction. The alternative medications also have significant negative side effects and cause more deaths annually than doctor-prescribed opioids. Pain itself also has harmful side effects and causes many deaths due to suicide or other poorly documented causes. While the debate over compassionate care continues, pain patients today have little hope of rational and caring treatment.[123-125]

The Opioid Crisis Catches Up with Patient Z

At the time he started prescribing opioids for Patient Z, Dr. C was acting in accord with State Board of Health guidelines that state that "the Board is aware that the undertreatment of pain is recognized as a serious public health problem that compromises patients' function and quality of life." Prior to the opioid crisis, doctors were being encouraged to prescribe doses appropriate to relieve persistent pain in accord with the above guidelines. However, during the seven years from his first opioid to the time he received a diagnosis, a change in attitude was swiftly transforming the medical community, medical policy, and law enforcement. As deaths because of opioid overdose rose further to unprecedented levels, attitudes toward opioid prescribing hardened. About a year before Patient Z finally received his diagnosis, Dr. C found himself caught in the middle of a changing regulatory climate brought about by a surge in public indignation over the overdose crisis. He had always put his patients first, and his prescriptions did not result in harm to any patient. Yet the punitive climate demanded some kind of action to appease an aggrieved family who had lost their son. It was a tragedy, but Dr. C was not responsible for the heroin overdose. During the investigation, Dr. C told Patient Z that he would need a second opinion to continue to receive pain medication. Dr. C did not even hint to Patient Z that he was under investigation or that his medical license was under any kind of threat. Patient Z was not even aware that his visit to a second pain clinic was a referral. There was no return to Dr. C's office after that. Thus began a process that would lead him to understand how difficult life has become for people living with persistent pain since the overdose epidemic began. He became what Dr. Thomas Kline has termed a "pain refugee."[121] His dose of opioids was higher than any pain clinic would permit in the new regulatory climate, Patient Z still had no diagnosis. This fact clearly hurt the evaluation of Dr. C in the investigation. Historically, doses in excess of 200 MEDD have been used for patients with conditions like Patient Z's.[113,114] However, the reaction of the medical board and the DEA had changed considerably because anti-opioid advocates had been given a free hand to reformulate the prescribing guidelines.

The meaning of the unit MEDD is that each opioid drug is assigned a strength relative to morphine. Using the concept of a morphine equivalent, the total daily dose of multidrug prescription can be calculated as one number. According to most US pain clinics and sources, one milligram of morphine is 1 MEDD, while one milligram of oxycodone has a value of 1.5 MEDD. However, the EU guidelines published in 2017 rate one milligram of oxycodone as 2 MEDD. This illustrates the subjectivity of the equivalency units, which has been noted in several recent papers.[126,127] There have been no studies to determine whether these equivalencies are accurate, or to examine individual differences in metabolism, the effect of body surface area, and so on.

Once the investigation was complete, Patient Z had to rely on the pain clinic for his medications. Without the knowledge of his personal history and understanding of his particular condition that he had from Dr. C, Patient Z became another statistic, another patient whose dose was considered too high by every pain clinic. Thus, he was gradually forced into a position where his life became one of constant pain. Our society had turned its back on a pain patient's human rights.

Patient Z Is One of Millions Who Respond Well to Opioid Therapy but Is Denied Relief

For many years, experts in the field of pain medicine had observed that there are many people with chronic illnesses who would benefit from opioid therapy. Cancer and sickle cell anemia are two diseases that have been accepted as being so painful in certain stages that opioid therapy is warranted.[28,67] Why have inflammatory arthritis, arachnoiditis, bone remodeling diseases, and genetic degenerative diseases not been included on the list of extremely painful medications? While autoimmune diseases are not as lethal as cancer, for the most part, they can be extremely painful. In 2014, a study was published on the connection between the pain and the inflammation of rheumatoid arthritis. The study used the temporal summation of pain scores and ultrasound Doppler activity as measures of pain.[128] In addition to the direct pain of joint and tendon destruction, there are secondary effects of the pain of inflammation such as hypertension.[129] Severe rheumatoid arthritis can rival cancer pain. Patient Z's condition is considered to be more painful than rheumatoid arthritis. Patient Z's disease is both debilitating and painful; unless he gets relief from opioid therapy he cannot function at all. He is in too much pain to stand. When patients testify that a medication has helped them to function for a decade, an expert's claim that the medication has no efficacy is puzzling. Regardless of the opinions of a few experts, there is an ethical requirement to treat pain, which used to be felt deeply by the medical community.[5,130] Yet today many patients remain in pain because of the policies imposed by the CDC with the DEA always present to remind the clinic director of the consequences of failure to obey the hard limits.

CHAPTER 3

⁓

What Your Doctor Never Told You—Pain Is an Antidote for Opioid Addiction

Opioids are the safest, most effective medicines known for treatment of acute pain.[131] They have low organ toxicity, and contrary to popular belief, and even to some expert opinion, they are "safe when used as directed."[132] For many years, starting in the 1980s, there was a growing consensus that those properties that were well-established for acute pain could also be extended to chronic or persistent pain.[21,22,133,134] However, the outcome of expanding compassionate care had unintended consequences because of the fact that addiction was not considered a central issue by the medical community or professional organizations.[14] Worse yet, a few opioid pharmaceutical companies had a plan to aggressively advertise the push of the product to expand their sales. Those companies hijacked all good intentions. While both chronic and persistent pain had been under-treated, addiction has been practically ignored as a social and medical problem, until quite recently. Even the Comprehensive Addiction Recovery Act (CARA) of 2016 allocated few resources to address the enormous population of users and failed to bring addiction into the mainstream of medicine. The lesson of the series of failed policies is that we need to have well-funded programs for prevention and treatment of addiction in order to make progress in the treatment of pain. Nonetheless, we should advocate for humane treatment of pain patients irrespective of whether they have a tendency to become addicted. Since the advocacy coalition that had written current medical guidelines had also suggested that pain patients were vulnerable to addiction, it is important to examine the scientific evidence to understand the effects of pain. This evidence shows that pain patients have a fundamentally different neurophysiology and neurochemistry than healthy, pain-naive people. This evidence had led many medical researchers to conclude that persistent-pain patients had a significantly smaller tendency to become addicted compared to pain-naive people. This important medical difference is either ignored or misunderstood by the anti-opioid advocates. The ethical consequences of this willful ignorance have been devastating to many hundreds of thousands of people.

There is one major, indisputable danger to opioid use. An opioid overdose can be lethal because of respiratory suppression. This has been known as morphine poisoning since the nineteenth century. It is reversible if a person receives an antidote in time. Naloxone, sold commercially as Narcan, is the current antidote. Naloxone competes with morphine for binding to an opioid receptor in the body responsible for respiratory suppression. Prior to naloxone, for the previous one hundred years, the antidote had been atropine, which is derived from deadly nightshade, also known as Jimson weed. Remarkably, pain is also an antidote to morphine poisoning. It has been known for 140 years that a person in pain is much less susceptible to morphine poisoning than a person who is not in pain.

There is a universal consensus in the medical community that a person who has severe acute pain needs relief, and most doctors would agree that morphine is the most appropriate medicine in an emergency. For many years, the standard of care was to give morphine until the patient reports that the pain had gone. The dose was determined mainly by the pain, although in medicine one must always take individual factors into account. However, morphine and similar opioids are unique medications because they have no ceiling dose if properly administered for pain. But of course, proper dosing means properly assessing the pain. The difficulty arises because of the subjectivity of pain and the fear of addiction. Because of the overwhelming concern for addiction,[11,12] it is crucial to understand that scientific and clinical research supports the hypothesis that persistent pain reduces the tendency toward addiction. Addiction rates are relatively low (<10% in most studies, but as high as 14% in one) for pain-naive people, provided they have no history of substance abuse, and they're lower still for people with persistent severe pain (<1% in most studies, but as high as 4% in a few).[62,133,135–144] Irrespective of the risk, we should treat each patient with risk of addiction in a responsible manner. When a drug can literally either kill or save a patient, depending on how it is used, there is bound to be controversy over its use.

My concern for Patient Z became a starting point in learning about pain management. As I look more deeply at the issue, I realize that there is no way to separate treatment of pain from the issue of addiction. How do we balance the need for public safety and protection against those who might harm themselves while providing medication to those who need it? This problem demands a medical solution for both the pain and addiction aspects of opioid use. Yet the United States government has permitted an advocacy coalition to implement a solution that does neither. The current policy is a version of abolition. The arbitrary limit on dose may provide relief for some people, but it certainly is not sufficient for every patient. Patient Z has been stable for years on a higher dose. He is very sick, and on many days, he suffers from many problems more serious than his pain. But even when he has a good day, he still has pain.

The doctor's mantra should be "listen to the patient." Treatment of disease should be a decision between doctor and patient. If we want good evidence to help determine efficacy, side effects, and addiction rate, study design and patient selection are critical. In the meantime, until the information is definitive, studies can provide guidance for treatment decisions in general, for the entire population, but they should not determine the treatment for any individual patient. There are many individual factors. The greatest individual difference in this field is whether a person has persistent pain or not. This chapter describes why opioids work for persistent-pain patients and how their experiences differ from pain-naive persons. I am not claiming any originality or novelty in this hypothesis. Rather, I am presenting the scientific evidence that exists to make a case that is well-known in pain medicine. It was the main point of Melzack's 1990 article "The Tragedy of Needless Pain," and that was a summary of one hundred years of experience treating patients with morphine.[134]

No one doubts that opioids can provide relief for *acute* pain. Those who argue that this pain relief does not last over the long term are not basing their claims on evidence, but rather the fear that addiction is inevitable. On the other side of the issue, it was naive for medical professional organizations to start a compassionate care movement without a plan to treat addiction. Furthermore, it is medically irresponsible not to differentiate between patients with severe, persistent pain and other patients. For both populations, medical evidence shows that there are vast individual differences, but the majority of patients are not prone to addiction. The vulnerable minority can be identified today using genetic testing, and follow-up can help to stop addiction before it starts.[145] There is no intrinsic or medical reason that prevents the medical community from treating pain patients who have a proclivity toward drug use, but as one author has put it, pain patients who have a substance-abuse issue are "guilty until proven innocent."[146] Studies of the treatment of pain in addicted persons reveal the challenges that doctors face.[147] Once a pain patient crosses over and shows aberrant behavior, the clinician should work with the patient and give the person a chance to demonstrate that they can manage their medication properly.[147] However, recent pressures have made this procedure less likely. Once a patient has left a doctor or pain clinic because of inability to follow the prescription appropriately, the only treatment options are those for a person with a diagnosis of opioid use disorder (OUD). Once a person has been diagnosed with OUD, more commonly known as addiction, the treatment options are limited. They include state methadone clinics and opioid treatment programs. Only recently has there even been a possibility to treat addiction as a medical matter. The medication-assisted treatment (MAT) program permits treatment, but there is still the barrier of the needed training and DEA waiver, as well as the associated greater risk. Consequently, the vast majority of doctors (>95%) lack the experience to treat addiction when it arises during the treatment of pain. We need to both distinguish the vast majority pain patients who use their prescriptions responsibly and provide a way to treat the aberrant pain patients in a humane manner. Treating pain properly requires understanding that patients with severe persistent pain have a different physiology than pain-naive patients. The response to opioids is as varied as the types of pain, but the general rule that is reported in many studies is that genuine, persistent pain decreases tolerance and also the likelihood of addiction.

The Different Meanings of Tolerance for Pain Patients and Pain-Naive Drug Users

The effect of tolerance is quite different in a pain patient compared to a pain-naive person. Colpaert summarizes the experience of many doctors that "chronic nociceptive stimulation [pain] acts to antagonize the apparent tolerance."[148] While some opposing clinicians have challenged the idea that tolerance is absent,[11,149] many studies have provided evidence that pain significantly lowers tolerance to analgesia and antinociception (inhibition of pain).[62,150–152] The effect of tolerance does not reduce analgesia to zero, but rather to a steady state. There is significant pain relief that is stable over the long term.

The two terms, *antinociception* and *analgesia*, refer to pain inhibition in the spine and brain, respectively. *Analgesia* is defined as "insensibility to pain without loss of consciousness," whereas *antinociception* is "the blocking of painful stimuli by neurons." The consensus document of the American Pain Society (APS) defines *tolerance* as follows[21,22,153]:

> Tolerance is defined as a decreased subjective and objective effect of the same amount of opioids used over time, which concomitantly requires an increasing amount of the drug to achieve the same effect. Although tolerance to most of the side effects of opioids (e.g., respiratory depression, sedation,

nausea) does appear to occur routinely, there is less evidence for clinically significant tolerance to opioids—analgesic effects (Collett, 1998; Portenoy et al., 2004). For example, there are numerous studies that have demonstrated stable opioid dosing for the treatment of chronic pain (e.g., Breitbart, et al., 1998; Portenoy et al., 2007) and methadone maintenance for the treatment of opioid dependence (addiction) for extended periods.

There is a different density of receptors for opioids in different parts of the body and regions of the brain. The tolerance to side effects, such as respiratory suppression, constipation, and nausea, is high while the tolerance to pain inhibition (analgesia and antinociception) is much lower. There is also a high tolerance for the euphoria that a drug user seeks. Stated in plain language, a person may take opioids for pain relief over a long time with relatively little reduction in effect (tolerance), but the pleasure-seeker taking drugs will find it increasingly difficult to recreate the euphoria that they seek unless the dose is escalated.[154,155] Opioid therapeutics have provided sufficient relief that many thousands of patients have maintained a constant dose over many years in observational studies.[141,156,157]

Some observers claim that opioid pain medications will lose effectiveness because of tolerance, in spite of the evidence. They describe tolerance as an absolute effect that abolishes the analgesia of opioids.[18] This is a misunderstanding of tolerance as it is observed in millions of patients who have reached a dose that gives them relief. In such patients, tolerance does not lead to a need for uncontrolled dose escalation to manage pain. Nonetheless, for patients with severe persistent pain the dose may need to be quite high in order to achieve relief. The dose required to manage pain should be a matter between doctor and patient. Unfortunately, in the legal framework of American medicine, the DEA can effectively terminate patient care by rescinding a pain clinic's license based on even a suspicion of diversion. The most damaging type of interference is when the DEA suspects diversion or illegal pleasure-seeking, merely because a patient's dose is high. Numerous patients have died when the DEA intervened and closed down a pain clinic.[158,159] Ironically, a doctor can be prosecuted if a patient dies under his or her care, while the DEA and other agencies that cause death by abruptly ending treatment are not held liable.

Physiological Differences in Opioid Effects of Pain Patients and Pain-Naive Drug Users

Given the attitudes of the advocacy coalition and the DEA, it is of central importance to establish the profound difference in the susceptibility to addiction between the patient in pain and without pain. Doctors know that a person experiencing intense pain after surgery will simply feel relief when given the proper dose of morphine. In this aspect, PROP makes a valid point that there was a tendency to give out too much medication in postsurgery settings during the compassionate care movement.[18] This occurred partly because of the active marketing of Purdue Pharma and associated companies who convinced some doctors that there was no danger. Postoperative patients are frequently healthy people who are mostly pain-naive. They need opioids for a limited time in cases where the pain of surgery is still intense, but the dose should be carefully monitored and opioids given as needed rather than automatically. With appropriate safeguards, there is still a very good reason to provide pain medication after surgery. It helps with recovery in many cases, aside from the aspect of humane treatment of the patient. Doctors frequently have had to reassure postoperative patients about giving opioids for short-term acute pain, but this has been done worldwide with little problem for one hundred years, and only recently in North America has anyone suggested that this practice has significant risk. There is a need to return to the protocols that worked for a century, not to abolish the use of opioids for treatment of acute postsurgical pain.

A patient given morphine before surgery may act a bit giddy, but the same patient given the same dose after surgery will be subdued. Many years ago, Patient Z's father was given morphine before a major surgery.

As a child, Patient Z saw his father briefly as he was being transported to the operating room after receiving a morphine injection. Presumably, the preoperative dose was to prepare for deep anesthesia since the surgery was to remove a growth on the kidney. Patient Z's father grinned and said in a boisterous voice, "Hi, Z, surgery is great. I am going to have surgery every day." It was the momentary euphoria of a completely healthy patient. While Patient Z's father was being wheeled into the operating room, he was *feeling no pain*. The next day, Patient Z visited his father in the hospital as he recovered from the surgery. His father had just received a morphine injection. He was subdued and said that he felt fine and that the doctors said that the surgery went well. There was no euphoria or giddiness. The pre- and postoperative difference in the psychology of the patient is of central importance to understanding the function of morphine in a persistent-pain patient.[154] If we can imagine someone who has the postsurgical pain on a continuous basis, then that is a persistent-pain patient. Giving that patient morphine every day will have the effect of relieving the pain. Any euphoria felt by a person in pain is short-lived owing to tolerance and perhaps a sign that the dose is higher than it should be. This is not to deny that pain relief has some degree of pleasure associated with it. But we must distinguish *euphoria* from *analgesia*. For many patients, pain relief is often reliable once the patient has adjusted to the opioid dose. There are some doctors, particularly those associated with PROP and its adherents, who contest this and claim that there is no long-term efficacy. When we get to the evidence, we will see how PROP has manipulated the published reviews to get the answer that they want.

If a healthy, pain-naive person took morphine every day, it would cause the euphoric giddiness for a while, but then tolerance would set in and the effect would be significantly less. A drug user who attempts to repeat a feeling of euphoria will often resort to dose escalation. The repeated drug use could lead to addiction if the healthy individual has a genetic predisposition.[160–165] A person chasing a feeling of euphoria is never quite satisfied, and certainly, if the ephemeral feeling is achieved, it does not last long. The only way to recreate the euphoric experience is to increase the dose, or wait a sufficiently long time until the tolerance has decreased. But the effect of withdrawal makes waiting impossible. On the other hand, a pain patient is trying to escape the constant assault of pain. Relief simply means that the pain becomes tolerable and the person can have somewhat normal function. Taking an opioid can give a greater range of function and decreases the intensity of the pain so that it becomes bearable. This pain-reduction effect is reproducible within a certain range of natural variation, just as the pain has some variation in intensity. This description is another way of saying that tolerance for analgesia and antinociception is relatively low and that opioid use can produce stable, reproducible relief as shown in more than one hundred medical studies discussed in chapter 6 and the appendix.

The drug abuser often seeks rapid delivery of the opioid to feel high. This is why injection is used and fast-acting heroin is one of the most frequently used drugs. Once a person starts on the path of wanting a euphoric high, the further problem is that the higher the high, the lower the low. A sense of loss and depression sets in when the opioid wears off. The low is known as an opponent process. A person who experiences the opponent process will have an incentive to take morphine again. The discomfort brought on by the chemical changes caused by morphine provides negative reinforcement. This opponent process puts the healthy person taking morphine on an emotional and pain roller coaster.

Some people, even some doctors, believe that pain patients are on a similar roller coaster.[167] This view suggests that euphoria masks the pain and therefore serves as analgesia. I believe that scientific evidence refutes this view. This chapter provides scientific evidence that the nature of the opponent process is qualitatively different for a pain patient compared to the euphoric experience of a drug user. Merely from a psychological point of view, relief and euphoria are very different experiences. Relief is almost never an absolute, pain-free state. Some patients have significant residual pain even on high doses of opioids. Most patients have variable relief: some days are good, and others are bad. When facing the alternative, patients are grateful that the medication works. It is important to establish this neurobiological foundation because it gives us a good understanding of why people who have genuine pain do not experience to the roller coaster of addiction.

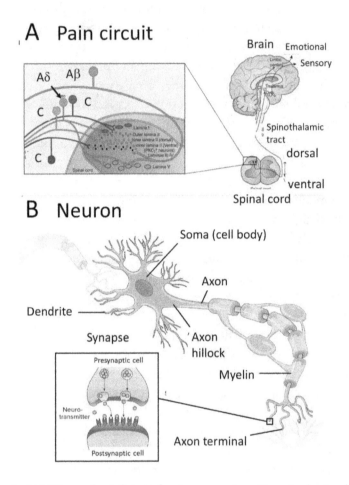

Figure 1. (A) Neurophysiology of pain messaging. Part A obtained from Ref. 225 used with permission from Elsevier Publishing. A message arrives from the periphery into the dorsal horn of the spine in either a myelinated Aδ or C fiber. Inhibitor cells control whether the message is sent on to the brain. The message is projected up to the thalamus and the process in the limbic center (emotional) and frontal cortex (rational processing). Opioid binding in the spine takes place inhibitor cells. (B) Nerve cell and synapse.[168] The neuron has dendrites on the receiving side and the axon that leads the length of the cell. The far end of the cell contains the axon terminal. Aδ cells have a myelin sheath, but C cells do not.

Electrical and Chemical Aspects of the Transmission of Neural Signals

Neurons provide two mechanisms to transmit signals—electrical and chemical. The electrical mechanism is controlled by ion channels, which permit positively charged sodium, potassium, or calcium to flow across the cell membrane. There is also a chloride ion channel, which permits negative ions to flow across the membrane. There are transport proteins that can return ions across by a pumping mechanism that requires energy. The fuel of the cell is a molecule called adenosine triphosphate (ATP) that can bind and release energy as heat by breaking a bond so that one phosphate (P) is removed: ATP $\rightarrow$ ADP + P + heat.

A pain signal, once initiated, moves along the cell by a series of changes in ion concentration that change the voltage across the cell membrane in a wave that travels from one end of the cell to the other. Figure 1B shows a typical structure of a nerve cell with an inset that shows the gap between nerve cells known as the synapse. The resting voltage is polarized at −70 mV. A signal can travel the length of the cell as a wave of ions as ion channels open and close in succession to locally depolarize the cell membrane, changing the voltage to 0 mV or to as large as +30 mV. After the signal has passed, each section of the cell membrane resets to its polarized state. When the signal reaches the end of a nerve cell, it must send the message to the next nerve cell by releasing molecules, called neurotransmitters, across the synapse. There are six main neurotransmitters—namely, glutamate (most abundant), GABA (inhibitory), dopamine (reward, aversion, motion), noradrenaline, adrenaline (stress, fight-flight, breathing, heart rate), and serotonin (emotion, pain).[169] The neurotransmitters are produced in the nerve cell, collect into small spherical vesicles inside the cell, and are then released by a chemical trigger (mainly calcium) that converts the electrical impulse into a chemical message. The vesicles merge with the presynaptic membrane, and the molecules are released so that they may diffuse to receptors on either the postsynaptic membrane (chemical transmission) or on the same presynaptic membrane (feedback inhibition) as shown in the inset in figure 1A. The concentration is also controlled by transporter proteins that can actively remove the neurotransmitters when they have done their job.[170] Once a message has crossed the synapse and reached the next nerve, the body resets the synapse by sucking out the neurotransmitters. Glial cells that surround the nerve fiber can actively transport the neurotransmitters out of the synapse and into their cytosol, inside the glial cell.

There are also many specialized peptide (protein) neurotransmitters that are synthesized inside the neuron. We will focus on the natural opioid system with three specialized neurotransmitters that inhibit pain signals—enkephalin, dynorphin, and endorphin.[171] Endorphins are widely known because they are associated with pleasure and the positive effects of exercise. Two very short fragments of enkephalin (leu-enkephalin and met-enkephalin) are the most common natural opioids that inhibit pain. The mechanism of inhibiting pain is a secondary effect of leu- or met-enkephalin binding, which induces pumping of potassium (positive) out of the cell. In other contexts, the neurotransmitter GABA induces pumping of chloride (negative) into the cell. Either of these effects causes a decrease in the membrane potential to –90 mV, which is more negative than the polarized resting potential. This hyperpolarized state inhibits the neuron.

Neurons can be very long and are often referred to as projections. A pain signal that reaches the spine may project all the way to the brain in a single neuron as shown in figure 1A. The neurotransmitter that binds at one end of a neuron may convert to a different neurotransmitter at the other end. Glutamate is, by far, the most common neurotransmitter in the brain.[172] Dopamine, noradrenaline, adrenaline, and serotonin are active in pathways that give rise to reward or aversion, fight or flight, and emotional aspects of pain, respectively.[173] We will focus on transmission of pain signals initiated by natural opioid peptides and on how those projections give rise to other neural messaging in the brain that is transmitted via glutamate or dopamine. This is a great simplification but useful to illustrate the main points of the relationship of pain to addiction.

Dopamine is a neurotransmitter active in reward-motivational and motor control pathways in the brain. Dopamine is important in pleasure and in learned responses because of its effects on regions of the brain that are called hedonic (pleasure) hot spots.[174] The neurotransmitters need to be at the right concentration in the brain and properly regulated in order for the nervous system to function. Low levels of dopamine are associated with Parkinson's disease, low levels of serotonin with depression, and so on. Dopamine is produced in only about four hundred thousand cells in the brain, which are located either in the substantia nigra (SN) or the ventral tegmental area (VTA).[175,176] The SN has projections into the nigrostriatial pathway, which plays a significant role in motor function and learning new motor skills. The VTA projects to the cortex, limbic system, amygdala, hippocampus, and the nucleus accumbens (NAC).[169,177] The NAC is often called the pleasure center of the brain and is often cited as the site in the brain where dopamine release is responsible for the euphoria produced by drugs like heroin. To understand pain patients' response to opioids, we need to consider how pain itself affects these regions of the brain separately and prior to taking opioid painkillers. The evidence suggests that there are numerous effects on the cell receptors and cell chemistry that have long-lasting effects. Thus, taking opioid drugs can produce learned cell responses that are hard to unlearn (addiction), and pain can produce long-lasting changes to cells that make them less tolerant of opioids for pain relief but more tolerant of euphoric or mood swings caused by opioids. Each of these considerations depends on the particular individual, their genetic polymorphisms, level of pain, psychological stability, and of course, the dose of the opioid.

Sensory and Nociceptive Neurons—the Gate Theory of Pain

The neurophysiology of nociceptive pain begins with nerve impulses originating from pressure, temperature, or puncture that are initiated in the peripheral nerves and projected to the dorsal horn (back corner) of the spine as shown in figure 1A. Nociception is a "noxious capture" event, the registration of a harmful event by the human nervous system. There are two entry portals into the spine: the dorsal horn in the back side and the ventral horn in the front of the vertebrae. Once in the spine, the pain message may either be inhibited by one of the many types of inhibitory neurons inside the spine or projected up to the brain (figure 1).[225] Inhibitory neurons are located between input neurons coming from various parts of the body and projecting neurons inside the spine that carry information to the brain.

A signal initiated by a harmful or painful event to the body can be transmitted by either fast or slow fibers, Aδ or C nociceptive fibers, respectively. Aδ fibers are larger and have a myelin sheath, while C fibers lack a sheath shown in figure 1A. In addition, sensory fibers, called Aβ fibers, are larger still and have a more rapid transmission compared to either of the pain fibers. The gate theory of pain[178] holds that an input signal can have sensory or pain contributions or both. The various input nerve cells also interact with inhibitor nerve cells in the spine. We can think of the sensory Aβ fiber acting as a gate for the nociceptive, Aδ or C, fibers. Opening the gate means that the brain receives the message of a pain input, and closing the gate inhibits the message from reaching the brain. Inside the spine, the signal is processed in a manner that is somewhat like a logic gate in an electronic circuit: (1) There is no pain signal if there is no input on either fiber, neither Aδ nor C (gate closed). (2) There is a pain signal if Aδ or C has pain input (gate open); or (3) there is a sensory input if Aβ sends the signal (gate closed).[179] (4) If both a pain (Aδ or C nociceptive) and sensory Aβ signal reach the dorsal horn, there is an inhibition interaction that cancels the pain signal by closing the gate.[73] The Aβ sensory fiber is dominant and that input goes through.

One physiological consequence of the gate mechanism is that the sensory Aβ neuron can distract the organism from the pain by shutting the gate. For example, the gate could be closed by a person rubbing their leg after stubbing a toe. The sensation of touching the skin elsewhere distracts from the pain. The gate model shows that it is more than just distraction and that the sensory signal can inhibit the pain projection to the brain. Shutting off the message may not entirely eliminate the pain, which is why the body has a natural opioid system with neurotransmitters (the natural opioid peptides) and receptors.

Opioid Receptors—the Natural Switches for Pain Inhibition

There are three nerve cell receptors that control transmission of a pain message—the mu-, delta-, and kappa-opioid receptors (MOR, DOR, and KOR).[180–183] The MOR is the most important since two natural opioids (leu- and met-enkephalin) and exogenous opioids (morphine, oxycodone, methadone, fentanyl) used as pain medications bind to this receptor. They may bind to other receptors in addition, but they all are MOR agonists. An agonist is an activator or stimulator for a receptor. It triggers the membrane-bound receptor to send messages inside the nerve cell. Receptors can either turn on or off internal messaging pathways in the cells. The messaging can affect ion channels or nuclear transcription factors (see below). Antagonists also can bind to a receptor, but they are blockers, meaning they bind but do not activate the receptor. The opioid receptors are inhibitory, meaning that they turn off internal messages. This is a bit confusing since an agonist (like morphine) binds to the MOR, causing it to inhibit the cell and terminate the pain message. The job of the inhibitory cells where MOR is found is to stop the pain messaging in the spine (antinociception). However, in the brain, MORs are also involved with dopamine receptors, either because they are both found on the synapse or because the opioid message can result in dopamine signaling.

The dopamine receptor is the same general type of receptor with similar structure and internal cell signaling. However, the dopamine-receptor agonist is dopamine, and the opioid peptides would have no direct effect on that receptor. The complex set of events in the brain can both yield pain relief (analgesia) but also send descending messages to the site of the pain signal and elsewhere to respond to the pain using motor control to react. The DOR and KOR receptors have more complicated functions. For example, the opioid peptide dynorphin is a KOR agonist that produces anxiety and depression.[181] Buprenorphine is a KOR antagonist, which is an important property for the treatment of addiction because it reduces anxiety, which is a side of effect of withdrawal.

Nerve cells can have MOR on the membrane surface at different densities, which are controlled from the nucleus of the cell by other proteins called transcription factors. Transcription factors control which genes are activated, transcribed, and translated into proteins in the cell. We could think of transcription factors as master switches in a cell. They determine the long-term development of a cell. The transcription factors are often the target of internal signaling. For example, the spinal neurons receive signals that affect transcription factors to induce MOR production when a pain signal has reached the brain and then returned to the spine.[184] The MORs are needed to inhibit the pain signal, but they are only produced in significant quantity when a pain signal exists and the thalamus has sent a descending signal to the origin of the pain transmission. At the same time there are also natural opioid proteins generated that can bind to the MOR and inhibit the pain signal. Together, these proteins comprise the natural opioid system (also the endogenous opioid system). Using various chemical challenges and gene manipulation, rodents can be tested for their response to pain and to morphine antinociception, which is pain inhibition by morphine at the level of the nerve cells in the spine. Morphine analgesia refers instead to morphine pain relief in the brain. Experiments suggest that both should occur simultaneously.

The Role of Dopamine and the Dopamine Receptors under the Influence of Pain and Opioids

Dopamine—which is simulated by drugs, including alcohol, cocaine, and opioids—plays an important role in reward processes. Dopamine binds to one of five different receptors—D_1 through D_5—on the synaptic membrane. The dopamine receptors are chemical receptors of the same type as opioid receptors, but the ligand is dopamine instead of opioid peptides. There are two classes. The D_1 class, which includes D_1 and D_5, stimulates or activates neurons. The D_2 class, which includes D_2, D_3, and D_4, is inhibitory. The density of receptors is quite different in various regions of the brain. The receptor density on the synaptic membrane can change. The receptors can be recycled, and they can interact with other receptors, including glutamate receptor ion channels and opioid receptors in the synaptic membrane. The changes in receptor density and connectivity in the synapse is called synaptic plasticity. The change in synapse structure accommodates learning and other conditioned responses.[185]

Opioid Tolerance

Tolerance has been studied in mice using a variety of methods.[186] One important set of experiments compares genetically modified "knockout" mice that lack the MOR genes to normal mice.[187] The MOR-knockout mouse can be studied using a normal mouse as a control. There are two different knockouts corresponding to a 50% and 100% elimination of the MOR.[188] Mice that lack the MOR survive and show normal behavior in routine situations. They can be exposed to a pain stimulus and given morphine to test their reactions in comparison with the control or normal mice. In MOR-knockout mice, morphine is much less effective, but it still has some residual effect. The MOR agonist function of morphine is only part of its mechanism of pain relief, but it is the dominant mechanism.

Using MOR-knockout studies, scientists have concluded that naturally occurring opioid peptides bind to the MOR to dampen the pain signal, but morphine and other exogenous opioids can replace those peptides.[187] Morphine and other opioid drugs bind to the MOR because they have a shape similar to the natural opioid peptides, the enkephalins.[189] Since the effective concentration of morphine can exceed that of natural peptides, morphine can bind to the MOR with greater effect than the natural opioid peptides and reduce the pain response beyond the ability of the natural opioid system.[187,190] If the MOR is absent, morphine has only a very small effect of inhibiting the pain signal based on the behavior of mice in response to the hot plate test.[191] The effectiveness of blocking the pain signal scales with the number of active MORs on the nerve cell membrane. Tolerance to side effects has also been observed and can be quite different because the MORs that give rise to those effects are located in other regions of the body. For example, constipation is caused by opioid binding to MORs in the gastrointestinal tract. For the majority of patients, the tolerance for side effects is higher than tolerance for pain. This is fortunate because it means that negative side effects, including respiratory suppression and euphoria, are less likely to be a problem as a patient becomes accustomed to a given dose. Euphoria is not usually mentioned as a side effect, but it is actually one of the factors that can lead to addiction, so it is an important side effect. In a patient who lacks genetic polymorphisms and environmental factors that predispose them to addiction (>90%), euphoria is a harmless side effect when it occurs. It usually does not occur in pain patients, or it is very short-lived when it does. If a patient has a high tolerance for euphoria, then it means that the patient will only experience that state at a high concentration of the opioid. This is precisely what happens to drug users when they repeatedly use an opioid (often heroin) and find that it is increasingly more difficult to feel the same level of absolute pleasure. They must escalate the dose to reach that same level. Pain patients have a different situation since their natural opioid system has been operating in response to pain and their physiology will have been altered prior to ingesting opioid medication.

Dose-Response Curves

The effectiveness of opioid binding is a function of the concentration of the complex of the messenger, O for opioid, with the MOR on the cell surface. The MORs are found in the synapse, the gap between two neurons where chemical signal occurs to project a neural signal. If we denote the surface density of MOR-agonist complex as [MOR(O)] and we assume that pain reduction is proportional to the product of the receptor and opioid (*pain reduction* $\propto$ [MOR(O)]), then we see that the intensity of pain reduction depends on the concentration of [O] in the synapse, surface density of the [MOR], and the affinity of O for MOR. This is a simplification of the complex biology of a synapse, but it is useful for illustrating the concept of the dose-response curve in figure 2. The dose-response curve could apply to any drug that has a single binding site in a protein or receptor. For example, dopamine and dopamine receptor have the same general considerations. The shape of the dose-response curve is the same as a curve showing the fraction of sites that are bound at equilibrium:

$$Fraction\ bound = \frac{[MOR(O)]}{[MOR(O)] + [MOR]}$$

Each curve in the plot in figure 2 has a constant MOR density on the cell surface, while the concentration of [O] is increased. We assume that the effect, in this case antinociception, is proportional to the fraction of bound sites on the cell. The response is plotted in figure 2 as the percent of the maximum possible effect or %MPE. In a simple model we could imagine that we reach 100% MPE when all the sites are bound—that is, when *Fraction Bound* = 1.

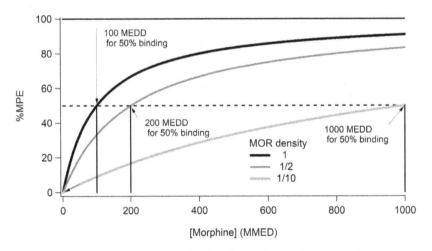

[Morphine] (MMED)

Figure 2. Dose-response curve for binding of morphine to a MOR. The effect is represented as the percent of maximum effect (%MPE), and the concentration of morphine is represented in terms of the milligram equivalent daily dose (MEDD). The curve is also proportional to the fraction of bound sites on the MOR receptor. The bound form is MOR(O), and the unbound form is MOR.

Morphine tolerance occurs because of either desensitization or downregulation of the MOR.[192,193] The loss of effectiveness because of desensitization or downregulation leads to a new lower steady state value for the active bound complex [MOR(O)]. For repeated use of a given dose of opioid [O], the steady state surface density of bound receptors [MOR(O)] tends toward a constant value.[94] Figure 2 shows that the curve never reaches 100% MPE, which tells us that it is impossible to completely eliminate persistent pain even at the highest dose of [O]. Therefore, treatment with any painkiller is a matter of reducing the pain to a tolerable level. Patients often accept a lower-than-optimal dose based on a personal compromise involving physical issues, such as side effects. The compromise leading to undertreatment of pain often arises from the stigma of opioids and concerns about addiction.[194] Patients often recognize that there is no such thing as absolute pain relief. In a sense, pain is always undertreated but it can be controlled. When pain is controlled, patient feels a sense of hope just because the pain can be reduced when it begins to become excruciating.

After sixty years of experience treating chronic malignant cancer pain using opioids, the WHO has standardized treatment in an analgesic ladder, consisting of three rungs: (1) acetaminophen, NSAIDs; (2) tramadol; and (3) morphine.[62]

> Opioid medication, commonly oral morphine, is the third step on the "analgesic ladder" and has been widely used for the management of acute and chronic cancer pain for many years, providing excellent analgesia without respiratory compromise often for months or even years.

The third rung involves getting the morphine dose right for the patient. However, there is no consensus regarding the appropriate dose for a long-term pain management. Medical research has still not determined the quantitative effect of tolerance on the morphine dose-response curve. If the number of MOR receptors is decreased, then one possible result would be that the dose-response curve is shifted as shown by the gray and light gray curves plotted assuming that the MOR surface density is one-half or one-tenth as large as the original density. Evidence shows that the active MOR surface density decreases and then reaches a steady state. The active [MOR(O)] density decreases but reaches a constant value and does not continue decreasing to zero. There is a common misperception, even among some experts, that tolerance leads to a complete lack of effect. This is simply incorrect, based on many laboratory experiments with mice and studies of patient reports of their pain level over time at given opioid doses. Psychologically, having some control over the pain is very valuable. Even when relief is not complete, a patient's morale is improved even by the knowledge that the pain can be reduced. Uncontrolled pain leaves a person with a sense of helplessness and a fear that the pain will simply take over. This sense is what causes pain patients to lose the will to live.

The Pharmacology of Opioid Medications— Differences in Potency and Mode of Action

There are three classes of pharmaceutical opioids. The first one synthesized and still one of the most used today, morphine is a simple derivative of opium. Opium is an extract from poppy flowers. Any molecule with a shape that appropriately mimics the natural opioid peptides, known as enkephalins, can bind to the MOR. The three classes of opioids are (1) phenanthrenes, (2) phenylpiperidines, and (3) phenylheptanes. The phenanthrene opioids (morphine, oxycodone, oxymorphone, hydromorphone, heroin, codeine, etc.) are full MOR agonists. The phenylpiperidines (fentanyl, carfentanyl, remifentanil) are also full MOR agonists and have extremely high binding affinities and very short half-lives. The phenylheptanes (methadone) are partial MOR agonists, tend to have high binding affinities, and have long half-lives. Doses of different opioid pharmaceuticals are usually compared using the unit of morphine milligram equivalent per day (MEDD). A patient who takes 1 milligram of morphine every day has a dose of 1 MEDD. One milligram of oxycodone, oxymorphone, or tramadol is equivalent to 1.5, 4.0, or 0.1 MEDD, respectively. A typical dose might be 90 milligrams of morphine and 20 milligrams of oxycodone, which gives 90 MEDD + 30 MEDD = 120 MEDD. The unit of MEDD is subjective, for the same reason that pain is subjective, and different researchers, different countries use significantly different estimates for these values.[126,127] However, there is no other system for estimating the relative strength of opioids in the United States. Doctors use MEDD units, and therefore they will be used in this book.

The relative strength of various opioid medications has been measured and tabulated in opioid rotation tables. These are not necessarily accurate because different opioids have different mechanisms.[126,127] According to an analysis of the various factors that determine the strength of the drugs, different opioids have significantly different tendencies to elicit tolerance. Studies in a mouse model show that fentanyl is approximately seventy-five times more potent than morphine.[195] Fentanyl is usually dosed for patches in units of micrograms released per hour. Using the above conversion, 120 MEDD would correspond to 67 micrograms of fentanyl per hour.

The pharmaceuticals in the same class as morphine have similar properties and are much easier to rotate but also have a high cross-tolerance. If the two opioids have precisely the same effect when they bind to the MOR, they are interchangeable, and they have a high cross-tolerance. This means that the tolerance of one also functions for the other, and a rotation will not give any extra benefit arising from a pre-existing tolerance for the new drug. On the other hand, low cross-tolerance means that one drug does not lead to tolerance for the substitute. Substitution gives a patient much more relief for some time until a new tolerance is established. The cross-tolerance is explained by the effect each drug has on opioid receptor internalization by endocytosis or desensitization following drug or natural opioid binding. Studies of opioid receptors (MOR, KOR, DOR, and others) reveal a complex pattern of binding and receptor uptake.[196–199] Methadone and other phenylheptanes have a relatively low cross-tolerance with morphine.

Signal Processing in the Brain—Neural Circuits

From the point of view of natural pain control, pain is a circuit with a starting and ending point in the spine. Although nerve cells are not wires, intuition about how electricity travels in wires can help to understand the speed and connectivity of neural circuits. A pain signal from the periphery is first projected to the spine where it passes through connecting interneurons to spinal neurons that project the ascending pain signal to the thalamus. From the thalamus, the pain signal projects to the limbic region and frontal cortex, where emotional and rational responses to the pain will result. Both brain imaging and animal studies provide structural and chemical evidence for a descending pain control signal.[220] After reaching the thalamus and projection to other brain regions, there are descending projections through the hypothalamus, which project back to the spine leading to the release of enkephalins, which bind to MOR receptors to inhibit the signal in interneurons in the spine.[221] Opioid receptors MOR, DOR, and KOR are upregulated by descending projections from the mid-brain.[222,223] The natural opioid, enkephalin, is released there so that it can bind to the MOR in the spine.[224] The natural binding of opioid peptides occurs both in the spine and brain of a pain patient and may have a continuous presence in a person who has persistent pain.

A pain-naive drug user who takes opioids has few MOR in the spine and experiences no analogous experience to antinociception, or pain relief in the spine. However, a persistent-pain patient experiences relief because of opioid binding to the high density of MOR produced by the neural pain circuit. There are many different types of inhibitory neurons in the dorsal horn of the spine shown in figure 1. Although the physiology is complicated, the Gate Theory that Melzack and Wall proposed in 1965 still describes the big picture correctly.[225] Adding an exogenous opioid, such as morphine, to this existing circuit produces both antinociception and analgesia, but the low cross-tolerance discussed in the preceding section means that these effects are different from the effect the same drug would have on a pain-naive drug user.

The brain must sort through the messages it receives to determine which stimuli to avoid, which are indicative of imminent danger, and what maneuvers are needed to escape a bad situation.[226] As an organism ages, it has memories of pain. These serve an important physiological function helping the organism to avoid harmful stimuli. These pain memories are part of the neuromatrix. The neuromatrix is a separate idea that Melzack proposed to describe the pathways that have already been traversed by a pain impulse in the brain.[73] It is recorded, and this may help prevent a future occurrence—for example, recognizing a thorn on a tree as a threat—or it may also cause phantom pain. Phantom limb pain has perplexed pain scientists. This is the significant pain that a person may feel coming from a limb that has been amputated. It is clearly "in the person's head," but it is not a fictional pain. The neuromatrix is that memory, and it is a physiological collection of nerve cells. One could think of chronic pain as arising, at least in part, from structural and chemical modification of the brain. In some cases, the neural pathways have been etched by a primary pain that has vanished, such as a wound that healed. Much more common is the case where there is joint and tissue damage from disease that persists, while constant pain messages reaching the brain alters the neural pathways, which is what we call persistent pain. By using MRI it is possible to see thousands of different images of the modifications of the brain because of chronic pain.[78,227] Using various cell biology methods, one can determine changes in cell chemistry that have occurred.[209]

Pain and Pain-Naive Patients Have Different Cross-Tolerances for Analgesia and Euphoria

We can also use cross-tolerance to compare how exogenous opioids (pharmaceuticals like morphine) compare to natural opioid peptides (leu- and met-enkephalin) in persistent-pain patients, who have an activated natural opioid response. If the cross-tolerance is high, then the pain patient will already be conditioned and will not be as strongly affected by the exogenous opioid. As discussed above, the cross-tolerance of analgesia and euphoria are very different. We often use analgesia to describe the overall effect of pain inhibition in a pain patient, which includes antinociception as well. Evidence suggests that cross-tolerance of natural opioids with morphine are relatively low for analgesia. This is why morphine works well for pain relief. However, the cross-tolerance for euphoric effects and respiratory suppression is much higher. One reason for the difference is that the opioid receptors giving rise to these various effects are in different parts of the body, which also includes different regions of the brain. There may also be different cellular effects, such as combined effects of opioids and dopamine, opioids and adrenaline, and effects of calcium, which each produce specific differences. As a consequence, the euphoric effect of morphine on the pain patient is diminished relative to the pain-naive person because the pharmaceutical and natural opioids have a high cross-tolerance. When a side effect is harmful, tolerance is a protection. The fact that the cross-tolerance of natural opioids and morphine for respiratory suppression is high means that a person in pain has some natural protection against respiratory suppression. For more than one hundred years, doctors have been taught that pain is an antidote to morphine poisoning, which means that a patient in pain can withstand a higher dose of morphine without danger of respiratory suppression. It is not clear that medical schools teach this today since the education in pain medicine has been phased out of many programs.

The fact that euphoria also has a high cross-tolerance suggests that pain is also an antidote to euphoria and therefore to addiction. This is one way to explain the observation made by clinicians that pain patients have a lower tendency to become addicted compared to pain-naive patients. These effects all scale with pain. Greater and longer-lasting pain increases the concentration of natural opioid peptide and the tolerance of receptors to those peptides. The greater the pain, the higher the dose that can be tolerated, and yet pain relief still increases with the dose. These properties explain why morphine and other related opioid drugs are the most effective pain medicine known.

Imaging and Chemical Studies That Support the Cross-Tolerance Hypothesis

Persistent pain causes permanent structural and chemical changes to the brain.[200] Based on data from rodent studies, we can infer that neuronal proteins associated with addiction[201–204] are significantly downregulated in the reward center of rats with a neuropathic pain model.[205] Pain patients' brains have some deterioration in the gray matter and spiny projections from the reward center.[79,206,207] The pain response upregulates proteins associated with depression in the reward center in a manner similar to opioids in pain-naive patients.[208,209] Chronic pain leads to downregulation of transmission of pleasure signals in the core part of the reward center, but not other parts of the brain,[201] which is partially caused by the decrease in activity of D_2 and D_3 dopamine receptor activity observed in positron emission tomography (PET) studies.[210,211]

PET imaging can be used to locate the position of a specific type of radioactive tracer in the brain to see the location and density of receptors. Using a spared nerve injury (SNI) model in lab rats, researchers showed that functional connectivity of the NAC (the reward center) to the dorsal striatum and cortex was reduced and levels of D_1, D_2, and KOR in the NAC decreased twenty-eight days after SNI.[212] In a separate experiment, a neuropathic pain injury model was used to observe selectively increased excitability of the NAC shell indirect pathway spiny projection neurons.[213] Each of these changes induced by pain gave rise to long-term changes in the brain's reward center that precluded the achievement of a euphoric state by opioid use.

Contradictory evidence based on the formalin test had been interpreted to mean that exogenous opioids and natural opioids are synergistic, leading to analgesia without necessarily reducing the intensity of the pain.[214] The interpretation of that dated experiment is that euphoria is simply masking the pain. Such thinking predates modern neurochemistry and imaging methods that show the effects of opioids on dopamine receptor levels, the desensitization, effects on glutamate receptor ion channels and transcription factors. These long-term changes, arising from neuroplasticity, are the explanation for the high cross-tolerance of natural opioid peptides with morphine in the reward center of the brain. The aversion to pain and the constant barrage of the stress cause the reward center of the brain to have less responsiveness to dopamine than a healthy pain-naive person would have. We can formulate these ideas as a hypothesis: persistent pain activates the natural opioid and stress responses, which cause chemical and structural changes in the reward center similar to opioid drugs. Consequently, there is a high cross-tolerance between natural opioid peptides and opioid drugs for the reward center in the brain and a much lower cross-tolerance for pain relief that involves an entire pain circuit from spine to brain and back again.

The low cross-tolerance of morphine and natural opioids for pain relief has been shown by a variety of methods. PET studies of binding to opioid receptors in rheumatoid arthritis patients found that pain decreased as binding of opioid peptide analogs increased.[215] One test for a common mechanism of action by the natural and exogenous opioids is treatment with the antagonist naloxone.[216] Naloxone displaces both the naturally produced opioid and the opioid drug bound to the MOR.[217] Both are ineffective when naloxone is administered.[218] Naloxone competition experiments found that natural opioid peptides and opioid drugs had different ranges of action. The low cross-tolerance for the natural and exogenous opioid treatment of mice for pain relief was found to be consistent with the high-cross tolerance in the reward center.[219] Although notoriously subjective, patient accounts suggested different experiences of morphine for pain patients and drug users as well. Drug users reported a feeling of pleasure and sense of euphoria, while pain patients focused on relief.[154] In summary, pain relief competes with euphoria as an effect when patients are treated with opioid drugs. The greater the pain, the greater the competition and the less likely a patient is to have any of pleasure experienced by pain-naive patients or the associated risk of addiction.

The Neurobiology of Analgesia vs. Euphoria

Both pain itself and non-pain-related drug use affect the central nervous system in parallel because the natural and exogenous opioids both target the same receptor, the MOR. However, that similarity is only part of the story because the brain on pain has a different distribution of opioid and dopamine receptors (MOR, D_1, D_2, and D_3) as well as different transcription factors. If we think of the DNA in the cell as a library of the code for proteins, the transcription factors are the librarians that decide which proteins will be selected to be produced by the cell. The transcription factors can remain in the cell and control protein production for months. Thus, they are master switches that control the state of neural plasticity. They determine which receptors are produced and what kinds of interactions are possible. For example, opioid, dopamine, and glutamate receptors interact with one another in complex ways to determine whether receptors will be desensitized or taken into the cell by endocytosis and then recycled in active form. Because of these changes, the state of the reward center of the brain in the presence of pain is similar to its state in a depression; the concentration of neurotransmitter tends to be lower than average because the receptor signaling is abnormal in pain patients.[228]

We have already seen that pain itself can reduce the concentration of dopamine receptors. Basically, it lessens the activity of dopamine. A pain-naive person who wants to experience the euphoria of an opioid ends up desensitizing dopamine receptors and changing neural plasticity in the VTA and NAC in a way that mimics the effects of pain. These similarities lead to similar changes in transcription factor concentration, which further explains the high cross-tolerance for the euphoric effects in pain patients.[229] The fact that opioids produce the same effect tells us that the long-term drug user will also have a high tolerance for the euphoric effect. Initially, the dopamine surge from the VTA into the NAC in the pain-naive drug user will be larger and have a greater impact than for the persistent-pain patient. When the drug user is first trying heroin or other injected preparation, the physiological starting point is quite different from the pain patient. However, by creating an imbalance in the nerve cells of their brain, the pain-naive person who overuses opioids also causes an opponent process that produces anxiety and depression once the effect of the drug has worn off. After repeated use, the drug user finds that tolerance to the euphoria has built up. This tolerance is similar to the pain patient's tolerance, but it has a completely different origin. The pain-naive drug user needs to keep increasing the opioid dose to get the euphoric feeling. But this also increases the feelings of anxiety and depression. These experiences are fundamentally different in a person whose starting point is severe, persistent pain. The pain patient (who has an appropriate dose) does not feel the oscillatory swings of the drug user.[230] Instead, the pain patient experiences a cycle of relief and pain. Since the pain patient is not chasing a euphoric feeling but trying to maintain relief by both analgesia (brain) and antinociception (spine) mechanisms,[231] the pain patient does not typically engage in dose escalation. Patients who have chronic diseases may experience worsening pain and require a higher dose for that reason, but that is distinct from dose escalation due to tolerance. One indication of the difference is evident in studies showing that pain patients try to cope with the minimum possible dose.[94,194] The reticence to escalate the dose and concern for the stigma reflects a physiological process that is not driven by irrational pleasure-seeking but by rational aversion of pain.

In an interview, a leading addiction specialist commented on how opioids relieve pain. Dr. Kolodny's description suggests that effect of opioids in a pain patient is to mask the pain with a euphoric feeling.[168]

> It isn't clear exactly how opioids relieve pain. They create a surge of the feel-good chemical dopamine in the brain, and one idea is that the resulting euphoria masks pain. For short-term pain, such as in post-surgical situations, opioids can be very effective. But the dopamine release also "reinforces" the drug-taking behavior, as it does for eating or sex.
>
> But the real driver of addiction, says Kolodny, is that "people feel really bad without

the opioid." Opioids inhibit the locus coeruleus system in the brain, which regulates fight-or-flight hormones. That's why opioids are relaxing. But as the drug levels drop, the locus coeruleus begins to wake up, until it's operating on overdrive. "Your brain is responding as if there's a lion in the jungle ready to tear you to pieces," says Kolodny. The sense of impending doom, combined with other withdrawal symptoms—pain comes back with a vengeance too—makes people desperate for relief, and for that next dose.

When the academic who has led the fight to limit medication for millions of pain patients claims in a magazine interview that pain patients are like addicts in their mental experience of the opioid, he is ignoring the science. The constant assault of pain on the various regions of the brain have made changes in neurochemistry that dramatically change the effect of opioids. For the pain patient, the opioid moves the pain patient closer to the original pain-naive equilibrium. These physiological tendencies do not exclude addiction, but they suggest that pain is an antidote to addiction. Studies have been conducted since the year 1925 examining the percentage of heroin addicts who began their addiction using prescription drugs.[62] The values ranged from 4% (1925) to 9% (1954) to 27% (1980) for Whites and 1% for Blacks for this entire period. A series of studies found percentages of addiction for pain patients ranged from 1% to 4% from the year 1980 to 2010.[62,133,135–142] The large range indicates different definitions of *addiction* and some differences in the patient population.

The Ethical Responsibility to Understand Patients' Pain and to Treat Suffering

Clearly, if pain patients take opioid medications to relieve pain and not for a euphoric high, then the meaning of *dependence* is very different from the psychological definition used in studies of mental disorders. Pain patients are aware of dependence on their medication, which is a natural consequence of the fact that the patients' function and quality of life depend on relief from pain. When clinicians write that dependence is essentially the same as addiction, the implication is that the pain patients are taking the medication for a reason other than alleviating pain.[11] This reasoning ignores the origins of persistent pain, which most often comes from a disease that has a somatic cause. The doctors are also presuming to have deep insight into the mental state of patients. Pain is a symptom, but it is also a disease that can cause harm to the body. In what other context would doctors simply dismiss a symptom of a disease as fictitious? Pain is in a category by itself. Because of the legal pressures and the mistakes that were made, the medical community today focuses on opioids as drugs of abuse rather than thinking about pain as a treatable symptom of disease. This misguided focus is clearly forced by circumstance. Many doctors would like to treat pain, but they are concerned about the possibility of addiction, of being fooled by a patient, and of the legal consequences that may be practically beyond their control. Understanding the neurobiology of pain helps us think about objective ways to identify pain that present a solution to the problem of patients taking advantage of doctors. By far, the best practice is for a doctor to take the time to get to know the patient.

The articles in medical journals focus almost exclusively on a population of people with low back pain or osteoarthritis.[10,11,51] There are tens of millions of people in that category, and a certain fraction of that population has become overmedicated during the compassionate care movement. That is an issue that requires a humane solution. There is also a small minority in that group who fake or exaggerate their pain to obtain opioids. There is no excuse for that behavior, and we need to find reasonable ways to confront it. A self-assessment by medical interns suggests an urgent need for better training to identify pretenders, deal with the psychological issues, and provide appropriate treatment for the rest.[232] However, there is another category of patients whose number is estimated from five to eight million people whose pain is much more serious.[2] People with inflammatory arthritis; genetic, degenerative diseases; and accident victims can have pain that most of us could not imagine.[1] To cut these people off or to limit their dose so severely that they live in intolerable pain is inhumane.[233] We should use science wherever possible to detect and treat pain, which means also taking the same approach toward addiction. However, stating that all pain patients are at risk for addiction is an extreme reaction to overprescribing.[10–12,51] This point of view simply does not agree with the overwhelming evidence that aberrant use and OUD comprise a small percentage of patients in any group studied.[133,137,138,140–142,144] This is why claims and policies advanced by zealots are being contested by many doctors, and the treatment of pain patients is a flashpoint for debate in the medical community.[1,3,121,234–236] For patients who have severe, persistent pain—if no other options alleviate the patient's pain and the patient tolerates opioids—there is no ethical justification for denying treatment. Nonetheless, an advocacy coalition that believes in hard limits appears determined to find a justification. Their leaders have been developing the case against efficacy of opioid treatment for chronic pain. If they could only prove that opioids have no efficacy, then they would no longer be ethically bound to treat those with persistent pain.[4,6–10] However, the only way to prove that "evidence is insufficient to determine the effectiveness" is to discount thirty-five years of clinical and observational studies that demonstrate efficacy.[141,156,157] There was no debate about efficacy from 1997 to 2009 when standards had been revised to permit higher prescriptions. Regardless of one's point of view of the issues that arose because of mistakes made during that period, medical researchers have a duty to adhere to honest debate and unbiased analysis. There has been a debate over the tradeoff between the risk of addiction and the benefit in relief of pain. That is an honest point of contention that has never been adequately resolved. The major reason is that addiction is not treated as a medical condition, but mainly as a law enforcement problem in the United States. This is still true despite recent legislation and some small steps toward a medical treatment approach. Rather than advocate inclusion of addiction into the realm of medical treatment, the advocacy coalition began a process of reinterpretation of published studies to question the efficacy of opioid therapy itself. Creating a debate in order to cast aside a scientific conclusion is scientifically dishonest.

CHAPTER 4

⁓ℨ⁓

An Advocacy Coalition Carries Out a Medical Coup d'État

Public perception of the relationship between prescription drugs and the opioid-overdose crisis has been heavily influenced by the news media narrative, which is steeped in the perspectives of the DEA, CDC, vested politicians, lawsuits, and expert opinion.[33,37,54,237–257] All stakeholders want an easy target, a way to explain the entire crisis that also presents a clear solution. Prescription opioids have been presented as the cause of the overdose problem. The governor of Vermont went so far as to state that the crisis could be ended by snapping our fingers, implying that all that needs to be done is to limit prescribing opioids and the problem will be solved.[258] He apparently believes the experts most often interviewed in the media, who advocated for and obtained restrictive prescribing guidelines.[37,168,259] Although the language in the final CDC guidelines sounds flexible, the original intent was not flexible. For reasons that must have to do with DEA enforcement, the CDC guidelines have been implemented without flexibility for prescribing doctors. Communication and lobbying behind the scenes have shaped policy in a way that has hidden conflicts of interest. A small group of academic medical professionals ignored professional ethics and used their authority to write articles and evidence reports that redefined the criteria for validity of clinical studies by government agencies. These same academic professionals formed an advocacy coalition that successfully rewrote opioid-prescribing guidelines. Some members of that advocacy coalition are also well-paid consultants and expert witnesses in the lawsuits against the opioid manufacturers.[260-262] Furthermore, politicians have received large campaign contributions from the law firms suing the pharmaceutical industry.[263] The rest of the medical community has been excluded. Despite the response of hundreds of doctors and the AMA[1,3,264] calling for a more humane medical policy, the situation for pain patients has grown dire, and there is no sign of a reprieve.

The pendulum has swung away from compassionate care. The rapid and haphazard change in policy has caused many problems for people with severe pain as they are forced to taper down suddenly or even lose their medication altogether. The logic of blaming overprescribing for the crisis inherently involves blaming doctors. The advocacy coalition claims that doctors were *duped*, but deftly shifts the major blame to the pharmaceutical companies since that fits nicely with the simple claim that the entire problem is caused by prescription drugs.[168,265] The crusade against opioids began in earnest once certain medical professionals realized that pharmaceutical companies have deep pockets and they, too, stand to get a share of the proceeds. In thinking about whether doctors were *duped*, it is instructive to read the report by the Institute of Medicine of the National Academies entitled "Relieving Pain in America."[266] The humane and thoughtful approach of the panel favors individualized treatment, the opposite of the PROP approach. This document does not mention overprescribing but does talk about the ethical and medical responsibility doctors have to treat pain. There is clearly a deep division in the medical community. Given the number of doctors who appear to have a deep concern for pain patients, it is hard to understand how hard limits could have been implemented without external pressures. The explanation lies in the role the DEA plays in policy implementation.

As an indication of how much treatment of pain has regressed, even patients with terminal cancer are now being denied prescriptions by some doctors, insurers, or pharmacies under the new regulation.[121,267] Only hospice for terminal cancer patients is still a refuge where pain is treated with compassion and until the patient feels a sense of relief. The punitive approach to illegal drugs has been extended to prescribing in a way that has effectively stopped the majority of the medical community from engaging with pain patients. Documents such as the Institute of Medicine report[266] suggest that many in the medical community would prefer to have the freedom to treat pain in a medically responsible way without the arbitrary limitations that resulted from the new policy monopoly, represented by Physicians for Responsible Opioid Prescribing (PROP).[3,5,120–122,158,251,268–270] However, most doctors do not have the time or want to take the risk to get involved with pain management any more. The legal and regulatory climate has dissuaded more than 80% of primary care doctors from prescribing opioids.

The PROP Advocacy Coalition

The advocacy coalition called PROP was founded to address the *poor prescribing practices* identified by them as endemic to the compassionate care movement.[8] Drs. Ballantyne, Kolodny, and Lembke are the president, executive director, and member of the board of directors, respectively. All three have been outspoken critics of the movement, having written extensively to promote an alternative viewpoint on the treatment of pain[10–12,18,51,52,124,132,271–276] and served as either consultants or expert witnesses in the legal cases against pharmaceutical companies.[260,261] PROP has promoted setting a maximum opioid dose that may be prescribed to *any patient*.[122] This proposal is based on the notion that the overdose fatality rate is dependent on drug prescribing. PROP claims to have found a simple solution for a complex problem: stop prescribing and the drug problem will cease. In chapters 8 and 9, evidence is presented that prescribing is not the main cause of this epidemic. By carefully distinguishing between criminal diversion and prescribing, we show the fallacy of the argument that reducing the prescription dose for pain patients will reduce the heroin and fentanyl overdose rate. This in no way defends the corruption, mistakes, or incompetence that accompanied the compassionate care movement as implemented from 1997 to 2010. But we must distinguish between the well-intentioned movement initiated by doctors, on the one hand, and the unscrupulous companies, irresponsible agencies, and criminal enterprises that hijacked it, on the other. We have an ethical responsibility to find a solution that addresses the problems of both those suffering in pain and those who are addicted to opioids. The solution will not be found by blaming pain patients for the addiction and overdose crisis, although that narrative is convenient for those in government who would like to avoid scrutiny for their role in the crisis and for those in academia who would like to profit from the demise of the opioid manufacturers. The arbitrary dose limitations effectively put the onus of the drug problem on the pain patient. That is unethical and violates human rights.

While PROP claims to promote a commonsense approach to dose limits and monitoring to prevent overdoses,[277] the effect of the guidelines they have promoted has been extremely harmful to patients like Z. PROP has published articles to attempt to justify the restrictions of the new guidelines by making the case that the harms of opioids outweigh any benefits.[4,10,51,52,124,132,278] Based on very weak evidence, they have added new safety concerns such as hyperalgesia, fall risk, and automobile accidents in recent studies.[4,7] These relatively new side effects appear to be a campaign to find new adverse side effects to add to the negative side of the ledger weighing against opioid use. Members of PROP have claimed that a major reason for patients continuing with their medication is not their pain but the fear of withdrawal,[11] or even that they are being paid by the opioid pharmaceutical industry.[279] PROP's message is molded to emphasize the adverse consequences and eliminate mention of any benefits of opioid prescribing for chronic pain. The doctors who have spoken out against this point of view have suffered consequences, including losing their practices. A North Carolina doctor named Dr. Thomas Kline was an outspoken critic of PROP on the internet.[121,280] He had a small practice of thirty-four patients, all of whom had serious diseases. Dr. Kline came under the scrutiny of the state medical board, and the DEA withdrew his license to prescribe opioids. While Dr. Kline continues his advocacy for pain patients, he is no longer able to medically treat pain patients. I could not find a doctor willing to go on the record concerning the validity of PROP's claims, but many will say anonymously that PROP has not based their advocacy on sound science. PROP has ignored the criticisms of reviewers, patient rights groups, and the hundreds of doctors who have spoken out for a more humane approach. There is fear in the medical community because the DEA has the ultimate power to ruin a doctor's career without warning and with draconian tools, such as asset seizure, turning patients against doctors as witnesses, searching Medicare and Medicaid databases for any errors in coding in the past ten years, any of which may lead to evidence in a prosecution.

The lack of concern for patient welfare in the articles written by the highest officers in PROP is alarming. Regarding recent changes in law in Washington state, Drs. Ballantyne, Sullivan, and Kolodny wrote the following[11]:

> As the rule [implementing a statewide limit on dose of 50 MEDD] comes into effect, clinicians are beginning to taper high dose opioid therapy in their patients. In some cases, this tapering has occurred because the rule has been misunderstood, leading prescribers to taper doses in patients who have been stable for years, resulting in the reemergence of severe pain and extreme anhedonia, both of which are likely to be withdrawal effects. What we have learned from these attempts at tapering doses in patients who have been receiving established therapy for many years is that tapering may destabilize the patients, leaving persistent craving and aberrant behavior in its wake.

The authors admit that the pain and suffering they describe in such a clinical fashion is unnecessary. Rather than concern for the poor treatment of patients, the conclusion the authors draw is that pain felt by patients is a *withdrawal effect*. In 2016, the CDC published a guideline, written by the members of PROP, who were given special access to CDC staff and decision-making authority by ex-director, Thomas Frieden. The CDC guideline was supposed to be a recommendation, but in practice, it became a mandate for hard limits and forced tapers.[281] The limit on prescribing and actions taken in the pain clinics have occurred entirely because of the policy PROP promoted. Yet PROP fails to acknowledge its own complicity and ethical responsibility when "the rule has been misunderstood." The rule refers to the way that tapering should be conducted according to the CDC guidelines. It appears to be of mere academic interest to the authors that the effect of their policy is a potentially harmful taper. Of course, if the patient's *pain* can be explained as *withdrawal* and *craving*, then the authors may justify the taper in their own minds. How can the authors be so certain that patients are experiencing withdrawal? The evidence is mainly based on whether the patient claims to need more pain medicine. The notion that a request for more pain medication is an expression of unmet pain needs is a thing of the past. The prevailing attitude is that asking for more medication is symptom of a disorder rather than a response to uncontrolled pain. If the patient could be seen as having a use disorder, it may justify more drastic tapering and therefore lead to the apparent lack of concern for patient welfare evident in this article written by the leaders of PROP.[11] Since Dr. Ballantyne's publication does not specify the patient's disease or any other details, it is impossible to know whether these authors would have a similar attitude toward the same procedure applied to Patient Z or any patient who has ankylosing spondylitis, psoriatic arthritis, sickle cell disease, or any other disease that results in intolerable pain. The authors from PROP do not specify what baseline pain levels would justify treatment, but of course, this is difficult because of the subjectivity of pain. Withdrawal is unpleasant and involves nausea and intense discomfort, but a doctor who ignores the pain of a disease such as ankylosing spondylitis is not on a firm medical or ethical foundation.

The Battle Over PROP's Policy Contributions: The DEA vs. the AMA

The CDC guidelines have received pushback from broad coalitions of doctors and even the American Medical Association (AMA).[1,2,121,122,158,159,264,267,282–285] Doctors can see that there is a disconnect between the stated goals of "reasonable opioid prescribing" and the treatment that patients are actually receiving in pain clinics. Hundreds of doctors have petitioned to end forced tapers.[3,282] They have also pointed out that it is not a good medical practice that quality of care has been reduced to one number, supposedly valid for all patients.[286] The origin of the disconnect between the guidelines and practice is not explicitly explained in any document, but the above paragraph from Dr. Ballantyne's paper shows that the members of PROP are aware of it.[11] PROP has put all patients into one group and decided the dose that applies to all, irrespective of their disease. Pain clinics have become opioid distribution outlets that follow a strict legal formula.

Observers have pointed out that the CDC guidelines are reasonable as written. It is their implementation that is inhumane and cruel. The guideline of a limit of 90 MEDD is a recommended limit for PCPs who are starting a new patient on opioid therapy. However, today PCPs are seldom the ones writing new prescriptions since any new pain patients have been referred to pain clinics. In practice, many state medical boards and legislatures have interpreted the regulation as a hard limit of 90 MEDD. This leaves the possibility for state legislatures to decide, arbitrarily, that an even lower limit would be safer still. As the paragraph from Dr. Ballantyne and coworkers states above, in Washington State the limit set by law is 50 MEDD.[11] The National Committee for Quality Assurance (NCQA) set the limit at 120 MEDD and stated that any dose in excess was indicative of poor care because of the high risk involved.[14,48] The NCQA sets the standards for Medicare, Medicaid, and all medical insurance. When that committee states that any dose above 120 MEDD is high risk, not only is reimbursement in question, but legal liability as well. Clinics may set the limit somewhere between 50 and 120 MEDD, but they are all setting a hard limit. The guideline says nothing about what type of disease might justify a higher dose or what action is required for patients who are already above the limit when they arrive at the clinic. The most important aspect of the guideline is the implementation, and that depends on how the DEA interprets the regulation. The DEA does not publish any information about prescribing levels that might trigger an investigation or prosecution. Pain clinics are left to guess, which means that they must de facto assume that the only security can be found in the most conservative interpretation of the published regulations on the CDC and NCQA websites. As a consequence, it does not matter what disease the patient has. The dose limit is the same.

Using the articles and lawsuits against Purdue Pharma as support, PROP and the DEA both set out to lobby the FDA to put a hard limit of 100 MEDD on opioid prescribing in 2012. However, after a lengthy public debate, the FDA denied PROP's petition (see document FDA-2012-p-0818-0691 on the internet). The FDA's rejection of this request is very sensible. It points out that there are many different types of diseases, and it is not appropriate to regulate a one-size-fits-all solution. When PROP failed to convince the FDA, it turned to the CDC, an agency that ordinarily might regulate the use of medication in an epidemic, but is not normally the agency that would regulate routine prescribing. The CDC is concerned with epidemiology, but usually not pharmaceuticals themselves. Nonetheless, PROP managed to direct the attention of the director of the CDC, Dr. Thomas Frieden, to the prescription drug overdose "epidemic."

Using the lobbying campaign and support by the DEA, PROP has successfully forced their prescribing regime on American medicine. The doctors and nurses in the clinic may want to frame their decisions based on the pain patient's well-being, but regardless of what the patient needs, the dose cannot exceed the maximum set by the NCQA or by state law. For a patient who enters the clinic at a higher dose, there are many clinics where tapering is rapid, despite the dangers. The concern for the patient is subservient to the fear that the clinic will suffer if the guidelines are not followed. The clinics may frame their concern for the overdose fatality rate as a patient concern, yet many pain patients who have prescriptions for years are being told that they must drastically reduce their dose. Patients have also been abandoned, which would be considered malpractice in other fields of medicine. The statements made to justify these actions are fraught with inconsistencies. For example, the vast majority of overdoses (>80%) have heroin, cocaine, or fentanyl as the primary cause of death, yet media reports and pain clinic rhetoric emphasize the overdose rate as though it were primarily a patient risk. The danger to legitimate pain patients has increased in recent years because of the severe cuts to their medication that has led to loss of employment, broken families, disability, and death. One of the reasons for the growing suicide rate and skyrocketing overdose rate is that pain patients who have no hope of relief have taken desperate actions that they would never have considered if their pain had been properly controlled. If reduction of overdose fatalities is the criterion by which PROP and the DEA measure their success, then they both have failed miserably.

A Cross-Sectional View of PROP's Lobbying Efforts

A few years after the PROP petition to the FDA was rejected, in 2015, two members of PROP, Drs. Kolodny and Ballantyne, exchanged letters with FDA officials in the Journal of the American Medical Association (JAMA) to express their opposition to FDA approval for another time-released formulation of an opioid drug. The FDA officials pointed out their approval does not unilaterally decide the matter and they had set conditions that the manufacturers must meet prior to any final decision. Drs. Ballantyne and Kolodny wrote, "Despite the enormous public health price being paid for the increased use of opioids, no evidence exists that their use has been associated with improvements in outcomes for patients with chronic pain."[52] The crucial statement that "no evidence exists" requires clinical studies. By 2015 PROP had conducted a systematic review that excluded all the previous evidence, thus permitting the statement that "no evidence exists" for efficacy of opioids.[4] When we look back on seventeen years of meta-analyses and reviews, it is clear that PROP designed the acceptance criteria of their later publications in order to be able to exclude all the evidence, and thereby write the statement "evidence is insufficient to determine the effectiveness." [4,6–9,287]

PROP claims it wants to ban marketing of opioids for long-term daily use, but not prescribing for patients who need them. This sounds like a reasonable goal, but this not what PROP has implemented. On the one hand, PROP proposes common sense when they say that opioid pharmaceutical companies do not need to advertise opioid drugs, hold conferences to promote their product, or make visits to doctors' offices to promote them. [288] Payments to doctors in speaking engagements are one form of kickback shown clearly in the case of the company Insys discussed in chapter 10. The recent criminal conviction of Purdue Pharma for kickbacks to doctors shows a widespread network of illegal payments in return for prescribing. We can all agree that this corruption is deplorable, but these cases should not be used to interfere with legitimate pain patients' access to medication. On the other hand, PROP's letter to the FDA[52] surrounds the only reasonable contention with categorical statements that are a matter of opinion, although they are represented as clinically proven. Drs. Ballantyne and Kolodny proceeded to say that "opioids have been oversold. Patients with nonstructural low back pain, fibromyalgia, and chronic headache do not exhibit improvements in function and quality of life and are at high risk of developing dependence, functional deterioration, or addiction." This type of statement may have a kernel of truth, but it has neither context nor supporting evidence. It is precisely the type of statement that has been used to justify denying treatment to any patient who has severe pain. Drs. Ballantyne and Kolodny provide no definition of which patients might benefit from opioid therapy. PROP has not written any guideline, article, or commentary that suggests that we should think about persistent-pain patients any differently compared to someone with low back pain. Both may need pain management, but they clearly differ in their severity of disease. Where is PROP's statement that an extremely painful disease such as epidermolysis bullosa should be treated with compassion? Both the articles and government guidelines speak of pain patients without distinguishing the myriad origins of pain. The exception is for cancer, which receives cursory mention as being an exception in some publications by these authors. But PROP does not even mention sickle cell disease, which many doctors have placed in the same category as cancer in terms of potential severity of pain. It is a great oversight of pain management that diseases such as psoriatic arthritis, ankylosing spondylitis, Ehlers-Danlos syndrome, and many other extremely painful diseases are not treated with the same compassion as cancer pain.

The FDA officials responding to the critique in JAMA called for comprehensive solutions.[289] The FDA has authority to define permitted usage of a drug, but they are trying to balance that authority with other state and federal agencies who will also play a role in determining the actual policy. In fact, the FDA has taken numerous regulatory actions to reclassify drugs, such as hydromorphone,[290-292] buprenorphine, and tramadol in recent years largely under pressure from PROP. The FDA must always contend with unintended consequences. For example, the recent reclassification of hydromorphone has made that useful drug often unavailable in emergency rooms. Hospitals are worried about the legal implications of using it since it is now seen as highly addictive. What happens when a patient arrives at an emergency room (ER) who does not respond well to morphine or oxycodone? Patients who have already taken morphine and oxycodone, like Patient Z, would need an additional very high dose of those opioids for an acute pain, whereas the lower cross-tolerance of hydromorphone makes it a more effective option in the ER. Aside from its greater potency, this was a reason for having hydromorphone available. Actions to limit marketing of opioids are common sense,[293] but the push to change language and institute stricter rules has an insidious effect of threatening basic pain management in emergency rooms, as well as for long-term diseases.

The legal authority to prosecute for narcotics violations lies with the DEA. When DEA officials read that opioids have *no efficacy*, that the medication has been *oversold*, and will lead to *addiction*, the agency has the justification it needs to interpret the guideline in the strictest possible sense. PROP's commentary is part of a pattern of articles and commentary that equates of pain patient's *dependence* with *addiction*.[11] From an ethical point of view, there are two serious issues here. The first is an attack on a patient's right to receive medical treatment for pain, a fundamental human right. The second is an attempt to discredit thirty-five years of studies showing the efficacy of opioids for persistent pain and to exaggerate the risk of every conceivable side effect.

Public Policy and Law Enforcement Lead to Division of the Medical Community

The lobbying of government agencies ultimately gave PROP the opportunity to influence medical policy directly in the CDC guidelines. The lobbying of the FDA and the CDC ultimately ended up as lobbying of Congress by law firms who have a vested interest in PROP's narrative for their multibillion-dollar lawsuits against opioid manufacturers and pharmacies. The outcome has been a politicization of opioid prescribing. These efforts have divided the medical community and our society at large.[294] Given the already precarious positions that many pain specialists find themselves in, it is disturbing when members of the medical community define doctors as drug dealers, as is proclaimed in the title of Dr. Lembke's book *Drug Dealer, MD*.[18] This may sound like a catchy title for purposes of marketing, but it is painfully descriptive of the way that so many innocent doctors have been treated by the DEA and state prosecutors looking to make a name for themselves. Fundamentally, the issue of addiction is at the root of the issue that most concerns the public and law enforcement. The medical community is profoundly conflicted in its attitude toward addiction since there are significant obstacles for doctors who want to treat addicts in the United States. Under most circumstances, addicts can only receive treatment in an opioid treatment program, which is not a medical treatment option. Although a doctor can apply for a waiver to permit prescribing of buprenorphine to treat recovering addicts under medication-assisted treatment (MAT), few choose to do this because of the required extra training and the risk of liability if patients engage in diversion or are simply noncompliant.[295,296] Even if this waiver system is possible in the Comprehensive Addiction Recovery Act (CARA) of 2016, there are still significant obstacles to treatment of addiction as a disease, or an addict as a patient. In fact, the perverse logic of the American legal system makes doctors criminally liable if a pain patient with an opioid prescription turns to addiction and harms himself or herself. Doctors have faced long prison sentences for their patient's diversion or addiction, and subsequent death. Doctors in the field of pain medicine have been stigmatized as well. It is no small wonder that most doctors pass on the opportunity to help recovering addicts.

What Is the Point of Accusing Doctors of Being Drug Dealers?

The book *Drug Dealer, MD* calls the nature of persistent pain into question.[18] Dr. Lembke claims that much of the pain being treated today is not genuine physical pain. Rather, she suggests that the types of pain patients suffer from are indicative of psychiatric illness. Her examples include fibromyalgia and complex regional pain syndrome (CRPS), which are both unquestionably painful diseases, not hallucinations of pain. In fact, CRPS is one of the most painful diseases known. The general tenor of Dr. Lembke's discussion is that patients tend to exaggerate or even imagine their pain in order to get drugs. Dr. Lembke is a psychiatrist who has psychoanalyzed "well-heeled" substance abusers and sees pain patients through the lens of addiction. She has blamed the medical community for liberal prescribing as a major contributing factor to the addiction of her patients. Her account contains sad stories of people who were not well served by their medical providers, but also clearly suffered from tendencies toward addiction that had gone unrecognized for many years. Regardless of the specifics of these individual cases, the notion that prescribing opioids after surgery or a trip to the dentist is an excess on the part of the medical community is an extreme viewpoint. Dr. Lembke's view is that current attitudes toward pain have led doctors to have greater trust in patients than is warranted. Her dismissal of pain as imaginary is both unprofessional and inappropriate for someone who has received an MD degree.

Nearly every observer agrees that attitudes toward prescribing need to be reviewed in light of the experience of the past twenty years. I agree with Dr. Lembke that routinely treating depression and attention-deficit disorder in teenagers with pills has potentially negative outcomes. These drugs are not opioids, but the issue of overprescribing is a general concern that the medical community needs to consider seriously. The point is not that doctors need to stop prescribing, but that a multifaceted and individualized approach is crucial. Opioid medication should be dispensed with great care and "titrated" to the pain of the patient. Although a small minority of patients fit the description of a drug seeker, doctors are justifiably concerned about being deceived by those patients. In honestly confronting such problems, we need a balanced view, not an overreaction that leads to ignoring legitimate pain or accusing *all* pain patients of pretending, imagining, or exaggerating. There is no study that suggests that a majority of pain patients are abusing their prescriptions or are drug seeking. It is a small minority who do so, and those who generalize this to the population at large are doing great harm to the practice of medicine. Perhaps more important is what kind of compassion we show for the minority who do have psychological issues that lead them to substance abuse. Suggesting doctors are *drug dealers* does not address the actual problem in our society or our medical system; it does greatly harm the millions of people who have genuine pain and look to the medical community for help.

Medicine has an ethical mandate to treat addiction as a disease.[297] If every patient fits somewhere in the spectrum of medical practice, then doctors can begin to look at each patient to try to address specific needs. If a nurse in a hospital ward suspects that a patient is asking for excessive medication, there should be a procedure to intervene, ensure there is not excessive suffering, and if the person is feeling a little too good on the medication, to cut back on the medication and help the patient overcome internal issues to avoid a future problem. On the other hand, if we simply change our procedures and refuse to treat pain, we risk harming patient health. Treating acute pain after surgery with opioids has been part of medical practice for more than one hundred years with good reason. However, treating acute pain is not the central issue. The advocates of strict controls on prescribing have mainly focused on curtailing or eliminating long-term prescriptions for persistent pain.

Dr. Lembke's book is a weathervane for many of the attitudes of critics of the compassionate care movement. She describes the typical pain patient as a drug-seeking impostor. A small minority of patients fit this description, and it is damaging to the great majority to portray patients as *drug seeking* without qualification.[278] Dr. Lembke suggests that the American medical community celebrated pain in the nineteenth century and did not treat it aggressively. She cites Meldrum's history of morphine use. However, Dr. Meldrum writes the following[17]:

> European physicians did their best to relieve their patients' pain, most often through judicious use of opium or after 1680, laudanum made by placing opium in sherry, introduced by Thomas Sydenham. But they also inflicted it when necessary to relieve evil humors or to amputate diseased limbs.

Moreover, Dr. Meldrum described the widespread use of morphine in the United States in the nineteenth century, administered orally, and after 1855 injected by syringe. Morphine was legal, and it was an accepted treatment for essentially any kind of pain. Of course, the access to pain medication may not have reached the poorer segments of society, just as is the case today. Dr. Meldrum's article does not support Dr. Lembke's contention that pain was not treated aggressively by doctors in the nineteenth century.

Dr. Lembke's treatment of the evidence pertaining to the addiction rate of pain patients is another example of dubious scholarship. On page 22 of *Drug Dealer, MD*, Dr. Lembke criticized a letter published in the *New England Journal of Medicine* (*NEJM*) in 1980 by

Drs. Porter and Jick entitled "Addiction Rare in Patients Treated with Narcotics."[137] Dr. Lembke wrote that the letter contains "false evidence that the risk of becoming addicted to opioids [...] was less than 1%." This letter has received enormous scrutiny and been cited an excessive number of times given that it is a short one paragraph letter, written almost as a passing observation. However, it was the first statement of the low addiction rate among pain patients, which has been confirmed many times since.[133,138,140–142] Does Dr. Lembke really mean to say that Drs. Porter and Jick falsified their data when they wrote that of "11,882 patients who received at least one narcotic preparation [in a hospital], there were only four cases of reasonably well documented addiction"? If Dr. Lembke is not making an allegation, then her statement is pure hyperbole since there is no evidence to suggest that Porter and Jick's account is false or even inaccurate. On the contrary, there is a great deal of evidence that the addiction rate among *pain patients* is indeed around 1–3% depending on how one quantifies *addiction*.[133,137,138,140–142] The results one obtains in a study of addiction rates obviously depend greatly on the patient population, the clinical setting, and how one defines and determines patients who have opioid use disorder. For example, Cheatle and coworkers did a careful study eliminating any patients who had a history of any kind of substance abuse, but allowing patients with signs of depression or mild anxiety, and did a one-year follow-up after a person had a course of opioids for routine pain.[144] They concluded that even healthy, pain-naive people had a rate of substance abuse of <5%. A higher rate would be expected for a patient population who had a history of drug abuse.[143,298] For example, Boscarino and coworkers studied a random group, in which 33% had a history of some kind of substance abuse.[143] They found 10.3% addiction and 21.7% aberrant behavior at the end of the study period. Dr. Lembke's representation of the medical literature is misleading, both in her attack on Porter and Jick and in her selective choice of one study, whose conclusions she misrepresented.

It would have been reasonable for Dr. Lembke to say that Porter and Jick's article was used improperly by Purdue Pharma as part of their advertising campaign.[299] Purdue admitted in court that it falsely used that and other medical articles to claim that addiction rates are <1% in *the general population* for extended opioid prescriptions.[245] When we view the general population, mostly healthy and typically younger than hospital or persistent-pain patients, there is a different statistic and a separate set of concerns for opioid prescribing. As documented in the last chapter, the vast majority of pain-naive patients would not react to opioids the same way that a pain patient would. Various studies estimate the addiction rate to be as high as 4–8% for the general population.[4,9,139,141,300] The important distinction between serious illness and more common pain is not to be found anywhere in the writing of those who have advocated for radical changes to prescribing. Dr. Lembke's book lacks nuance to a degree that it misleads her audience into believing that chronic pain is a fiction created only by those who have a drug problem. This misinformation will not solve the drug problem as we see from the continued exceptionally high overdoses years after PROP's guidelines were implemented, but the attitudes promoted by the book hurt the most vulnerable in the population, whose very real pain is debilitating to the point that they cannot defend themselves.

Having set up a straw man using a single paper from 1980 without the context from the medical literature since that time, Dr. Lembke proceeded to select one study from the dozens of studies in the literature for her counterargument that the addiction rate is actually very high. She claims that the rate of addiction in patients is 56%, citing a study by Martell and coworkers.[301] This is wildly incorrect use of the data from this paper. In fact, the rate of substance abuse or addiction observed *during* the sixteen-week time frame of the ten studies analyzed by Martell ranged from 3% to 24%. The Martell meta-analysis of ten previous studies reported that 35–54% patients selected had admitted to a *prior* substance-abuse issue at some point in their lives, which means that they violated the terms of a narcotics contract. This could mean anything from getting medication for an oral surgery without permission to abusing drugs. The study design is poor since Martell and coworkers mixed ten qualitatively different patient groups with different histories in one meta-analysis. The Martell publication is a study of low back pain, which has become controversial since low back pain can mean anything from an excuse to get some pills to the most excruciatingly painful conditions known to humankind. There is a great deal of doubt about what the Martell study means since the editors actually took an unusual step of putting a disclaimer in the article that cautions the reader about potential bias. Nonetheless, this study became the sole evidence for Dr. Lembke's misleading statement that "as many as 56% of patients receiving long-term opioid prescription opioid pain killers for low back pain [...] progress to addictive opioid use, including patients with no prior history of addiction." The origin of the number 56% is unclear since there is no such value in the Martell paper. The only number that is close is the high end of the range of a *prior substance abuse* rate in one of the studies. The studies in the meta-analysis find opioid misuse rates from 3% to 24% with a weighted average of 7%, fully eight times less than the number quoted by Dr. Lembke. Before accusing others of false statements, Dr. Lembke should do a careful review of her own scholarship. She has made unsubstantiated allegations and has misused statistics. There are so many incorrect citations in *Drug Dealer, MD* it would take a separate chapter to document them.

Dependence vs. Addiction: There Is a Distinctive Difference

The leaders of the medical community should be promoting understanding of the distinction between dependence and addiction. However, a paper by Drs. Ballantyne, Sullivan, and Kolodny carrying the title "Dependence vs. Addiction: A Distinction Without a Difference"[11] does not educate, but instead it puts pain patients on the defensive. This publication sets the tone for one of the themes that PROP has consistently promoted since 2012—that pain patients are effectively addicts and that they know it, but their doctors are in denial. The authors put it this way[11]:

> For pain patients, drug-seeking behaviors are different from behaviors that are listed by standard

criteria and are focused on obtaining opioids from prescribers. Aberrancy in pain patients may include doctor shopping, frequent lost prescriptions, and repeated requests for early prescriptions, while the behaviors listed in the fourth or fifth edition of the *Diagnostic and Statistical Manual of Mental Disorders*, e.g., "failure to fulfill major role obligations at work, school or home," tend to be attributed to pain rather than to addiction. In fact, pain patients who are treated continuously with opioids may not manifest any aberrant behaviors because they are effectively receiving maintenance therapy, which suppresses craving. However, when opioids are suddenly not available, tolerance occurs, or attempts are made to taper, craving and addiction behaviors emerge. Recent teaching has been that this should be thought of as *pseudoaddiction*, a misleading term that suggests that aberrant opioid seeking is predominantly a consequence of inadequate pain relief and should be addressed by increasing opioid dose. The concept of *pseudoaddiction* implies that opioid seeking ends when an adequate dose is reached, but this is not apparent in the long-term treatment of chronic pain. It is noteworthy that patients are often more willing to diagnose their own addiction than are their providers, who have been taught that addiction to prescribed drugs is rare.

This depiction of the persistent-pain patient as a drug dependent who is more concerned about withdrawal than pain and is consistently trying to increase the dose is indeed a description of an addict. The description also portrays a hapless doctor who is unable to see through the masquerade of the pain patient, which is apparently common enough that no qualification is required in the description. The statements are, in fact, allegations made by archetypal doctor and patient. Ballantyne and coauthors make no effort to differentiate the persistent-pain patients from the general population of patients whose pain is less severe or patients who have histories of substance abuse.

The article does not discuss the pain of specific diseases, such as cancer, sickle cell disease, or the many rare diseases that can be equally painful. Instead, the theme is that all pain patients who rely on opioids are drug dependent and that dependence is functionally the same as addiction. This type of reasoning harms all pain patients but is particularly egregious toward those who have serious, incurable diseases. Patients with more serious disease often have greater pain. Although the data are inadequate, there are data and medical consensus that high doses of opioids have helped patients with rare and extremely painful diseases as even Dr. Ballantyne has documented in prior work.[113] Yet in today's climate, a doctor who treats that pain with a dose higher than the limit can be accused of pushing the patient toward addiction. The DEA cannot use that as an explicit reasoning for shutting down a pain clinic or pain specialist, but they can always suspect diversion or misappropriation and close down a clinic to investigate.[280,302-307] Suspicion alone is grounds for law enforcement action by the DEA. PROP's statements justify this type of action by suggesting that patients pulling their doctors along as they head toward dependence and addiction.[11]

Developing the Narrative That Pain Patients Are Not Really Suffering

If PROP had not been so successful at imposing their view on the entire medical community, the points I am making about their bias and sloppy science would be of merely academic interest. However, PROP has been successful in policy implementation and the analysis of their publications is not a pedantic exercise. Based on the new restrictions, hundreds of thousands of patients have been denied treatment or given substandard care, including sickle cell disease patients[68,69,308] and a host of other inflammatory or degenerative diseases.[159,233,251,283,309,310] A recent comment period in the Federal Register that ended in July 2020 received more than five thousand patient statements concerning how the CDC guidelines had ruined lives and created miserable conditions.[279] The attacks by the leadership of PROP on both doctors and pain patients need to be scrutinized for accuracy and objectivity.[269]

Articles written by the members of PROP espouse the conviction that "evidence increasingly suggests that gains from long-term opioid therapy are small and may not justify the risk."[273] The journal discussion in "Why Doctors Prescribe Opioids to Known Opioid Abusers" involving Drs. Ballantyne and Sullivan on the one hand, and Dr. Lembke on the other, is easily resolved between them because the authors agree that there is an ethical imperative to help drug users. Most pain patients, on the other hand, are simply out of luck, since according to Dr. Lembke "opioids are not a very effective treatment for chronic pain that is not related to cancer."[278] In mentioning cancer, Dr. Lembke makes a blanket dismissal of many diseases known to cause severe pain. As a trained medical professional, Dr. Lembke should be aware of other painful inflammatory or degenerative diseases. The example of sickle cell disease is prominent case where the pain has been undertreated for years but is now recognized to be persistent and often severe.

The members of PROP do not discuss the origin of pain or negative consequences of living with persistent pain in any of their recent publications. Their concern focuses on side effects, risks of overdose, hyperalgesia, and self-deception that leads to abuse. Whether one considers pain as part of the disease of a symptom, persistent-pain patients are often people with serious diseases. Pain causes its own symptoms that further damage the cardiovascular and endocrine systems in ways that shorten life spans. It is disturbing that doctors would have so little to say about pain itself but feel confident stating that the patient's motives are drug seeking. It is one thing to doubt an individual who presents him/herself in an office visit. If a doctor feels that there is something peculiar about the request, it is legitimate to question, doubt, or refuse to write a prescription. But to doubt that the categories of pain in the literature are real is a violation of clinical ethics, which say that in the absence of overwhelming evidence for a course of treatment, one should treat each patient individually.[5] Persistent pain is bad enough. To have the notion that the disease is painful be doubted and to be accused of drug-seeking behavior is humiliating to the patient who actually has pain.

The suppositions and prejudices present in the articles written by members of PROP were not sufficient to convince anyone that there is a need to modify prescribing practices. These articles built the case that pain patients, those with severe pain and a need for high-dose opioids, are actually suffering from opioid use disorder. The complement to this case is to delegitimize the more than one hundred clinical studies that show opioids have efficacy for the treatment of chronic pain. However, there was no push to question those studies. Therefore, the members of PROP created the conditions for a change by redefining the criteria for valid studies. After all, if none of the studies is valid, then clearly there is no evidence for efficacy. Using connections within the government agencies, PROP managed to change the criteria for evaluating scientifically valid studies in government-evidence reports. This change made in a government report that is seldom scrutinized laid the groundwork for new rigid prescribing guidelines that affected millions of patients. With the threat of law enforcement action behind them and pushes in state legislatures and other government agencies, such as HHS and NCQA justified by their actions, a few doctors managed to execute a medical coup d'état that radically changed opioid prescribing. In the short term, this change appears irreversible despite the thousands of doctors who oppose it.

CHAPTER 5

⤜⤙

The Inherent Limitations of Clinical Studies and Meta-Analyses of Pain Relief

Essentially every clinical study agrees that long-term use of opioids for chronic noncancer pain (CNCP) has not been studied sufficiently. Despite this consensus, there are many individual studies indicative of efficacy of opioid therapy. Policy statements by the American Pain Society[21] and the American Geriatric Society[22] in 1996 and 1997 were based on clinical experience, but they have now been completely disregarded because of the opioid addiction and overdose crisis. There have been studies of side effects, abuse, and addiction for many years as well. Despite the reality that some patients have been harmed by opioid use disorders, many more patients have received benefits of long-term opioid therapy that outweigh the disadvantages. Many thousands of patients have continued to work and take care of families because opioid prescriptions permitted them to control their pain. Many more thousands with incurable conditions have had an improved mobility and some relief from the ravages of inflammatory or degenerative diseases. One need only look to the evidence in the thousands of patient testimonials of the destruction to lives caused by the implementation of the CDC guidelines in 2016 written in the Federal Register to see a cross-section.[279] These patients have clearly suffered from the reductions in prescribing, and they have made that suffering public in their commentary to the CDC. Hopefully, this information will contribute a more humane prescribing guideline in future policy considerations. But patient accounts are subjective, and medical researchers may object that this is simply a large amount of anecdotal evidence. I counter with the question, Are these medical researchers able to do better in the area of pain management?

PROP claims we cannot treat pain using opioids because some people may fall prey to addiction. I believe we must confront the dangers of addiction honestly, but refusing to treat pain is medically indefensible. There is a large divide in the US because many people were harmed by the environment created by the mismanagement and corruption of the compassionate care movement. However, that is not a reason to abandon millions of pain patients, or to give up finding a humane, medical solution for millions of addicts. The current posture taken by PROP is to propose prohibition and treat all patients who take opioids as dependent, thereby unifying pain treatment and addiction by ignoring the medical problem of pain. The medical treatment suggestions are uniformly focused on the peculiar suggestion that all pain patients should be encouraged to admit that they have a "dependence" and encouraged to use buprenorphine. The notion that buprenorphine is the best substitute for morphine and oxycodone requires sound clinical data as the authors admit themselves.[588]

Given the subjectivity of pain, the biases in this socially and medically complicated area, and the lack of appropriate measurement methods, how can a research scientist be certain they have an objective and methodologically sound approach to the treatment of pain? In this chapter, we examine the inherent problems of clinical trials and meta-analyses in the area of pain medication. Each meta-analysis can choose from among thousands of articles, but the selection is restricted based on search terms and criteria such as the type of study, whether it has proper control experiments and so on. By changing the criteria for inclusion of studies in the metal-analysis, one can affect the outcome.

In order to have a real impact on prescribing practices, PROP decided to attack the consensus that opioids have efficacy for long-term care, particularly for those who have seriously painful diseases.

That consensus was what led to the compassionate care movement. Thus, in parallel with the kinds of commentary in the publications discussed in the previous chapter, there has been a concerted effort by the members of PROP to reinterpret thirty-five years of randomized controlled trials (RCTs) and observational studies, finding that opioid treatment has efficacy for chronic or persistent pain.[40–47,141,311–342] If financial gain were not a consideration, one could imagine that PROP's motive is a concern for how advertising by the pharmaceutical companies and poor training of some doctors contributed to the addiction and overdose problem.[260,261] However, the financial stakes in this field have changed dramatically. In the 2000s, there were billions to be made by selling opioids. Since 2007, with the guilty plea by Purdue Pharma's executives, it has been clear that there are billions to be made by suing pharmaceutical companies.[343] Suddenly the doctors involved in treating chronic pain patients have become a valuable asset to the law firms leading the legal campaign against pharmaceutical companies, pharmacies, and even professional organizations. The articles written by the members of PROP provide academic cover that strengthens expert witness testimony. We would not be so concerned with that testimony if it did not play so directly into the narrative that pain patients are addicts.

A critical examination of study design reveals the severe limitations on studies of pain and function that all clinicians must acknowledge at the outset. First, pain is essentially impossible to quantify. Second, studies that attempt to quantify function have also foundered on subjectivity and the inherent impossibility of proper quantitative methods. Third, defining a proper patient group that represents the types of severe pain found in the population is impossible, because human beings are not lab rats and we cannot conduct studies that result in great human suffering. Fourth, bias is very strong in this type of research. The inherently subjective nature of pain puts a special ethical requirement on any studies done or statements made with reference to those studies. Consequently, the National Academies have stated that use of RCT studies for dosing policy of opioids in pain management is not ethical.[344] Nonetheless, the medical literature appears not to recognize this, and one reads that RCT studies are the "gold standard." Policy changes have been justified by meta-analyses of RCT studies. One of the astonishing facts is that the federal agencies have relied on only a few medical researchers for twenty years to lead many of these federally funded meta-analyses and evidence assessments that are used to set policy. The lead author on many studies is Dr. Roger Chou. Dr. Chou's view of this field is evident from his actions. Dr. Chou championed the effort to taper all opioid patients on Medicare in the state of Oregon to a dose of zero.[345,346] Those with ability to pay could obtain medication, but the poor were to be abandoned. Fortunately, that policy was not implemented, but the appalling lack of ethics in this approach is being propagated throughout the pain clinics of the United States. Dr. Chou and the leaders of PROP have used their bully pulpit to justify the tapering of an entire population based on a series of meta-analyses and evidence reviews that are contradictory.[4,6–9,11,281,347] When authors contradict their own findings by introducing unprecedented methodological changes, we can suspect that bias has been injected into the process. To be precise, over time these authors have changed their viewpoint and have found ways to shape the conclusions of their meta-analyses to match their bias.[7,11,113,132,287] The conflicts of interest of some of the authors are also evident.[260,261] It is scandalous that the members of PROP hid their conflicts of interest during the crucial period when they were given access to policy-making bodies.[262]

What Can Be Learned from Studies on Pain in Human Subjects?

Clinicians ideally follow a scientific process in studies with human subjects to develop hypotheses, test them, and solve medical problems. One of the most difficult issues in a clinical trial is the design of appropriate controls to distinguish between the treatment and control groups. The treatment group receives the active medication, and the control group most often receives a placebo, a pill, or other medication that looks identical to the active medication but lacks the active agent. We cannot treat human beings as laboratory animals, so doctors are quite limited in the types of pain that they can study. Clinical studies of opioids have focused mainly on two very different groups (cohorts): first, cancer patients, and second, patients with low back, osteoarthritis, and neuropathic pain. Persistent-pain patients with serious autoimmune or degenerative diseases can hardly be found in published studies on long-term opioid use. This is, in part, because those diseases are relatively rare but also to a greater degree arising from the difficulty of conducting a controlled study on subjects who have such severe pain and debilitating conditions. This is one of the major inherent shortcomings of every study of pain. With the exception of cancer, one cannot study directly those patients who have the most severe pain because of ethical and practical constraints. Even in cancer studies, it is very difficult to properly assess placebo effects. We cannot justify letting a control group suffer horrible pain. This fact leads to one of several inherent methodological flaws in every single study of pain medications. PROP has simply ignored these fatal weaknesses in their quest to reinterpret the entire body of work using the tools of meta-analysis and evidence review. With regard to methodology, neither proper interpretation of the placebo effect nor the subjectivity of pain has received mention in PROP's publications. There seems to be no recognition either here or elsewhere of the need for a systems approach to dealing with these complicated and inherently subjective issues.[344] The systems approach is one alternative for policy changes needed to combat the massive diversion problem, which led to over sixteen thousand overdoses annually in 2015.[348] This is an alarming figure, but we must keep in mind that over twice that number died from heroin, fentanyl, and other illegal drug overdoses in 2015. The prescription drug-overdose wave occurred in a culture where drug overdose has been escalating for decades.

An Institutional Review Board (IRB) scrutinizes studies of mice or rats and any other laboratory animals to determine whether there is unnecessary pain and suffering. Studies on human subjects are subjected to a similar process but are much more stringently scrutinized for ethical considerations. This limitation means that the normal placebo-controlled experiments are impossible for the most severe persistent pain. In an RCT, both groups, medication and placebo, must be randomized as well as possible. In most studies, the treatment group receives an opioid to relieve their pain and the placebo group would receive identical pills without any pain medication. An RCT is possible only for minor pain, because it would be immoral to give a placebo to patients who are suffering severe pain for a significant period. In a single-blind study, the patient does not know whether they are receiving the treatment or the placebo. In a double-blind study, neither the patient nor the physician knows whether the patient is being provided the treatment or the placebo. These considerations are important for the applicability of studies to a patient population. Unfortunately, the patient population is poorly described in many of the studies on opioids. However, we can be sure that patients such as Patient Z were not covered by any of the RCT studies discussed in this chapter. Their pain was too severe. One might have thought that this was one of the issues that concerned Dr. Ballantyne in the 2008 paper cited above. However, she later held up RCTs as the gold standard and advocated excluding observational studies, despite the inherent weakness of the RCT approach for persistent pain.

The other type of study that can be done is an uncontrolled observational study where one tracks different patients over time and uses the data to draw conclusions about the efficacy of drugs and side effects.[141,156,157] While these have been reported for many years, PROP's recommendation has been that we should discount them entirely despite the fact that many of these studies involve patients who have lived for years, even decades, using opioid medications to manage their pain. The claim that the studies of human pain must meet the gold standard of the double-blinded RCT in order to have any validity is a fiction created by those who want to discount thousands of patient years of experience demonstrating that opioids have brought relief to patients. Obviously, it is desirable to conduct high-quality RCT studies wherever possible, but where it is impossible, the obstacles should not be used to the detriment of patients who need treatment. The consensus that has existed for nearly thirty-five years that opioids have a role to play for severe noncancer pain as well as cancer pain should not be simply ignored because of a new criterion for what constitutes a valid study. The criterion of study duration was not debated or openly discussed, but merely changed in a government evidence review by a few authors contracted by the NIH. The statement that has been made repeatedly that opioids have *no efficacy*[349] for long-term chronic pain is being used to dismiss patients and entire research efforts to treat pain as *a failure.*[37] Since the conclusions by the members of PROP have changed over time, we must ask whether the origin of the change is improvement in methods or response to political and legal pressure.

Methodological Limitations of Meta-Analysis and Evidence Review

Both meta-analysis and evidence review involve conducting a computer database literature search with selected keywords to retrieve a collection of published studies on related topics from a database in order to extract any useful or high-quality information. Individual studies are often too limited in the number of control conditions possible, may contain methodological flaws, or have become less reliable as statistical standards have become more reliable over time. Both meta-analysis and evidence review are methods to collect and simultaneously analyze the results of many studies, along with the various treatment methods and controls. A meta-analysis further permits an appropriate statistical weighting based on quality of evidence and homogeneity of conditions allows researchers to determine which factors are significant in ways the original clinicians may have been unable to detect. The data in various studies are often too heterogeneous to permit a meta-analysis. In that case, the analysis must be a systematic review or an evidence review. Meta-analyses themselves must also be rigorous, but the range of possible individual study designs can limit their scope. For example, Patient Z and millions like him have diseases that fall outside of the range of any pain management study that has ever been conducted. To generalize any meta-analysis or review of pain studies to the entire population is, by definition, biased. There are other biases that can be introduced in study selection and statistical choices concerning how to combine disparate types of information that may omit data. For example, while RCT studies are preferred, observational studies may have much more utility for diseases like Patient Z's. The extreme pain of his condition makes it impossible to measure a placebo effect. Since the patients with extreme pain are outliers in the population, and simultaneously are extremely vulnerable, special ethical considerations should apply. For this very reason, many cancer studies have been observational studies. In this context, the abuse of meta-analyses to exclude observational studies or specific patient populations is unethical.

The rules of meta-analysis have been standardized.[353] The method has been given the acronym PRISMA, preferred reporting items for systematic meta-analyses. We should not lose sight of the fact that a meta-analysis adds yet another layer between the actual observations and the final interpretations. A collection of studies that meets search criteria is combined in a network, and an observer needs to read dozens of publications in order to determine that the basis for the analysis is sound. The reader must trust that the authors have done a proper job and fairly represented the body of work in the medical or scientific literature.

Meta-analyses provide a method for evaluating, comparing, and quantitatively synthesizing the evidence from prior research in individual studies. The pressure to publish is sufficiently high that research groups sometimes publish sloppy studies. They may be poorly written, mistaken, or even fraudulent. The philosophy of the meta-analysis is that a collection of studies will provide more accurate information than any of the individual studies. The poor studies may be discarded, and the preponderance of studies will still provide a reasonable result. However, for many of the studies accepted into the meta-analysis, the concerns over data quality, design, or bias may still limit the interpretation. Ultimately, the conclusion is only as strong as the weakest study, and if studies are at variance with other studies, there can be obstacles to interpretation. It is frequently the case that one or a few publications are the most significant, and there are such serious differences in experimental conditions that comparison between the studies leads to exceedingly weak conclusions. Therefore, the result of the meta-analysis is often inconclusive. This invites authors to reach different conclusions from previous studies. At this point research ethics is crucial. A researcher may succumb to the narrative that science is getting better, old studies were flawed, and we now have more experience so we can see the significance more clearly. The new conclusion supersedes the old one. In other words, it is possible to use the meta-analysis format to change the emphasis or range of validity of certain findings. There are ongoing safety concerns about drugs, even drugs like aspirin that have been on the market for more than 120 years. Meta-analyses on aspirin may change prescribing despite extensive experience. Aspirin is not controversial, and bias is less likely to interfere in such an analysis. However, the efficacy, safety, and addictiveness of opioids is far more controversial than other drugs. Therefore, appropriate precautions must be taken to avoid bias.

Each meta-analysis begins by reporting how many studies met the criteria of the search. Often the number of studies that meet the acceptance criteria is somewhere in the range from ten to sixty. It is difficult to generalize given the large number of variables in the more than one hundred studies that have been done on long-term opioid treatment for noncancer pain. The meta-analyses in the field of pain medicine have compared RCTs and observational studies. The RCTs usually are conducted as single-blind studies with placebo. The placebo effect is significant in pain medical studies. Across dozens of RCT studies of opioid efficacy, which control for the placebo effect, have found a 20% reduction in pain for placebo and 28% reduction for the opioid in round numbers.[354] In aggregate these studies give a reproducible pain reduction of 8% with a 95% confidence of ±2%.[40–46,312] The interpretation of these numbers is subjective, as are the numbers themselves. The fundamental design issue for every single study of opioid efficacy is that pain itself cannot be quantified. Using zero-to-ten scale or the VSA, which is a line from 0 to 100, could be interpreted in different ways by patients. This fundamental methodological weakness must be acknowledged by those who make the claims that there is "no efficacy." The most recent study by Chou and coworkers, conducted in 2020, has attempted to assuage the critics by stating honestly that on the zero- to six-month time scale there is efficacy and on the twelve-month and longer time scale there are no data, and therefore we cannot say whether there is any efficacy.[345,347] Since they weight the greater-than-twelve-month period as the only valid study, they have not changed their conclusion, but at least they honestly acknowledge that the rest of the academic world sees things differently. However, the damage has already been done. The review from 2015 permitted members of PROP to use the phrase "no efficacy" to convince those in a position of authority and to change the CDC guidelines.[4]

Consensus on Neuropathic, Low Back, and Osteoarthritis Pain

For many years, clinicians thought that opioids had no efficacy for neuropathic pain. However, McQuay conducted some preliminary trials showing that neuropathic pain responded to opioids in 2001.[355] The Ballantyne and Shin review includes six RCT studies[337–342] that showed efficacy for various kinds of neuropathic pain, diabetic, postherpetic, and mixed neuropathy.[287]

> The randomized studies also make it clear that contrary to traditional belief, neuropathic pain is opioid responsive, although larger doses are required than those needed to treat nociceptive pain. It should be noted that the randomized trials are conducted only over the short-term (usually weeks, although 1 trial reached 32 wk), and that the doses used in these trials are generally moderate (up to 180 mg morphine or morphine equivalent per day).

The review discusses the issue of tolerance, claiming that the basic science is still not settled. This was discussed in detail in chapter

3 where possible mechanisms discussed were MOR desensitization and downregulation by endocytosis or degradation in lysosomes. After pointing out the tolerance to opioids in hedonistic use is well-known, the authors state,[287]

> Tolerance to the analgesic effects of opioids is far less obvious, to the extent that some clinicians argue that there is no pharmacologic tolerance to the analgesic effects of opioids. This is on the grounds that after initial titration, there may be stable analgesia with no need for dose escalation.

However, the authors of the review note that there are exceptions to this behavior. These can be overcome by opioid rotation[356] or use of extra opioids for breakthrough pain. Normally once the dose has been *titrated to effect*,[357] which means until the pain is controlled, there is a period of adjustment, after which the dose tends to be stable. Dr. Ballantyne's 2008 review presents scientific data that disagree with her own subsequent studies and commentaries. There has not been a methodological change or other reason to discount the previous work. It is still cited in the most recent analysis sponsored by PROP.[345,347] Dr. Ballantyne's statements today are in contradiction to her own review of the evidence of efficacy presented in both studies prior to 2008.[113,287]

Understanding the Distribution— Not All Patients Are the Same

It has been a problem from the beginning of pain medicine research that studies have avoided drawing nuanced conclusions that take into account the actual distribution of patients and their diseases.[358] PROP's proponents mention that others have neglected to account for the diversity of patients, but sadly they proceed to do exactly the same. The conclusions of individual studies are often applied to the average rather than looking at the implication of the range of outcomes for different patients. Side effects may be a problem for one subpopulation, but not for all patients. Addiction is a pernicious problem for a small subset of patients, but not for the majority.[359] These differences are crucial when conclusions from studies are used to justify policy or treatment guidelines. In general, it is obvious that observations that are accurate for a majority of patients are not accurate for *all* patients. The exceptions are crucially important to the design of appropriate public health policy.[360] As an example, fifty years ago we did not have handicapped parking spaces and all the aids that exist today for people with mobility issues. They are clearly a minority, but finally our society realized that we have a social responsibility to be inclusive. Today many pain clinics are dispensing opioids with the same limit for all patients no matter how painful and disabling their disease. This protocol is cruel and discriminatory. It is leading to a great deal of personal tragedy. The failure of medical commentaries and meta-analyses of clinical studies to carefully define the patient population, and to ensure that results are not used inappropriately because of vague or incomplete information, is a sufficiently general deficiency that it warrants harsh critique.

The distribution of symptoms or reactions to medication are an important aspect of statistical analysis for diagnosis and treatment in clinical research. Diseases have many symptoms, but not all patients present in the same way. Making a diagnosis depends on being able to recognize the collection of symptoms that indicate a particular disease, even when some common symptoms may not be present because of natural variation. Many doctors missed Patient Z's diagnosis because they were confused by a somewhat unusual presentation of symptoms. The weakness in understanding statistics is a recognized weakness of medical training.[361] Doctors have to assimilate so much information that they sometimes memorize the most common profile of symptoms for a disease, the textbook case, and miss important details that might occur in a rare form of a disease. To a certain extent, this is unavoidable. No one can remember everything. But we would hope that a doctor would be curious enough to follow up on observations that do not quite add up the same way a detective tries to solve a case. This means the doctor must keep an open mind, consider cause and effect in a logical flow chart, and understand small probabilities for rare symptoms (or absence of symptoms). Doctors also have an obligation to read the current medical literature in their field of practice. Above all, doctors must see the patient as an individual who may be in the tail of the distribution, not presenting as a textbook example. By understanding the effect of disease and pain on function, a doctor can better assess how great the need is for pain relief.

Work and Pain—What Metrics Are Being Applied to Function?

Although clinicians tell us that function is an important criterion, in practice the attempts to assess function in RCT studies have been fraught with difficulty. Assessment of the effect of pain on function is as subjective as assessment of pain itself. It is remarkable that the medical community has failed to acknowledge the methodological problems associated with any assessment of the efficacy of opioids (or any pain medication) on pain and function. New paradigms are needed. Observational studies that directly examine the lives of patients on opioid therapy could potentially give us a window on the value of these treatments for patients and society. However, doctors who have tried to include function as a treatment goal and a criterion for opioid prescribing have not been rewarded for their efforts. The case of Dr. Geller is a striking example. His methods for a holistic approach to opioid prescribing included function, but the state medical board rejected his approach. Dr. Geller understood the fear some observers have that opioid prescriptions would interfere with function and, specifically, ability to work. He was vocal in opposition to PROP's implemented guidelines and decided to justify opioid prescriptions for persistent pain by pointing to enhanced patient function, as measured by their gainful employment in the following[362]:

> Sullivan and Ballantyne appropriately scorned indiscriminate long-term opioid therapy, since

considerable numbers of patients receive these potentially dangerous agents but only rarely return to work. Characteristically, patients with high psychiatric comorbidity self-select as "requiring" opioids as well as disability from work, and the authors correctly report that most are not viable opioid candidates, given greater abuse and death risks. However, rather than discarding 50-plus centuries of experience with a highly potent clinical tool to ameliorate incurable persistent pain, judicious opioid dosing should be embraced if properly prescribed to clinician chosen patients demonstrating enhanced productivity, objectively working full time.

Ironically, Dr. Geller was reprimanded by the medical board in his state in 2018 precisely for using the definition of work as a measure of function used to prove the efficacy of opioid treatment. The article in the *Nashua Telegraph* states that the state medical board reprimanded Dr. Geller's use of work as a measure for opioid efficacy and as evidence of compliance. One would think that his view that opioid therapies can relieve pain and lead to rehabilitation in the workplace would resonate with law enforcement and politicians. At a time when there are work requirements for federal programs such as food stamps, emphasizing how opioids can permit people to work seems like a powerful argument. This is not a recommendation for a work requirement as a prerequisite for opioid therapy, but rather to observe the effects of opioid therapy on work history. Dr. Geller's evidence that opioid therapy would provide relief from pain that would help able-bodied people to be productive appears not to have resonated with the medical board. Dr. Geller was fined $2,000 by the medical board, and he was told that he must seek oversight from a professional.[363] Here we see the response of the current system to a doctor who was trying to carefully justify the treatment of pain using a functional criterion. He is the one reprimanded, not the experts who are writing that patients should simply go to work regardless of their pain. This example shows the absurdity of blindly using traditional types of studies for pain, which is both subjective and potentially debilitating.

Inability to Objectively Measure Pain as a Fatal Flaw in Pain Medicine Research

A quantitative measure of pain, known as the Brief Pain Inventory,[70,71] has been implemented for cancer patients.[364] Yet this widely used model and all other attempts to quantify measurement of pain rely solely on patient reporting. Thus far, no proxies have been validated, such as blood pressure, biomarkers, or imaging methods that might corroborate the patient's subjective report. Pain research in humans would not exist if researchers honestly confronted their inability to measure pain. Thus, in RCTs and other studies, the zero-to-ten scale is used for rating pain because no researcher has an objective way to measure pain. Other methods discussed in chapter 2 are also used, but they all rely on patient reporting. For therapeutic approaches, clinicians use a similar subjective approach based on a reduction in pain score of (1) slight, (2) moderate, (3) lots, and (4) complete, on the scale from zero to ten. The average reduction in pain score in many studies is approximately three points in the opioid arm and two points in the placebo arm. There has been no methodological discussion of how to evaluate the large placebo effect in studies of pain medication. However, the pain studied using these methods is always relatively minor pain, not pain like Patient Z's. Both the reporting and interpretation of pain scores is subjective, which gives rise to bias. This bias combined with the inherent limitations in the range of diseases that can be studied for pain treatment should force an ethical physician to seek an evaluation grounded in the etiology of a specific disease. PROP's enforcement of draconian measures based on poor science, over the objection of hundreds of doctors and the AMA, is scandalous.

CHAPTER 6

⟿

Sowing Seeds of Doubt That Opioids Can Relieve Persistent Pain

P ROP and their allies have intentionally used evidence reviews to change the conclusions regarding long-term opioid prescribing for persistent pain. The initial studies in 2003 focused on which opioid formulations are most effective, time-release, or short acting.[6,113] Efficacy was assumed in those studies, and the conclusion was that there is no significant difference between immediate-acting and slow-release medications. From a starting point of meta-analyses in 2003, when efficacy was self-evident, the academic conclusions evolved until by 2015, PROP's review conclusions denied that opioids have any efficacy at all.[4] Using evidence reviews, PROP has reevaluated the body of over one hundred existing studies and to make conclusions based on expert opinion about the combined information content of those studies.[4,6–8,113,287,347] The series of meta-analyses changed the conclusions of the entire field of pain medicine. Simultaneously, studies have proceeded in EU countries, in the UK, Canada, and Australia. It is an important task to compare PROP's studies and conclusions to the numerous studies in the medical journal literature from other countries that have demonstrated modest but reproducible efficacy.[40–47,141,312,318–320] An evidence review has scientific legitimacy if the assumptions are carefully stated in advance and the synthesis of the studies is conducted in a bias-free manner.

Intentionally changing evaluation criteria in order to exclude data is not a scientific way of proceeding.

There has been a profound shift in attitude in just a few years. In 2008, Dr. Ballantyne had an empirical and open-minded approach to examining the patient's situation and needs. She concluded,[287]

> The complexities of pain and opioids, and the significant biopsychosocial influences on pain and pain relief, make assessments on the basis of simple pain measures less useful for predicting overall treatment success. Analgesic efficacy, as demonstrated in randomized trials, does not necessarily predict effectiveness in terms of the larger real-life goal of providing helpful pain relief that is not compromised by adverse drug effects. Differences in handling opioids between patients often confound opioid trials. These factors are not fully understood, but could be related to pharmacogenetic effects, sex effects, concomitant medications, or the opioid responsiveness of the underlying pain conditions.[365] Finally, one must ask if the randomized trial really is the best form of evidence for assessing opioid treatment of chronic pain given the artificiality of the trial setting, the tendency of trials to select "ideal" patients, and the lack of generalizability to the wider population that is being treated outside trials.

This introduction to the 2008 review acknowledges that the RCTs and meta-analyses in the field of pain medicine have several inherent shortcomings.[287] Since most RCTs over the years have found some efficacy, this paragraph supports individualized treatment of pain patients. Dr. Ballantyne correctly cautions that general conclusions from a particular RCT may be irrelevant for the general population of pain patients. For example, an RCT on patients with low back pain has no relevance to Patient Z, who has a serious incurable inflammatory disease. Within a few years, Dr. Ballantyne had changed her mind and led PROP's effort to use meta-analyses to prove that opioids have no efficacy for any patient.

Dr. Ballantyne explained in an interview that she had changed her mind about the efficacy and appropriateness of opioid therapy and decided that she no longer believed that prescribing opioids at high doses was a good idea for any patient.[265] While that is a judgment that any doctor is free to make, the literature that supports dosing recommendations and community opinions about what is safe should be based on community consensus and scientific studies, where data are available. The point of the analysis that follows is not to deny any of the authors their right to an opinion. However, the research record of these various articles, commentaries, and meta-analyses reveals an attempt by the doctors in PROP to change a consensus conclusion based on science. Moreover, their concern that opioid prescribing has led to a public health emergency coincides with their own agenda of blaming both the pharmaceutical companies and pain patients for the crisis. The leadership of PROP points fingers at pain patients and doctors who speak out in favor of compassionate treatment of pain as being in the pay of the pharmaceutical companies. Meanwhile, PROP's president and executive director have been paid lavishly for expert testimony in the court cases against those companies.[260,261] PROP has tapped into the public's deep distrust of large corporations and the pain of those families who have lost loved ones. The modus operandi has been to scapegoat prescriptions written for pain patients as the origin of the overdose crisis. Blaming all that has happened on *overprescribing* leaves out a massive amount of evidence that explains the trends in light of a failed *war or drugs* and unchecked drug *diversion*, as the major causes of the continuing problem of skyrocketing drug-overdose rates. The data presented in chapters 8 and 9 show that pain patients are being blamed for a much bigger problem that is not of their making. The evidence shows overprescribing was twenty times smaller than the role of illegal drugs, including diverted prescription drugs. The fact that PROP, the DEA, and government agencies got this wrong is evident in the continuing high overdose rate despite major cuts to prescribing.

While there are tragic examples of people who were harmed by overprescribing, the drastic solutions being implemented today are making the problem worse. Those who have become habituated to unnecessarily high doses need a compassionate solution, but many have been force-tapered or abandoned. Patients like Z who have a real need of relief from severe pain are suffering, as doctors worry more about their jobs than about patient welfare. It is a violation of human rights to take pain medication away from persistent-pain patients or curtail their dose to the point where they are miserable. Legitimate pain patients are seldom drug abusers. But the leaders of PROP have a vested interest in portraying pain patients as addicts. Pain patients are useful as pawns for Drs. Kolodny and Ballantyne to make the case that the societal harm caused by Purdue Pharma is addiction of the population at large. Of course, that portrayal plays better in a courtroom compared to use of the actual clinical data that greater than 92% of patients do not turn to addiction, according to conservative estimates.[9,139,141]

From an intellectual point of view, there is no simple way to make a rapid change in the collective research results in a field like opioid therapy. There are already thousands of papers, and many of the basic topics are available as Cochrane database meta-analyses. The totality of the clinical research effort is like an oil tanker steaming in a given direction. For many years, the consensus has been building that long-term opioid prescribing can play a role in pain management for serious inflammatory and degenerative diseases. That is still the case in England, Germany, and de facto almost the entire European Union where policies toward pain patients are humane. Therefore, when PROP wanted to insert a different conclusion into the research results, they needed to take decisive action. Instead of doing research and obtaining new data, which would have taken many years or decades, PROP worked instead to redefine the field by reinterpreting the existing data. Prior to 2017 the longest RCT on pain medicine had an observation periods of sixteen weeks.[9] Observational studies of patients who received opioid prescriptions had been conducted for years, even decades.[141,156,157] While RCTs are considered the most rigorous type of study, we have discussed significant weaknesses arising from a lack of measurement methods and ethical limitations in study of severe pain. Despite the fatal flaw in the studies, the entire trajectory of meta-analyses proceeded with the assumption that these studies have the potential to measure reductions in pain that have clinical significance.

The Moving Target—How the Consensus on Opioid Efficacy Was Buried

As the focus of an investigation into how meta-analyses were used to change consensus, we will examine a series of papers with common authors who are members of PROP or collaborators. It is remarkable that a single clinician, Dr. Roger Chou, has been the first author or a prominent author on an entire series of meta-analyses that we consider here, over a period of seventeen years. Clinical research is expensive, and Dr. Chou and the members of PROP have been well-supported by government funding to conduct studies for government agencies. It is my experience that government funding panels often function like a club. Those who belong have an excellent chance of getting their grant proposals funded and renewed. Outsiders, or scientists who have iconoclastic points of view, face much greater adversity in obtaining funding. Dr. Chou is clearly an insider. Dr. Chou's bias is rather evident both in the trajectory of the review conclusions and in his other actions as a panel expert in the state of Oregon. Dr. Chou was the head of a state committee in Oregon that recommended cutting the opioid dose of all Medicaid recipients to zero.[345,346]

The conclusions of meta-analyses authored by Dr. Chou have changed significantly between 2003 and 2020.[4,6–9,287,347] The consensus viewpoint that long-term opioid therapy had efficacy was implicit in conclusions in 2003[6] and supported again in a review in 2008,[287] gaps were observed in 2009,[7] results were questioned in 2011,[8] a new set of criteria was proposed in 2014,[9] and the conclusion was downgraded to "evidence is insufficient to determine the effectiveness" in 2015.[4] By 2015, none of the previous studies were included in the efficacy portion of the review because of the requirement of a minimum duration of >1 year. However, the more recent studies also included more side effects than ever despite a paucity of evidence. Using arbitrary selection criteria to eliminate studies is not a scientific approach. Adding a laundry list of new side effects supported by poor evidence is also a transparent attempt to bias the evaluation of efficacy. The details are provided in the appendix for those who would like to see more of the evidence.

Starting at the beginning of the process that led to the change in an entire field, the first in a series was the review by Chou and coworkers conducted in response to a bill passed by the Oregon Legislature in 2001 (Senate Bill 819).[6] Because of the new opioid prescription practices at that time and also Medicaid expansion, the legislature mandated the development of a Practitioner-Managed Prescription Drug Plan (PMPDP) for the Oregon Health Plan (OHP). One irony is that "the Oregon Health Resources Commission (OHRC) required that an evidence-based review of the state's most expensive drug classes be performed." Most common opioids are inexpensive to manufacture. The reason that the drugs were considered among the most expensive is not known. Could it be because of the expense of the patented formulation, OxyContin, that has gotten so much attention? The study questions were indicative of the time, in the sense that the issue was not whether opioids have efficacy, which was accepted in 2003, but rather which type of opioid works best. In their conclusion, the authors wrote[6]:

> There was insufficient evidence to prove that different long-acting opioids are associated with different efficacy or safety profiles. There was also insufficient evidence to determine whether long-acting opioids as a class are more effective or safer than short-acting opioids. A subgroup of three studies on long-acting versus short-acting oxycodone was more homogeneous and provided

fair evidence that these formulations are equally effective for pain control.

The issue that the state of Oregon wished to consider was to find the best methods to deliver opioids, long-acting or short-acting. The conclusion was that there is no significant difference between the two formulations, but the efficacy of short-acting opioids had been studied previously and found effective for pain control. Obviously, society's view of this has changed, but the basic scientific studies are as valid today as they were when they were conducted over twenty years ago.

Defining Gaps in Knowledge as a Strategy for Redefining Review Criteria

The efficacy of opioids was so well accepted in 2003 that Dr. Ballantyne proposed guidelines indicative of confidence in opioids to treat severe pain, with discussion of doses as high as the gram range (>1,000 MEDD).[113] Her published review and recommendation agreed well with another leader in the field, Dr. Joranson, in a paper published in 2000.[114] Yet later Dr. Ballantyne felt that the message needed to change, and it did so abruptly sometime around 2009.

In 2009, Dr. Chou, Dr. Ballantyne, and other authors published an article entitled "Research Gaps on Use of Opioids for Chronic Non-cancer Pain."[7] This paper is a first step away from the compassionate care movement. This article is focused almost exclusively on harms of opioid therapy. The "gaps" are largely related to harms, some of which were widely known (addiction, constipation, nausea, pruritus, and sex hormone reduction) and others that have been added more recently to make the case better that opioids should be highly restricted (falls, insomnia, heart attack, auto accidents, and loss of mental acuity). To be clear, the harms in the latter category are far from established, but the proposal is to study them and look for statistical correlations that might link them to opioid use. The purpose of the studies is not to address a solution for side effects, but rather to present them as insurmountable obstacles that should prevent opioid prescribing. For example, if one wanted to help patients and provide constructive solutions, one might determine which laxatives relieve constipation or investigate treatments for hormonal deficiency using replacement therapy. Rather, the point of the studies is to weigh harms and benefits to arrive at a negative conclusion about the overall appropriateness of opioids for long-term persistent pain. As time progresses the scales have tipped further in the direction of harms outweighing benefits, not because of the evidence, but arising from changing criteria for how to include studies in the meta-analysis and what to consider as a harm. The paper on "research gaps"[7] used the 2006 evidence assessment of the American Pain Society (APS) and American Academy of Pain Medicine (AAPM). The gaps identified were shortcomings in the studies, including a pointed statement concerning the fact that no study had conducted controlled comparisons for more than sixteen weeks. While the "research gaps" publication could be useful criticism that points out many facets of therapy, patient monitoring, and care for adverse effects that should be studied further, from context it is clear that the authors' aim was not to carry out such careful studies themselves, but rather to build a case against opioids that could be used as evidence in making policy as well as in lawsuits.[7]

The published prescribing guidelines in 2009 still conformed to the ideas that pain should be treated with opioid therapy in a patient-centered way.[366] That meant that the doses were appropriately higher for painful conditions. The cutoff given between intermediate and high dose was 200 MEDD, which had been a standard for at least a decade prior.[113,114] However, by 2016 Chou and coworkers published the restrictive guidelines in the medical literature that followed the PROP proposal to the CDC.[281] Many of the same authors were involved in these various publications and guidelines. These authors were also party to the failed petition to the FDA in 2012 to put a hard limit on prescribing. One can understand the need to rethink what had happened during a period of overprescribing. I am not taking issue with commonsense prescribing for the many kinds of transitory pain or less painful conditions. However, it was inappropriate to disregard evidence that was already in the literature or to institute guidelines that completely ignored the needs of patients with serious diseases. Today the limitation of high-dose prescribing has become an end in itself, irrespective of the condition of the patient.[367] The harm of these clinical decisions is immense.

The Announcement of PROP as the Pivot Point in a Series of Meta-Analyses

The changing viewpoint of the advocacy coalition is evident in the 2011 review entitled "Long-Term Opioid Therapy Reconsidered" by Von Korff and coworkers, also involving Dr. Chou as a coauthor. The conclusion of this commentary is that the risks of opioid therapy tend to outweigh the benefits and the patient's tendency to divert or misuse medication is substantial.[8]

> Perceptions that long-term opioid therapy typically yields long-lasting benefits for patients with chronic non-cancer pain are not supported by strong evidence. Controlled trials lasting 1 to 6 months suggest modest pain relief relative to placebo, but no long-term studies have determined whether analgesic efficacy is maintained.

The qualifier in this 2011 study is that there is no "strong evidence" for efficacy of long-term opioid therapy. The study creates the impression that the dozens of studies conducted over the past thirty years prior, including the eighteen studies cited in the 2003 Chou review should be discounted. However, the basis for discounting those older studies was not presented until later. The authors stated that opioid pain relief is modest and that we cannot be sure about efficacy because the study duration was too short. These vague conclusions may be helpful as talking points for a commentary that suggests we need to change how we view opioid prescriptions, but they do not give us a lot of insight into what the real issues are.

This review is part of the evolution toward the stronger statement that there is no evidence of pain relief. Despite the paucity of new evidence, van Korff and coworkers make the blanket statement that long-term opioid therapy has no long-lasting benefits for noncancer patients.[8] There is no explanation as to why cancer patients are different than other patients. Recently, clinicians have even questioned whether cancer pain should receive opioid therapy.[368] The reduction of opioid dose for every disease is foremost on the clinician's mind.[268,369]

The 2011 article by von Korff, Chou, and others is an announcement of the formation of PROP. To explain their view of why this became necessary, the authors of the newly formed PROP wrote,[8]

> The original case for using long-term opioid therapy to treat chronic non-cancer pain was based on safety assumptions that subsequent experience calls into question. In 1996, the American Pain Society and the American Academy of Pain Medicine issued a consensus statement supporting long-term opioid therapy. This statement acknowledged the dangers of imprudent opioid prescribing but concluded that the risk for de novo addiction was low; respiratory depression induced by opioids was short-lived, occurred mainly in opioid-naive patients, and was antagonized by pain; tolerance was not a common problem; and efforts to control diversion should not constrain opioid prescribing. Unfortunately, experience regarding the risks for opioid addiction, misuse, and overdose in community practice has failed to confirm these assertions.

Here the words "community practice" are of crucial importance. There were plenty of errors made during the compassionate care movement. For more than ten years, there was no system in place to electronically connect pharmacies who prescribe opioids on a database that would make it impossible for a patient to obtain multiple prescriptions. There was no mandatory patient testing to ensure compliance. There was no plan for how to treat patients who did show signs of addiction. The dreadful state of opioid treatment programs for addicts was not addressed. There was little or no training or education of doctors. Instead, the vacuum was filled by companies such as Purdue Pharma who provided their advertising, which had distorted the meaning of the words of experts. However deplorable those mistakes and reprehensible the actions of corporations that corrupted the intent of the American Pain Society, it is unacceptable to deny that there was any validity to the original studies. Instead, we should learn from the clinical experience with pain patients, including the mistakes, to avoid making a second tragic misinterpretation of the needs of patients. Instead, the approach has been to deny care to millions of people who live with intolerable pain. Somehow, the compassionate care movement to help the patients in intolerable pain became converted into a movement to treat any pain from a toothache to a shin splint with an opioid medication. Clearly it was a mistake to permit rampant overuse of opioids for minor pain. Was this the fault of the leaders of the pain societies, the prescribing doctors, or the pharmaceutical companies? There is some blame for each, but the real story is sordid because government oversight was both incompetent and corrupt during this entire period. However, when corrective action was finally taken after ten years of unrestrained diversion and overprescribing, the patients with life-threatening conditions like adhesive arachnoiditis were lumped in with patients who had shin splints once again and all had their doses reduced together. The sudden new solution was a single limit for all patients and a campaign to frighten doctors so that they would stop prescribing altogether. PROP's success in changing the culture of prescribing resulted in record number of overdose deaths, suicides, and patient deaths from botched tapers.[121] The statistics for pain patients are much more difficult to obtain since there is no International Classification of Diseases-10 (ICD-10) code for dying of chronic pain. People are dying at a greater rate than ever, and misery index is as high as it has ever been. The mistake being made under the present guidelines is at least as large as the compassionate pain movement.

The Search to Find the Conclusion That "Evidence Is Insufficient to Determine" Effectiveness

Following the 2011 position paper and formation of PROP, Dr. Chou and other authors wrote an "Evidence Report for the Agency for Healthcare Research and Quality" in response to an NIH workshop called "Pathways to Prevention."[9] This report was the first occurrence of a requirement that the duration of studies should be longer than one year in order to qualify as long-term studies. The "Evidence Report" included many of the same sources included in previous meta-analyses. A total of thirty-nine studies met the criteria, but none of the studies addressed efficacy of opioids because none of them had greater than one-year duration.[139,152,298,334,370–403] The studies consisted of a mixture of studies of harms and side effects including falls, heart attack, sexual dysfunction, addiction, and abuse. The addiction rates ranged from 0.6% to 8.0%. The highest quality of evidence was rated low, with one exception of a study on buccal fentanyl, which was rated moderate. The studies were criticized for lacking risk mitigation strategies for overdose, addiction, or misuse. The evaluators in PROP wrote that "[e]vidence was insufficient to evaluate benefits and harms of long-term opioid therapy in high-risk patients or in other subgroups." Since none of these objections to opioid prescribing had sufficient seriousness to warrant the changes sought, the members of PROP came up with an idea to eliminate previous studies from consideration. Their evidence review in 2014 required a time duration of greater than one year for an efficacy study to be valid.[9] It was obvious from the beginning that no studies would meet this new criterion set by PROP. Tayeb and coworkers pointed out that none of the existing pain medications in use today meet the requirement set by this "Evidence Report."[404] To make the point another way, none of the drugs used to treat pain—aspirin, ibuprofen, acetaminophen, lidocaine, etc.—would have been acceptable for use if the results of a random control trial of greater than one year duration were the criterion. They were all studied with twelve-week follow-up observations, which is what the FDA requires. No analgesics have ever required a one-year follow-up observation. This is not an industry standard. But it is a PROP standard.

Since 2014 there has been only one study on opioid therapy that met the criteria for duration of one year.[351] Unfortunately, the study was poorly designed since the researchers mixed opioid treatment in both the opioid and non-opioid arm. Moreover, the study cohort (patient population) was not opioid-naive, which was pointed out in letters to the editor.[350] These are two fatal flaws, either one of which invalidate the conclusions (see appendix paragraph on "the gold standard").

In 2015, a review was conducted by Chou and coworkers to reexamine the literature in light of the new requirements that doctors had agreed upon in the "Pathways to Prevention" workshop.[4] The concept for future guidelines had already been formulated, and it consisted of reducing opioid prescriptions for all patients regardless of their disease (except for terminal cancer). Sickle cell anemia patients have suffered because of these policies as well as many others.[68,69,308] The title of the study was "The Effectiveness and Risks of Long-Term Opioid Therapy for Chronic Pain." The review included thirty-nine studies considered the highest level available. The conclusion reads,[4]

> Evidence is insufficient to determine the effectiveness of long-term opioid therapy for improving persistent pain and function. Evidence supports a dose-dependent risk for serious harms.

This statement has a ring of authority, suggesting that the science supports the conclusion that the benefit is in doubt, and the harm clearly outweighs the benefit. The authors do not say directly that their conclusion is based on no evidence at all. It is absurd, but true, that they excluded every single efficacy study from consideration in making this conclusion. Based on the exclusion of all previous studies, it was possible to say that there was insufficient evidence of efficacy to draw any conclusion. Using PROP's reasoning, we should stop selling aspirin, acetaminophen, and ibuprofen, as well as morphine and oxycodone, since there is no evidence that any of them are effective either.

In Germany and other EU countries, the three-month follow-up criterion continued to be accepted, and recent studies found modest efficacy similar to those done for years previously in the United States. In the appendix, there is more information on the comparison of recent studies from Canada, Switzerland, Germany, and France that consist of well over one hundred studies in seven meta-analyses. In aggregate, these studies agree and conclude that the pain reduction from opioids was –0.8 points on the scale from 0 to 10 if one corrected for placebo by simple subtraction. Such an interpretation of the placebo effect is the most conservative way to look at the clinical result. This number –0.8 is a high-quality result with 95% confidence interval from –0.6 to –1.1. The patients for these studies had low back pain, osteoarthritis, or neuropathic pain and were typically given doses of 30 MEDD. The German, French, and Swiss authors conclude that this is a small benefit. They did not compare the benefit to the side effects, which were found to be minor. The Canadian study finding the same basic result did not endorse opioid therapy and was equivocal when considering the side effects. The US study found "insufficient evidence of effectiveness" because none of the evidence was included. It is interesting to consider how these differing opinions relate to the medical system, overdose rate, and other factors. Examining the same clinical data, the European doctors find a small benefit, the Canadians are equivocal, and the Americans find no benefit.

Observational Studies on Dose and Duration of Opioid Treatments

Observational studies are often carried out using insurance company databases that include hundreds of thousands of patients.[141,156,157]

These studies provide information on the duration of use and dose of opioids over a period of years. In a field of investigation where the definition of a scientific study provides zero hits in a database search,[405] perhaps we should reflect on what the goal is. If the question is whether people with specific medical conditions are benefitting at all from opioid therapy, it is possible that RCT studies are not in a position to even answer the question. For example, RCTs were not found to be particularly useful in determining the best treatment for sacroiliac joint pain.[406] For the most painful conditions, which are the ones in the greatest need of opioid therapy, an RCT study with a control group requires a placebo. No review committee would permit the control group to live in severe pain for a year.

An observational study can tell us what dose patients have been taking and for how long. That is important information. If the patients had bad side effects or the opioid was lacking in efficacy, then why would the patients keep taking them? Of course, a cynic's answer is that the patients are addicted to opioids. If the patient is functional, goes to work or works in the home, does not have aberrant behavior, loses their prescription, and so on, the patient functionally is not behaving like an addict. These items are in the record, and one could tell if opioids resulted in aberrant behavior. Using a functional definition for addiction leads to the inference that these insured patients, often in group plans obtained through their employer, are functioning as non-addicts who have persistent pain would be expected to behave.[156] Quoting from the TROUP study, "Opioids are widely prescribed for non-cancer pain conditions (NCPC), but there have been no large observational studies in actual clinical practice assessing patterns of opioid use over extended periods of time. The TROUP (Trends and Risks of Opioid Use for Pain) study reports on trends in opioid therapy for NCPC in two disparate, commercially insured (HealthCore Blue Cross and Blue Shield plans) and one state-based and publicly insured (Arkansas Medicaid) population over a six-year period (2000 to 2005)":[157]

> It is not possible to determine from our data whether this increasing use of opioids for NCPC

137

provides net benefit or net harm to patients.
Many aspects of benefit (pain reduction, functional improvement, distress reduction) need
to be carefully weighed against many aspects
of harm (opioid-induced hyperalgesia, reduced
function, increased depression, iatrogenic addiction). Future studies are needed to provide the
necessary information for making clinical decisions that result in net benefit to patients.

Sadly, the authors miss stating the obvious. People who suffer
from hyperalgesia, reduced function, and addiction often have trouble maintaining their job and insurance. The mere fact that many
thousands of people have taken opioids for years or even decades and
gone to work for that time tells us a lot about efficacy. This is not a
scientific conclusion, just common sense. The point is not to suggest
that observational studies are all we need, but they contain evidence
that should not be discounted.

Studies of the Safety and Long-Term Health Effects of Opioids

In the field of pain medicine, there are more than one hundred studies and there was a consensus for many years that long-term opioid
care was efficacious and that the side effects were tolerable for the
majority of patients. Opioid side effects are not tolerable for approximately one-third of individuals, and they usually withdraw from trials. Nonetheless, two-thirds of patients remain who potentially benefit from opioid therapy. The more recent meta-analyses in North
America emphasize a growing list of side effects that appear to be
intended to deter any doctor from considering opioid treatments.
The study of side effects such as constipation, pruritus, nausea, sedation, tolerance, and androgen (sex) hormone imbalance have now
been augmented with myocardial infarction, fractures, loss of mental
acuity, and depression.[4,407] If one is going to test for the effect of opioids on a range of such measures of health, then one needs to define

the disease state of the patients. Many patients with ankylosing spondylitis, rheumatoid arthritis, lupus, etc. tend to have their own serious health problems quite apart from the pain medication.[408,409] Since these are progressive autoimmune diseases, they tend to worsen during the study period. Side effects can be serious, but they vary from patient to patient. If the goal of the study is to improve patient welfare, then we need to consider the effects of denying treatment to patients with serious disease and extreme pain. Patients in pain have high blood pressure, stress hormone imbalance, a tendency to fall, inability to walk or exercise, insomnia, extreme mental distraction, nausea, and depression. The side effects of pain itself are in many regards similar to those of opioids.[410]

Safety can also apply to studies of alternative pain medications, such as nonsteroidal anti-inflammatory drugs (NSAIDs). Studies of older adults (ca. eighty years old) with osteoarthritis and rheumatoid arthritis compared the safety of NSAIDs versus opioids for the treatment of pain. The studies found that the hazard ratio (HR) was higher for opioids relative to NSAIDs for heart failure, fractures, and overall risk of safety events requiring hospitalization.[411] The study has major design flaw because it fails to separate patients into osteoarthritis and rheumatoid arthritis groups. The difference between osteoarthritis and forms of inflammatory arthritis, rheumatoid arthritis and psoriatic arthritis and other related diseases is enormous. The health consequences and pain levels of these diseases are dramatically different, which is why the diagnosis of a disease is so important. It is hard to say what the data mean since it is likely that there is a correlation between the stronger pain medicine and the more serious medical condition, which would bias the results.[411]

Supporting the Conventional Wisdom That Opioids Are "Safe When Used as Directed"

One of the most remarkable facts about opioids is how safe they are compared to other medications. Organ toxicity of opioids is low even compared to common drugs such as aspirin. Apparently, the leadership of PROP felt the need to challenge even this common wisdom in the new milieu of *responsible prescribing*. In the article "Safe and Effective When Used as Directed: The Case of Chronic Use of Opioid Analgesics,"[132] Dr. Ballantyne makes the case that long-term opioid use is neither safe nor effective. The negative message is not subtle. While the ostensible message that we need more responsible prescribing is one that any reasonable person would agree with, the real objective of the article is to argue against any prescribing for chronic conditions. The main new hazard Dr. Ballatyne introduces in the recent work is the risk of falls and fractures. While several studies indicate that elderly patients on opioids show a nearly two-fold higher risk for fracture,[397,411] the origin of the effect was not explained. Miller and coworkers suggested that the observation of falls had been made for short-term, but not long-term opioid use.[412] It may be that elderly patients are disoriented when they first take opioids, but this is abated with time. Elderly people often fall because of pain, which is something completely ignored in all the studies. This is an issue that is difficult to study because of the questions of environment and control group. The issue is yet another poorly-controlled and inconclusive excuse used by PROP to justify recommending against opioid therapy for any patient.

Clinicians outside the US took these observations as a challenge that needed to be resolved. A recent article by Coluzzi and coworkers, "The Unsolved Case of 'Bone-Impairing Analgesics': the Endocrine Effects of Opioids on Bone Metabolism," takes this a step further and suggests as an answer to the mystery.[413] In examining the possible explanations, one fact that appears to agree with Miller and coworkers is that fall risk on opioid therapy is short-term issue, a lack of balance that may arise in patients who are new to opioid therapy rather than a long-term symptom of a medical condition in the balance of patients. Geriatric patients have problems with balance that have numerous causes. A second aspect has to do with opioid binding to MORs on bone. The study points out that alternative medications that have multiple modes of action (e.g., tapentadol, tramadol, or buprenorphine) may be advantageous if osteoporosis is of concern for patients. Finally, hypogonadism is a known side effect.[414] Opioids tend to reduce testosterone levels, which decreases bone density. This problem can be overcome by steroid replacement therapy or an off-label prescription of clomiphene. Side effects can be regarded as inconveniences that we need to confront with solutions, rather than a reason to stop using a drug entirely.

Dr. Ballantyne's article reexamines the evidence for use of opioids to support an agenda to limit prescribing.[132] Coluzzi's group has a different "agenda," which is to overcome potential problems so that opioids can be used safely to relieve pain.[413] The point of view of EU countries is quite different compared to the United States' at present since they have a significantly smaller overdose rate, despite the fact that they are increasing opioid prescribing for persistent-pain patients. When articles are written with a subtext that dissuades clinicians from treating pain, they can negatively impact therapeutic decisions for patients who need help.

"Pay No Attention to That Man Behind the Curtain"

In the *Wizard of Oz*, the great and powerful Oz is revealed to be a mere carnival barker who uses a machine to control the hologram of Oz and shooting flames from behind a curtain. Similarly, in making one of the most pervasive changes to prescribing in the history of the United States, PROP has relied on an intellectual approach that is as false as the man behind the curtain. The internal contradictions of the meta-analyses and the arbitrary nature of the change in acceptance criteria provide strong direct evidence of the scientific dishonesty of PROP's approach.

Having eliminated more than half of the studies from consideration because they are observational, Dr. Ballantyne and her collaborators then used the study duration as a criterion to eliminate all RCTs from consideration as well. All studies have now been declared unacceptable for use, except for one sole study done in 2018, which itself has fatal design flaws.[350,351] The authors' claim that "evidence is insufficient to determine the effectiveness"[4] is disingenuous because they rejected all available evidence based on an arbitrary criterion.

Moreover, their conclusion is contrary to their own results twelve years previously.[6] Once the leaders of PROP felt confident saying that there is "no evidence," the next step was to write that there is "no efficacy" in as many commentaries and media reports as possible. The "no efficacy" slogan is a distortion of the published studies.

Now that PROP has declared all evidence invalid, and while we wait for the evidence they claim is needed, PROP has pushed strict dose limitations. These dose limits have already caused great suffering. Instead of recognizing that an overreaction may occur as an unintended consequence of reining in prescribing, which we could forgive and correct, PROP's articles proceed to state that there is high probability that patients are drug seeking, that patients are subject to "iatrogenic addiction," and that their pain is "withdrawal." The evidence presented for these claims is either weak or nonexistent. Having admitted that by their own standard there is no evidence, the members of PROP should know that it is unethical to base prescribing guidelines on suppositions that lack evidence. However, it has become the accepted standard in pain clinics throughout the United States where doctors insist to patients that cutting their dose is "medically necessary." This falls even harder on Patient Z and those like him who have the most severe and debilitating pain.

The one-sided debate in the US is not for lack of concerned doctors who care deeply about this issue. However, when the federal agencies favor one narrow viewpoint and permit that group to define the validity of evidence and use their subjective criteria to guide policy, the other doctors in the field who understand these issues have no option but write petitions and letters. For corroboration that honest intellectual inquiry still exists, I turn to the alternative viewpoints from other countries. The study by Noble and coworkers from Oxford, UK, in the Cochrane database is a meta-analysis of twenty-seven different studies with 4,893 patients. The rate of opioid use disorder was 0.27% in those combined studies. The studies own plain language summary states,[141]

> The findings of this systematic review suggest
> that proper management of a type of strong pain-

killer (opioids) in well-selected patients with no history of substance addiction or abuse can lead to long-term pain relief for some patients with a very small (though not zero) risk of developing addiction, abuse, or other serious side effects. However, the evidence supporting these conclusions is weak, and longer-term studies are needed to identify the patients who are most likely to benefit from treatment.

Referring to Dr. Noble and coworker's study,[141] Dr. Ballantyne wrote, "More recently, observational studies have expanded to include open-label continuation studies undertaken as part of the design for the growing number of RCTs [randomized controlled trials] being conducted to assess opioid efficacy in chronic pain. For these observational studies, again, useful short-term analgesic efficacy is established, but overall, no conclusions can be reached about COT's [chronic opioid therapy's] ability to improve function or quality of life."[132] Despite Dr. Noble's cautious but positive conclusion, Dr. Ballantyne concludes that "evidence that questions the dominant paradigm supporting COT [chronic opioid therapy] is accumulating."[132] Dr. Ballantyne's generic warning disagrees with the primary source.[141] Quality of life is an important consideration, but it is among the most difficult to quantify or to correlate with treatment. Recent publications by members of PROP have placed much greater emphasis on opioid side effects or issues such as quality of life, which are nearly impossible to measure as a means of discounting opioid therapy.

The recent extensive German studies on long-term opioid prescribing, reviewed in the appendix, agree with Noble and others that opioids have a role to play.[40–46,312,352] The recent studies from Germany reconfirm that opioid therapy has efficacy, with all the appropriate cautions and concerns. These studies have been ignored in all recent commentary by PROP authors. Those authors repeat the simple phrase "no evidence of efficacy" at every opportunity. Doctors and medical researchers in the United States have a hard time addressing

PROP's studies because of the pressures they face. The misconceptions in the media and the political forces that are calling for severe limitations on prescription opioids affect funding and support by medical schools. The medical community is aware of the importance of opioids in medicine, and there is no possibility that opioids will be phased out as useful medicine. It is a remarkable time when the title of a journal petition is "The National Imperative to Align Practice and Policy with the Actual CDC Opioid Guideline."[282] This petition is a clear recognition from hundreds of medical professionals[3] of the denial of basic human rights of pain patients in the United States. Today, it has become nearly impossible for those who have rare, painful diseases to get treatment appropriate to their condition. Hundreds of thousands of pain patients who have lost their medication are searching for allies or help online, or contacting their congressmen and congresswomen. But many do not know what to do and have simply given up, resigning themselves to a life of little or no activity because their pain is unbearable. The power of academic publishing gives credibility and an aura of authority to an argument. This is why it is so dangerous to abuse the privilege of academic publishing. Coopting the academic literature for personal gain in a lawsuit is an especially egregious abuse. The warning and proposed restrictions in articles such as Dr. Ballantyne's[132] are having a profound effect on the prescribing by doctors throughout the United States. Dr. Kolodny's threats against academics are supported by state attorney generals and the DEA, who have initiated investigations into medical schools whom Dr. Kolodny has identified as "collaborators" with the pharmaceutical companies. The climate of fear that pervades academia in the field of pain medicine has a profound impact on clinical practice as well. When combined with pressure from the DEA and state medical boards, many clinics do not follow the CDC guidelines. The CDC guidelines have, in principle, some flexibility for clinicians, but practice today includes hard limits on prescribing and harmful rapid tapering of all patients regardless of the disease or history.[415] The change has come in just a few years, and it is obvious that research on the effects of tapering is still lagging behind the massive medical experiment being carried out on the population of the United States.

CHAPTER 7

⤙⤚

The Modern Pain Clinic—a New Way to Fragment Treatment

A new system of pain clinics has been created in the United States, in which pain management focused mainly on the concern for an "epidemic of prescription drug abuse." [416] A patient's pain is a secondary concern of these clinics. The primary concerns today are controlling diversion and preventing addiction. The system of multidisciplinary pain centers that used to exist was dismantled in the 1990s as a cost-saving measure. [417,418] Subsequently, patients were prescribed more opioids compared to any time in history. While the compassionate care movement had intended to expand prescribing to include some new categories of patients, entrepreneurs of all types saw other opportunities that were possible because of more permissible prescribing. Just as suddenly, after twenty years of massive expansion, the decision was made to reverse course. The excesses of the pill mills and a number of highly-publicized prescription-drug overdose deaths caught the attention of the nation. The sensational reporting caused public outrage, which was used to justify a new policy for prescribing. The advocacy coalition behind PROP with support within the CDC and DEA successfully advocated for a drastic change in prescribing, ignoring the harm that would do to millions of people. Pain clinics have become the preferred medical facilities for opioid prescribing because they permit a standardized guideline to be implemented. Confusion reigned because the CDC guideline addressed prescribing by primary care physicians, while PCPs were simultaneously discouraged from continuing to manage pain and most patients were referred to the new pain clinics.

Doctors have been caught in the middle, attacked by patients for not treating pain adequately in the 1990s, and then by the families of overdose victims for prescribing too much to vulnerable young people in the 2000s.[419] They have also been under siege by the DEA when their prescribing exceeded certain bounds set arbitrarily by the agency, regardless of medical justification.[302,307] Some of the most egregious actions have been taken against doctors who have had the courage to take on the intractable pain problem or simply were vulnerable.[108,239,303,305,307,420] In the end, PCPs and individual doctors gradually lost the will, or perhaps we should say courage, to write opioid prescriptions. Patients were referred to pain clinics, which had a simple mandate not to overprescribe.

This chapter is dedicated to an overview of the context of these pain clinics. Here, we develop the main theme of this book—namely that it is inappropriate to blame persistent-pain patients for the mistakes of the past: the drug problem, the diversion, or the overprescribing. The reality that some pain patients have a tendency toward opioid use disorder or even addiction should be regarded as a separate medical problem. This concerns a small minority of patients, but they deserve compassionate treatment as well. The arbitrary limits on prescribing implemented by the CDC have the effect of punishing pain patients for problems that they had no role in creating. Those pain patients who still have access to medication are increasingly forced to follow the rules of pain clinics that are more directly responsive to the DEA than any medical institution has ever been.

The Modern Pain Clinic as Opioid Control

It is not good policy or medical practice to mix the law-enforcement function of opioid control with the operation of a pain clinic. The justification for doing this is that the crisis has been described officially as a "prescription-drug overdose crisis." But what is the drug crisis? For many years, the Mexican drug cartels and other international drug-smuggling rings had received the brunt of the blame for America's drug-addiction problems. In the 1970s when the *war on drugs* was initially conceived, the target was clearly the trafficking of illicit drugs from Mexico, Colombia, or other smuggling routes and, of course, domestic distribution networks. The passage of the Controlled Substances Act of 1970 furthered a trend to criminalize the possession and consumption of opioids, which has further complicated their use in medicine. The war on drugs has been pronounced a failure by quite a number of observers including the Office of Management and Budget of the Congress.[421–424] For many years people have been dying of drug overdoses in major urban areas because of these failed policies. But, after 2000, when it became evident that young people who were from middle-class neighborhoods were dying of overdoses and turning to heroin when the prescription drugs were no longer available, there was a sense in many parts of the country that something new and terrible had happened.[168] Indeed, something terrible was happening, but it was not new.

Addiction was not a new problem, and it did not suddenly worsen because of overprescribing starting in 1997. Addiction and overdose have been problems continuously for more than a century with the exception of World War II, when addiction rates were significantly lower than at any other time during the twentieth century. Since then, the addiction rate, including to heroin, cocaine, and crack cocaine, has been increasing gradually until 2011 when heroin addiction took a large jump. While it is true that heroin addiction was at a relatively low rate at the beginning of the compassionate care movement (about 0.2% of population), cocaine and crack made up the larger part, and overall drug use was as high as it had ever been. The notion that heroin addiction "came from nowhere" was a naive view that fails to see the way drug use had evolved in the United States.

The reason for the sudden increase of heroin use in 2011 was the restrictions on prescription drugs, which were implemented without any planning. While state and federal governments made no plans, the Sinaloa cartel ramped up heroin production in anticipation of the closure of the pill mills. The cartel bosses watched as the states slowly implemented prescription drug monitoring programs (PDMPs) after 2005, culminating in Florida's program in 2010. By putting all the pharmacies on an electronic database, it was possible to track each individual's prescriptions from all sources. It was no longer possible to obtain multiple prescriptions (doctor shop). The largest pill mills were put out of business. The restrictions, which culminated in the introduction of PDMPs in Florida in 2011, drove illicit users of diverted prescription drugs to use heroin out of desperation.[49,425–427] The policy of suddenly cutting off all prescription drugs from the pill mills without a plan to provide addiction services for the users was extremely ill-conceived.[428] But it was also unconscionable to permit the pill mills to operate with impunity for more than ten years. With too few methadone clinics and a dearth of counseling or services for addiction available, many of those who had become recently addicted had no idea where to turn.[429] The policy forced users to choose between heroin and a cold-turkey withdrawal with no support.[49,426,427,430,431] For persistent-pain patients the dilemma was far worse. They had real pain, and once they lost their prescriptions, some committed suicide, some chose heroin, and many toughed it out, but their pain was truly not something that a healthy person could comprehend. It was the advocacy of zealots that pushed the opioid crisis into its worst period yet.[270,432–436]

Overdose fatalities had been mainly an urban problem since the 1970s. The rise of drug use in rural areas of Appalachia, the rust belt, the four corners area of New Mexico, and Arizona were new phenomena.[437] Despite the evidence of an increase in heroin and, later, fentanyl, the easiest thing to do was to blame overprescribing for the entire scandal. Although Congress had supported the DEA's mission of a *war on prescription drugs*, diversion of prescription drugs grew significantly on their watch. The large companies and the DEA had the tools to identify diversion but took no action to stop it.[250] This trend had continued with the recent action by the Department of Justice (DOJ) to stop any kind of indictment against Walmart, despite evidence from Texas prosecutors that executives in the company had received hundreds of messages from employees reporting suspect prescriptions and wanting a company policy to prevent sales to customers who were coming directly from pill mills.[438] The DOJ tied the hands of the DEA in this instance. However, the DEA had played its part by increasing production quotas during the entire decade of overprescribing without taking a single action against the major pill mills.[252] The DEA had not taken any action against Purdue for more than a decade while evidence mounted of a prescription diversion scheme on a massive scale.[439–443] After years of inaction, state governments began to raid some of the pill mills.[428] The largest were in Florida, and their actions did not become serious until 2010.[49,444] As public anger rose, the easiest course of action for politicians at all levels was to blame pharmacies and pharmaceutical companies. That meant keeping the focus on prescription opioid medications as the cause. State attorney generals filed lawsuits and municipalities followed so that there are currently over 1,600 pending lawsuits against opioid manufacturers, pharmacies, professional organizations, and doctors.[31,33] None of this is helping to address the two major underlying problems of addiction and the undertreatment of pain.

It is clear from the attitudes and approach of the new pain clinics that they see their mandate as the first line of defense against *overprescribing*, which PROP and their adherents believe to be a major route to addiction. This is a fallacious argument. Examining the primary literature in chapters 4 to 6 has shown the inconsistencies, lack of evidence, and bias in academic articles that support these harmful policies. The message that patients are either addicted or on their way to addiction places blame on persistent-pain patients for a problem beyond the scope of pain management.[445] After blaming the problems entirely on *overprescribing*, many states repealed any law or special rule that permitted prescribing of opioids to pain patients.[446] Any legal or regulatory protection patients had gained in the past thirty years was erased. Following the backlash against overprescribing, pain patients were denied treatment or pushed into the new pain clinics where the rules were strictly set according to hard limits.[284]

Most citizens do not understand that there are people whose pain is so severe that they need high doses of opioids just to function.[447] Although there are many pain patients, they do not have a lobby and they have little energy to fight the injustice. There are concerned doctors and government agencies, but their voice has so far been drowned out by the focus on the CDC guidelines and the implications for pain clinics. Medicine should be individualized, and it should not take a special policy statement of the Department of Health and Human Services (DHHS) to get that message out.[448] There are millions of people who have serious conditions with debilitating pain that is poorly understood and undertreated by the new pain clinics. The focus on opioid control is failing to meet the needs of pain patients and looking increasingly like an extension of the punitive mindset that the DEA has employed to every aspect of opioid control. Society does not need opioid control; it needs opioid medical expertise.

The Importance of Treating Addiction as a Medical Problem

One's viewpoint on this controversy depends strongly on personal experience. The families of people who struggle with addiction have a different outlook compared to families whose loved ones are suffering from chronic inflammatory diseases or cancer. Both are valid and both require a solution. Recently, there has been some recognition of undertreatment of addiction. Although it is a small step forward, the Comprehensive Addiction Recovery Act (CARA) was passed by Congress in 2016 and was signed into law by President Obama. The law provides funding for a national program to provide treatment for addicts and treat addiction as a disease.[449] However, the funding is woefully inadequate for the scope of the problem, and it begs the question, What about persistent-pain patients who have also been harmed by these policies? In a free society, it is not acceptable to solve the problem for one group at the expense of another unless one can make the argument that the two are irreconcilable and some higher principle is involved. In recognition of this fact, CARA's first section requests the formation of an interagency task force led by the DHHS to develop guidelines for safely prescribing opioids to patients with acute and chronic pain.[449] In this context, PROP's successful lobby to immediately implement guidelines at the CDC in 2016 can be seen as an attempt to preemptively set the standard pain management for the United States. PROP and CDC Director Frieden effectively usurped the authority that Congress had meant for the DHHS in their writing of the CARA Act. The DHHS Pain Management Best Practices Inter-Agency Task Force released its final report in 2019 calling for "a balanced, individualized, patient-centered approach."[448] The United States clearly does not have such an approach today in its pain clinics. This document, like the revised CDC guidelines, does not directly affect the pain clinics' decisions or policies. Rather the enforcement agency, which is the DEA, set its priorities based on the perceived justification provided the CDC guidelines. The harmful policies promoted by PROP are evident in a microcosm in the poor treatment that sickle cell anemia patients have received in recent years since the new guidelines were published.[68,69,308] Like cancer, one would think that a painful genetic disease that often shortens life span by twenty years or more would be an obvious candidate for compassionate care using opioids. That is not the case today.

Overprescribing—What Went Wrong?

The recurring theme in the news today is that overprescribing is responsible for the massive problem, even for the entire epidemic. It is a matter of record that doctors began prescribing larger and more frequent opioid prescriptions after 1997, when it was encouraged both by the American Pain Society and American Association of Pain Medicine, as well as by several pharmaceutical companies, with Purdue Pharma leading the way. The issue of overprescribing is complicated by systemic issues in American medical care, the private insurance system, Medicaid, and poverty. There are so many real-world situations that doctors must confront, particularly if they are in a low-income area. If we imagine a situation where a physician opens a pain clinic and finds rapidly that dozens of patients cannot afford x-rays or tests to prove that they are in pain. Because of poverty, patients at the clinic often lack insurance or have issues with insurance denying coverage for certain medications. Patients have poor past medical records that would perhaps justify treatment of pain. Pain physicians may mean well, but they can quickly end up in a situation that would be considered criminal to the DEA merely because they are trying to be responsive to patient's needs and they have limited staff and resources to properly document care. It is difficult to read the accounts of doctors arrested and charged with narcotics violations whose main crime was poor recordkeeping. The kickbacks given to doctors and support given to pill mills by certain pharmaceutical companies led to diversion on a massive scale that is clearly criminal. Yet this diversion too is technically *prescribing*. As a consequence, there are relatively few doctors who will take on the risk to prescribe opioids. Education proposed by the AMA would likely help the matter. But such initiatives are underfunded, while DEA enforcement received a budget of $15.6 billion in 2018.[450] We must carefully differentiate criminals who run pain clinics as pill mills from doctors who are overwhelmed and do not have the office help to follow all the regulations. A compassionate pain specialist ends up swamped with patients because of the dearth of pain clinics. Those doctors frequently had to make a choice between denying treatment and believing a patient who has little medical documentation. Pain was considered undertreated in 1996 when the compassionate care movement began. Now, there are new guidelines and patient advocates,[159] lawyers,[450] patient news websites,[283] and Human Rights Watch[233] are decrying the extremely adverse effects of the new restrictions on prescribing.[451] Even after the changes in the revised CDC guideline in 2019, the situation remains dire for millions of pain patients.[159,309]

Those doctors who downplay the need for opioids in medicine should spend some time with a person like Patient Z who is struggling with chronic illness.[125] One viewpoint on the failures of our medical system over the past thirty years attributes the failures to overmedication. The fragmentation of care and lack of insurance coverage are not mentioned in the analysis. There is also the tendency to exaggerate the numbers in the United States to create the appearance of a tsunami of overprescribing. To make the case, the author, Dr. Tick, estimates that the United States prescribes fifty times as many opioids as the rest of the world combined.[125] Many articles and news reports present similarly inaccurate estimates of the consumption of opioids in the US. The United Nations International Narcotics Control Board Report states that the United States consumes 56% of the world's morphine with a 6% of the population, while Europe consumes 28% with 11% of the population. Thus, the European Union consumes approximately 3.7 times less than the US on average and Canada about the same per capita as the US. In fact, the consumption of opioids scales with wealth. That is not so much a statement about the intrinsically high consumption rate of the United States, but of the lack of pain medicine for the vast majority of the world's population. For many years increasing opioid consumption was viewed as a positive development because it meant better care for people suffering with pain. Clearly, there is a limit to such a correlation, just as there is an optimum dose for a persistent-pain patient.

We may examine the example of Germany for comparison. It has the largest population at 82.9 million, and it is one of the wealthier countries in Europe.[452] According to analysis of the prescribing rates, the US consumption rate is 50% higher compared to the German rate, not fifty times higher. This estimate agrees reasonably well with UN data showing that US consumption was 100% higher in 2018, but around 33% higher in 2020.[453,454] German medical administrators point out that a systematic approach to opioid prescribing means that rates of prescription are lower than in the United States, but persistent-pain patient needs are addressed by their universal health care system.[454] At the same time addiction rates are less than one-third of those in the United States and similarly lower overdose rates have not changed since 2006 despite a 100% increase in chronic noncancer pain prescriptions over the same period.[455] While the American medical literature appears to have strongly varying viewpoints steeped in financially-driven controversy, the European medical literature recognizes that opioids have a place in the treatment of pain and that pain was undertreated for many years.[311] These same ideas were prevalent in the 1990s in the US, and yet the effort to address the problem utterly failed; whereas, in many European countries, they addressed persistent pain needs of the population without increasing addiction or overdose rates. The United States has a long history of criminalizing opioids, which has created a contradiction in our medical system. A doctor who prescribes opioids for pain is always at risk of prosecution.[108,239,305,307,420] This circumstance has caused the vast majority of doctors in the United States to stop prescribing opioids.

We must carefully distinguish overprescribing from diversion, which we will consider in the next chapter. There is some overlap, and understanding that overlap is very important since sloppy analysis confuses the different categories, which is often to the detriment of pain patients. There were three types of overprescribing during the decade of the 2000s: (1) genuine concern for a patient's pain leading to a larger prescription than necessary,[456] (2) doctors being fooled by patients and writing a prescription that the patient could misuse,[457] and (3) pill mills that wrote prescriptions for profit and were surely aware that the patient's pain was fake and their goal was to divert the opioids.[442,444,458-460] Then there were cases such as Patient Z where the prescribed dose was relatively high, but it was not a case of overprescribing. The prescription was necessary for pain control.[461]

Understanding the scale of the pill mills is difficult, but that illegal activity skewered the perception of legitimate prescribing in a way that the medical community is still not recognizing. One pill mill could easily prescribe hundreds of times the dose in a normal pain clinic of the day. One example in the DEA records were shipments to one Virginia county of 74 million pills from 2006 to 2012, enough for 106 pills for each resident per year.[462] There was gross negligence[253,462] and significant corruption[250,458,459] on the part of the DEA and the federal and state governments.

Today's pain clinic focuses on the first cause of overprescribing to justify their policy. They suggest that pain patients' doses are too high. There are hundreds of accounts of patients who were stable on a fixed dose for years who were forced to taper because of this. For patients with minor low back pain or osteoarthritis, there is evidence for benefit from lowering the dose of overmedicated patients, but for the millions patients with persistent pain from chronic diseases, the results have been almost uniformly bad. It is unethical to reason that patient suffering is the price we must pay for opioid control. Of course, they do not want to admit this, but the policy has had the effect of limiting prescriptions regardless of the disease. Although they pay lip service to patient welfare, pragmatic pain clinic directors are well aware that limiting the supply of opioids is the highest priority.[367,463]

Dosing Guidelines, Tapers, and Hard Limits

The concern is frequently expressed that pain patients need continuous dose escalation to maintain pain relief.[278] On the contrary, many studies support the observation that consistent long-term pain relief is possible with a constant dose.[151,152,154] Patient experiences vary a great deal, and any generalization is fraught with peril. Nonetheless, the literature today is rife with categorical statements about how opioids will adversely affect patients leading to dose escalation.[132] Along with this statement, tolerance has been discussed as a necessary failure mode of opioids.[18] This is a misunderstanding. In practice, tolerance means that a new dose may need to be adjusted to account for the onset of tolerance, but then a steady state is reached that provides stable pain relief. Many patients experience consistent pain relief for years.[62]

Another concern is that every other method should have been tried before resorting to opioids. This is rather obvious, but it is repeated nonetheless. Each time Patient Z meets a new pain specialist, there is the obligatory set of questions about what has been tried in the past. In Patient Z's case, he passed through the three stages of the WHO ladder of pain medication more than a decade ago. Given a patient who has advanced-stage ankylosing spondylitis, it is a bit odd that the pain doctor wants to consider trying acetaminophen again. But they ask. For some diseases, certain types of pain can be mitigated by appropriate non-opioid medications. Chemotherapy or immunotherapy can stop or even reverse cancer progression, reducing any associated pain. Biologic drugs made from human antibodies can intercept immune-system messengers in the blood and thereby reduce the pain of inflammation in autoimmune diseases. However, even modern anti-inflammatory drugs do not alleviate the pain of an aggressive autoimmune disease. Opioid treatment is often the only option to control the persistent pain of incurable diseases.

The medical literature has documented that the pain of many inflammatory or degenerative diseases increases as a condition becomes systemic and increasingly aggressive. For years opioids at <200 MEDD were considered a moderate dose that could alleviate autoimmune inflammatory and cancer pain in many patients.[113,114] In hospice and some other rare instances, higher doses were given. Many articles written today justify significantly lower doses on the basis of a lack of quality-of-life data and concerns over patient safety.[464] It is rather ironic when a patient may have lived for a decade at a given dose without an incident of opioid side effect and is suddenly informed, by a doctor, that they are at great risk. Often these statements are made based on evidence contaminated with other risk factors such as alcohol use or benzodiazepines. Taking sedatives is a major reason for overdose fatalities involving prescription opioid medication. When physicians tell a patient that they are potentially at risk, they are often making a general statement to encourage a taper. Even accepting the premise that risk of respiratory suppression increases with opioid dose, it should a doctor-patient consultation that decides whether the pain relief is worth the risk. Today, patients are not given a choice. They must live with the pain on the lower dose based on "safety concerns." Despite the fact that Patient Z had the same dose for years, the new pain clinic insisted he taper for his own safety.

The Fear of Prosecution Dominates Prescribing in Pain Clinics

The DEA controls licensing and has broad authority to close down a doctor's office for the mere suspicion of diversion. The DEA can do so without warning in a single raid.[465] In 2018, without explanation the DEA took down its FAQ webpage that many physicians had relied on for guidance. This type of action adds to the anxiety doctors feel.[466] The last time an important document was taken down from a DEA website in 2003, it was because of the DEA's prosecution of a compassionate doctor who received an unjustifiable twenty-five-year sentence for "drug trafficking." Those events coincided with the DEA's decision to aggressively prosecute doctors for a number of years subsequently. Some have argued that a commonsense regulation would be to have all suspected overprescribing referred to the state medical board and thus remove the possibility of direct DEA intervention. The board would evaluate using medical expertise, and only if the medical board thought there was criminal negligence or intent would the case be referred to law enforcement.[467] But this is not an agenda item in the current climate. The threat of DEA action is significant enough to cause a pain clinic director to decide that hard limits for all patients are safer than permitting doctors to make decisions based on individual patient needs.[468] The clinics may justify this by saying that they need to stay open to help patients and the best way to avoid scrutiny is to be as conservative as possible. To hear the thousands of abandoned and traumatized patients tell their stories in news articles and internet websites, the compassionate pain clinic is a thing of the past.[156,251,469,470]

The medical boards should be supportive of patients. An extract from a typical mission statement is provided below:

> The [State] Medical Board recognizes that principles of quality medical practice dictate that the people of the State [...] have access to appropriate and effective pain relief. The appropriate application of up-to-date knowledge and treatment modalities can serve to improve the quality of life for those patients who suffer from pain as well as reduce the morbidity and costs associated with untreated or inappropriately treated pain.

There appears to be a disconnect between what pain specialists are saying in their clinics and the position statement of the medical board:

> Inappropriate pain treatment may result from physicians' lack of knowledge about pain management. Fears of investigation or sanction by federal, state and local agencies may also result in inappropriate treatment of pain. Appropriate pain management is the treating physician's responsibility. As such, the Board will consider the inappropriate treatment of pain to be a departure from standards of practice.

Inappropriate pain management could result from either too low or too high a dose. Despite this fact, most pain clinics are currently focused only on bringing all patients' dose down to a predetermined maximum opioid dose. The state medical board is a pressure point that could be responsive to patient needs, either by filing a complaint or petitioning for a policy.

The Aftermath of the CDC Guidelines—Never Mind What Is Written on the Website

The CDC guidelines, which were published online in 2016, and in the *New England Journal of Medicine*, stated that primary care physicians should justify any prescription above 90 MEDD for new patients.[281] Since this was the only quantitative statement and it was limited to a specific set of circumstances, there was ambiguity in the intent of guideline. In practice, the guidelines were implemented as a hard limit of 120 MEDD at Patient Z's clinic. This is coincidentally the same level set by the National Committee on Quality Assurance (NCQA) in 2017 as the dose cutoff for acceptable risk in prescribing.[48] The NCQA stated that it was building on the CDC guidelines in setting 120 MEDD as a limit, above which prescribing would be considered high risk for any patient. At Patient Z's clinic the 120 MEDD hard limit was called "clinic policy," yet no one at the clinic could explain the origin of the limit to Patient Z. The pain clinics interpreted the CDC guidelines to mean that patients who had a dose greater than the maximum should be tapered as quickly as possible to that limit. However, in Patient Z's pain clinic none of the doctors could explain the reason that the limit was set at 120 MEDD.

Many doctors thought that the limit set by the CDC was arbitrary and not supported by evidence.[471] There was great concern about the negative impacts of these interpretations in the medical community. In 2018, a panel of fifty-three experts assembled by the CDC registered concern that prescription benchmarking could result in providers being "incentivized against caring for patients requiring above average amounts of opioid medication."[472] In 2019, 381 health-care professionals wrote a letter to the CDC to press for a statement by the agency to guard against the interpretation of the guideline that led to hard limits.[1,285] There were at least twenty documented suicides and many deaths to abrupt withdrawal in very sick patients attributable to the implementation of the guidelines.[121,473] A detailed policy analysis describing the challenges of prescribers was published as well.[2] In 2019, the CDC issued revised guidelines.[474]

> **Misapplication of the Guideline's dosage recommendation that results in hard limits or "cutting off" opioids.** The Guideline states, "*When opioids are started*, clinicians should prescribe the lowest effective dosage. Clinicians should…avoid *increasing* dosage to ≥90 MEDD/day or carefully justify a decision to titrate dosage to ≥90 MEDD/day." The recommendation statement does not suggest discontinuation of opioids already prescribed at higher dosages.

This new recommendation could hardly be clearer in terms of how the clinics have misinterpreted the spirit if not the letter of the guidelines from 2016. When patients have serious illnesses, burns, or physical deformities caused by an accident or wound, the humane approach is to provide relief for the associated pain. That should be a decision between doctor and patient.

The concern for patient's health and protection of a physician's right to make an individual decision for a patient is also given in the American Medical Association's House of Delegates Resolution 235 issued in November 2018.[469] It reads in part:

> No entity should use MEDD (morphine milligram equivalents) thresholds as anything more than guidance, and physicians should not be subject to professional discipline, loss of board certification, loss of clinical privileges, criminal prosecution, civil liability, or other penalties or practice limitations solely for prescribing opioids at a quantitative level above the MEDD thresholds found in the CDC Guideline for Prescribing Opioids.

None of these policies change the fact that patients are being tapered and the hard limits are being enforced on many patients. The fear of prosecution or loss of license weighs so heavily in a physician's mind that they weigh patient pain against the need to stay within the perceived prescribing limits already set in 2016. Patient pain is not their pain, and they have a very real anxiety about losing their livelihood or worse.

The End of the Intractable Pain Laws and Prescribing by Primary Care Doctors

The impetus to increase the dose of opioid drugs began in the 1990s as awareness of so-called "intractable pain patients" reached a wide swath of the medical community and beyond.[134] These are patients who have such severe pain that they need palliative pain management despite the fact that they may live for decades. The need for a new medical approach that permitted use of high-dose opioids was recognized and specifically permitted by statute for patients who met that standard in certain states (California, Oregon, Washington, Texas, Iowa, Florida, Tennessee, Arkansas, Colorado, and Louisiana).[475] A number of other states gave a prescriber reassurance that he or she would not be prosecuted for providing opioid medications to patients for purely medical reasons.

The implementation of the intractable chronic pain treatment concept was corrupted by the greed of relatively few people. Rather than recognize the specific nature of the greed, the failures in legislation, monitoring and enforcement, and the role played by the fragmentation of medical care, the response had been to blame *all* prescription drugs and *anyone* associated with producing, prescribing, or selling them. In 2015, Tennessee repealed its Intractable Pain Patient statute unanimously and began a rigorous enforcement of new, strict limitations on pain medication for persistent-pain patients.[446] Other states followed. As a federal authority, the DEA had made it impossible to practice medicine according to the states' Intractable Pain Statutes in recent years.

New state laws discourage or even prevent patients from relying on their PCP for pain medication. Today doctors will usually refuse to treat pain, citing the restrictions that they face. They may refer a patient to a pain clinic, but there is no certainty that a pain clinic will accept a patient. Nor is it certain that a pharmacist will fill a prescription. A recent report summarizes the state of affairs today[267]:

> During the recent Interim Meeting of the American Medical Association, the organization's president, Dr. Barbara McAneny, told the study of a patient of hers whose pharmacist refused to fill his prescription for an opioid medication. He had prescribed the medication to ease his patient's severe pain from prostate cancer, which had spread to his bones. Feeling ashamed after the pharmacist called him a "drug seeker," he went home, hoping to endure his pain. Three days later, he tried to kill himself. Fortunately,

McAneny's patient was discovered by family members and survived.

Does the pharmacist lack empathy? Or is this a reaction to the pervasive fear of opioid prescribing and sales that has accompanied the new guidelines? Either way, in this climate, the brunt of the rejection of opioid prescribing falls on the patient. The patient is made to feel shame for taking an opioid, even if it is prescribed. Since there are dishonest people who fool doctors, the patient in pain with a genuine need feels even more shame at the thought of being identified as a con man. The level of suspicion and intolerance for any deviation is so high that patients are afraid to speak their minds. Recognizing that this is not a healthy environment for pain management, there are numerous medical experts who advocate a return to a multidisciplinary approach,[476] because pain is not being treated adequately at present.[471]

The Tragic Policies of the Veteran's Administration

Once the prescription of pain medication is decoupled from other medical considerations, it becomes more difficult to evaluate who really needs treatment and who is seeking a high dose because of a use disorder. The challenges of pain patients were better documented in the Veteran's Administration (VA) than in the general community arising from a willingness to confront issues such as gender discrimination in care, the role of depression and posttraumatic stress disorder (PTSD), and a frankness about the need to communicate and take patient wishes into account in decisions to taper.[477] There used to be a vestige of an integrated approach to pain treatment at Veteran's Administration (VA) hospitals. However, the policy was changed, and veterans were forced to taper en masse a few years ago, which led to thousands of suicides and a great deal of pain and suffering.[478–480] The overall picture for persistent-pain patients is bleak because, in addition to the change in structure that disfavors working with patients on the sources of their diseases, there is a shortage of pain clinics, which is particularly acute in rural areas.[481]

CHAPTER 8

⁓

Patient Z's Encounters with Pain Clinics

When Patient Z arrived at the first pain clinic of his life, he could see that the point of the visit was not going to be to try to find a diagnosis or treat his symptoms. The pain clinics actually have a difficult task if they take it seriously. They are the ones who need to determine how to take care of pain when every other medication in the modern arsenal has been used and the patient is still miserable. If the pain clinic really looks at the patient's pain, the medical staff needs to first use every possible alternative to make sure there is no other way to control the pain, but then if opioids are required, the task is to "titrate" the medication to try to alleviate suffering. But when the multidisciplinary pain clinic was replaced with the new generation of pain clinic, the goal clearly changed from treatment of disease to ensuring that patients do not abuse the prescribed analgesics.[416] The pain clinic today is mainly an office to evaluate whether a patient is reliable enough to trust with an opioid drug prescription and to ensure compliance. Patient Z called it "opioid control." The pain specialists had sympathy with Patient Z. They seemed to believe that his pain was real. But they apparently had no choice. "Clinic policy" dictated the same limit for all patients. The doctors and nurses had to tell themselves that tapering down really was in the patient's best interest. There were a few journal articles to help them justify their work.[123–125] But to convince themselves that their treatment option was the only one, they must avoid reading medical

163

journal articles that describe the injustice being done to an entire population of pain patients.[3,120–122,158,251,270,282]

Patient Z went to a pain clinic to see a pain specialist for the first time about three months before he received his diagnosis at the NIH. Dr. C was under investigation by then, and he had asked Patient Z to make an appointment at the pain clinic to get a *second opinion*. Dr. C was not permitted to tell Patient Z that the second opinion would actually be the only opinion because he was no longer permitted to write prescriptions for Patient Z.

The pain specialist, named Dr. L, immediately told Patient Z he was *overprescribed*. Instead of asking about his pain or trying to understand his illness, his only concern was that he needed to reduce his dose of opioids as aggressively as possible. Patient Z asked him why this was essential, pointing out that he was relatively comfortable since he had started taking opioids and that he had been miserable before.

Dr. L opined, "We need to reduce the narcotic dose to increase your function." He enunciated the word *function* with a great emphasis as though it were a foreign concept to Patient Z. As far as Patient Z could see, his function was increased because of the opioids, since he finally could walk without being in constant pain. He could go to the store or cook a meal without feeling completely miserable.

Patient Z challenged Dr. L. "What specific function will be enhanced by decreasing the opioid dose?" he asked.

"Look," he replied, "what I am telling you is based on a study from Harvard."

"I see," he replied, "can you tell me the reference so I can look it up?"

Dr. L gave him a hostile look. Perhaps he thought that Patient Z was trying to be arrogant, but Patient Z read and thought about evidence. Perhaps Dr. L thought that saying that the study was from Harvard would mean that it was beyond question. Patient Z knew that the authors of the study were more important compared to where the study was done. Dr. L did not know the name of the corresponding author, so Patient Z never had a way to look up the study.

Dr. L's response instead was to pull out a piece of paper and to make a drawing of a figure showing some data. He wrote the word *function* on the horizontal axis and the word *drug* on the vertical axis. He drew a curved line increasing and then leveling off relative to the horizontal axis. The drawing looked a bit like figure 2 except that the labels on the axes were switched. Patient Z recognized his drawing as a dose-response curve, a standard pharmaceutical representation of drug effectiveness. Many drugs have an efficacy that increases over some range of drug concentration and then levels off at high concentrations. However, Dr. L had reversed the axes such that his drawing was not a correct representation. He seemed not to realize that he had done this and continued speaking to Z in a condescending tone. He said that function may be helped by low doses of opioids but that high doses show no further increase.

In fact, he said triumphantly, "Your function is probably worse at the higher dose."

Patient Z responded, "It seems that the Harvard researchers reversed the axes on their dose-response curve. This figure shows function increasing without bound at constant dose of the drug."

Dr. L looked flustered and embarrassed as he realized his mistake. He wrote the prescription very hastily for the same dose Patient Z had been taking and said, "I have to go. Try to reduce your dose on your own. Next time, we will discuss how to bring down the dose more aggressively."

He left the room in a great hurry without any further discussion. He deserved that humiliation for disregarding Patient Z's disease and lecturing him about "function" without even taking the time to understand his symptoms. This "Harvard study" was clearly a standard phrase that he used to shut down discussion since most patients probably would not know what to say when a doctor justifies his decision invoking a study from a prestigious university. Sadly, patients need to be ready to answer such pretentious nonsense, which is used to intimidate them and to force them to accept that there is no way to treat their pain. Dr. L's pronouncement was not true for many patients. It certainly was not true for Patient Z. He thought it was an easy way to force Patient Z to accept a taper.

That was Patient Z's first encounter with a pain specialist. Between that initial visit and the following visit many months later, Patient Z had visited the NIH and obtained the diagnosis of ankylosing spondylitis. Dr. L was informed of the diagnosis. Moreover, Patient Z had voluntarily reduced his dose from 420 MEDD to 320 MEDD. He did this mainly because he had started taking a biologic drug for his inflammation and the antibody had decreased the inflammatory component caused by a protein known as tumor necrosis factor (TNF). Only once he had received a diagnosis could he obtain a prescription for the biologic antibody drug. Patient Z said that the pain of inflammation was different from the pain for grinding bone on bone, which we might call mechanical pain. There is also a separate pain from muscle spasms. Technically, the bone and joint pain and muscle spasms are classified as nociceptive pain. For many patients, nociceptive pain is greatly reduced by opioid therapy. The inflammatory pain is not helped as much by opioids. The class of antibody biologics (for example, Humira, Remicade, or Enbrel), which bind to TNF, can alleviate inflammatory pain. TNF causes a disruption in the uptake of glutamate in astrocytes, which causes an excess of the neurotransmitter to build up in the synapses.[482] This keeps the pain signaling active. TNF is produced as part of the immune response in attacks against the patient's own tissues, and it effects neural transmission by increasing the intensity of the signal, including the pain signal. This is one of origins of inflammatory pain. Opioids alone can help, but the combination of the biologic drug and 320 MEDD of morphine and oxycodone had brought Patient Z the greatest comfort in many years. Thus, when Patient Z returned to the clinic, he had voluntarily reduced his dose by about 25% over a period of six months. This slow taper was possible for Patient Z to implement himself, because his pain was well controlled by the biologic and opioid working together.

On the second visit to the pain specialist, Dr. L's tone changed substantially. He seemed genuinely concerned for Patient Z's welfare. He walked into the room and said warmly, "Hello, Z, how are you?" and began asking about his symptoms with genuine compassion. He encouraged Patient Z to continue to reduce his dosage, but on his own terms. He did not issue threats or suggest that there would be any repercussions if he continued at the same dose. He seemed genuinely impressed with the reduction he had already achieved. Although it had been a rough start, Patient Z felt that he had a good working relationship, and he resolved to try to reduce his dose further. The doctor-patient relationship was based on trust and positive reinforcement. Patient Z was more inclined to taper further when he felt that the doctor was supportive rather than scolding him and forcing him. He could tell that the biologic drug had made a difference, and he believed that the lowest opioid dose possible was the best dose, as long as the pain was well controlled. Unfortunately, Dr. L decided to move west shortly after his second visit. Patient Z had gained Dr. L's trust and compassion, but because of Dr. L's move, Patient Z had to start over. Other pain specialists would not be so sympathetic.

Patient Z's Transition from Shame to Indignation

In the beginning, Patient Z felt shame about taking opioid drugs. By the time he entered the first pain clinic, he had taken them for seven years without any problems or significant side effects. He had realized that, in this sense, he was one of the lucky patients. Some patients had side effects so severe they could not continue with opioid medication. However, he felt a sense of shame as though there was something wrong about having to rely on an opioid for his condition. Sometimes he would be in pain, and after taking opioids, he would feel such relief that he genuinely felt good. At that moment, he would suddenly feel guilty as though there were something wrong with feeling relief from pain. This is a common reaction. There is such a fear of addiction in our society that the mere idea of taking an opioid and deriving benefit from it as medication makes people feel ashamed.[483]

It is interesting to reflect on how we feel no shame about taking non-opioid prescription medications. No one would feel bad about taking blood-pressure medication and feeling a relief that the tight hypertensive feeling has gone away. Opioids are still taboo, and many people misunderstand their effects and use. Later, when Patient Z reached the point in a forced taper where he was miserable from the pain, he finally became angry enough at the insensitivity of the doctors that he felt no shame at all in saying he needed to rely on opioid painkillers. But on the way to the realization that the drugs were helping him and were essential for his quality of life, he had to go through all the stages of self-doubt that almost all patients experience. When Dr. L left the pain clinic, his replacement at that pain clinic was a nurse who was completely insensitive. Her reaction to Patient Z's dose made him feel as though he were drug seeking. He felt shame for having to rely on opioids for survival. Despite the diagnosis of ankylosing spondylitis and evident disability, the nurse practitioner showed no concern for Patient Z's symptoms or welfare, but merely pointed to the need for aggressive reductions in the dose to save him from the dangers of opioids.

It was as this juncture that Patient Z discovered that his rheumatologist had prescribed the incorrect dose of the biologic. The rheumatologist had not written the prescription but had entrusted that to a subordinate who made a mistake. For months, Patient Z had been on a dose of one injection of the antibody protein per month. That dose was half of what it should have been. Patient Z felt frustrated with the poor care. He searched online and found that a new rheumatologist had moved to the area. He decided to switch rheumatologists. He also had the opportunity to go to the pain clinic where his new rheumatologist practiced. After his only meeting with Dr. L's draconian successor, it seemed worth the risk to switch to a new pain clinic as well. The new rheumatologist made sure that it was not a problem to make the switch.

At first, the pain clinic at the new practice seemed more openminded compared to the previous one. The new pain specialist, Dr. N, did not insist on dose reductions. On the appropriate dose of anti-inflammatory medication, Patient Z was able to slowly taper his dose to 260 MEDD. He stayed at that dose for three more years. He had three operations during this period, which occupied his mental and physical energy. Back surgery and knee replacements are taxing even on a healthy person. He had begun to realize the limitations of opioid treatment. At the new pain clinic, he could have asked for a higher dose, but he understood that the marginal benefit decreased as the dose increased. He also sensed that the nurse at the new pain clinic regarded him with disdain. He never met the doctors, and the only nurse there treated him like a child. Patient Z found it very demeaning. He had asked about alternatives to opioids, and he was told that there was no point in considering them. This may have been correct, but the way the information was delivered made him feel bad for even asking. He asked about an opioid rotation, and the nurse just smiled and said that it was not something they did. When Patient Z's rheumatologist unexpectedly decided to return to the northeast, Patient Z was once again forced to seek a new rheumatologist. Given the limited choices, he returned to the university medical system where he had seen Dr. J. Patient Z's new specialist was a young intern. Given the attitudes in the pain clinic, he decided to move to a pain clinic in the university medical system. It was here that Patient Z was first confronted with a demand that he taper down to the maximum allowed level for the clinic, which was 120 MEDD. By this time, Patient Z had moved to his third pain clinic in five years.

Coming to Terms with the Realistic Goal and Expectation of Pain Control

Patient Z was given a series of rationales for the required taper. However, he found many articles in medical journals indicating that tapering a stable patient could be dangerous and that it should be voluntary. Patient Z asked many questions and pointed out that he was stable. After discussion, they reached a compromise. The taper was forced on Patient Z, but at least the nurse agreed that the taper would be done in two stages. First, he would taper to 180 MEDD and then after a few months he would complete the taper to 120 MEDD. Although the pain specialist promised that the taper to 180 MEDD would be done slowly and with consultation, the clinic set up a forced taper to 180 MEDD within three weeks. They had done this quickly and with poor planning so that the insurance company did not have time to approve the new time-released morphine medication at the lower dose. Because of the poor coordination, Patient Z spent twenty-four hours without any medication at one point in the process while waiting for insurance approval. It was very distressing and painful. Patient Z was so miserable that he could not sleep or have a pain-free moment during the day. Every movement was painful, and the idea of leaving the house caused him such distress that he rarely had the stamina to do it. He was discouraged from activity even when he had stabilized on the new lower dose. Going to church became something he could only muster the strength for once a month at most. Walking from the car to the building seemed like an eternity. Even getting into a wheelchair was a painful ordeal. He could find no comfortable position to sit. He was under stress, and his blood pressure was elevated.

Patient Z wrote a letter to the clinic director and informed that the forced taper he had experienced was not in accord with the CDC guidelines. He received an appointment with one of the doctors. The doctor seemed surprised by Patient Z's knowledge of the CDC guideline. The doctor admitted that they had handled the taper poorly. During the conversation, the doctor also admitted that he had never previously treated a patient with ankylosing spondylitis or any autoimmune disease. The doctor told Patient Z that he could see that Patient Z really was in pain but that he could not change the clinic policy. The doctor suggested that Patient Z should find a new pain clinic, but he was quick to qualify that was only because his pain was genuine, and the pain clinic limit would clearly not be sufficient for Z's pain level. The nurses and doctors actually did show compassion, but they also repeated several times that their hands were tied by clinic policy. Patient Z looked into the possibility of changing to another pain clinic, but no one wanted to consider a patient who had a dose higher than 120 MEDD. Every clinic wanted to know why he was looking to leave. Some clinics said openly that their dose limit was also 120 MEDD, but most simply said that they had no openings for a new patient. Patient Z explained that he was not looking to increase his dose but merely to stay at the current dose. He understood the climate and was clinging to any pain relief he could get. A pain patient begins to feel grateful for any relief as disease progression and clinical pressures combine to threaten well-being. Physicians are under enormous pressure to reduce the dose regardless of the consequences for the pain patient. Even a series of patient deaths documented in newspapers seem to have had little effect on the overall trend toward rapidly forcing pain patients to live in constant pain.[158,233,305,484]

Pain patients generally understand that pain management does not mean the elimination of pain. The goal of treatment is to control pain and reduce it to tolerable levels. Sometimes in a resting position, a persistent-pain patient may be comfortable, but most patients with chronic inflammation will feel discomfort as soon as they move. The higher the opioid dose, the greater the relief, but it is not a linear scale. As the dose is increased over time, the marginal benefit decreases. The pain relief from 0 to 100 MEDD may be enormous, but the relative increase in relief from 100 to 200 MEDD is much smaller. For each increase, there is an immediate effect, which feels more effective than the long-term average effect. This is a result of tolerance. Over time, the pain relief stabilizes at the new dose, and it is relatively constant after that. For the vast majority of patients, it is still true that 200 MEDD gives greater relief than 100 MEDD over an extended period.

For someone with intractable chronic pain, the opioid dose may need to be high in order to provide acceptable relief. In Patient Z's case, it was only when forced to taper did he come to understand that there really was a difference between two dose levels. His pain was significantly greater over a long time at the lower dose of 180 MEDD. The fact that a patient could document the difference of a twelve-month period of differences in pain and function before and after refutes the notion that Patient Z's pain was actually withdrawal disguised as pain, as some doctors in PROP have suggested. But Patient Z knew better than to protest or even mention his higher level of discomfort. He had mentioned the guidelines, and that was as far as he felt he should go in telling the pain clinic about how bad the taper was for him. Asking to return to his original dose could be seen as drug seeking and perhaps would earn him a diagnosis of opioid use disorder (OUD). If his situation was difficult at present, an OUD diagnosis would make his life unbearable.

The "Narcotics Contract"—a Matter of Life and Death

Every patient who enters a pain clinic signs a document that specifies the strict rules for following the prescription and not having any outside prescriptions. This document is the pain management contract. However, many pain clinics blatantly call them "narcotics contracts." The word *narcotics* is a reminder that the medication the patient relies on is an illegal drug in the eyes of the DEA. The pain clinic has a constant preoccupation that patients could be drug addicts and could be diverting their medications, selling them for profit. Any aberration no matter how small will be considered suspect. For example, Patient Z once received a Vicodin prescription from a dentist after oral surgery. He had simply gone to the pharmacy with the prescription given to him by the dentist that included antibiotics and Vicodin. He had not asked for the Vicodin, and while he filled the prescription as a precaution, he did not take the Vicodin. Patient Z had filled the prescription only because he had recalled how unpleasant his experience had been after one of his knee surgeries when he did not have enough pain relief. At the time, he did not dare ask for more pain relief for fear of being accused of OUD. When he went to the pain clinic a week later, they knew about the Vicodin and explained to him that he had violated his narcotics contract. They had grounds to terminate him. Patient Z explained the situation. The dentist had prescribed the Vicodin in case of oral pain. Patient Z had not taken any of the Vicodin. The nurse insisted that he prove that by bringing the bottle of Vicodin to the clinic for disposal. Patient Z brought the full bottle on the following visit, and the nurse counted the pills in front of him. The nurse made a point of explaining that they were being very reasonable this time but that such an infraction could not happen again. In current circumstance, a minor incident or misunderstanding can be interpreted as a violation of the agreement and grounds for termination.

Patient Z Comes to Terms with Opioid Therapy

No one wants to be sick. Certainly, no one wants to be in pain. Very few people would want to take opioids if they did not have pain. That statement must be qualified since some would say that many people—namely addicts—would take opioids. But addicts are a small percentage of the population even in our distorted system that makes treatment difficult and creates an underclass of addicts. If we treated addiction as a disease, as some other countries do, the numbers would likely decrease as people could seek treatment with some privacy and dignity. Many drug users who have experienced addiction for a while become disenchanted but feel that they have no way to stop. Many would choose the option of safe treatment if it were available. But society is constantly putting addicts in a difficult situation by the barriers in place to getting treatment.[485] Many institutions and many people make pain patients feel like they are drug seeking and therefore just like addicts. Therefore, it is hard for a person to accept that opioid therapy is necessary. Patient Z certainly resisted it, then tried it only when he could not stand the pain any more. Finally, he came to understand that he could live a full life, given the limitations of the disease, with some comfort and sense of purpose once he could control the pain. Part of the sense of purpose came from the realization that there are millions like him. There were many other people who have had to make the decision to take opioids for pain. Once Patient Z realized that opioids really did control his pain, his course of action was clear. He began to advocate for all those like him who benefitted from opioid medications. It took Patient Z some time to realize that he would have to stand up for his rights as a patient and that there are powerful forces at work trying to take those rights away. Indeed, once Patient Z began to see the forces behind the denial of care, which constitutes a threat to his health, he found a reason to get involved in the advocacy for patients' rights.

The year Patient Z got his diagnosis was a watershed. Receiving the diagnosis was a bit like accepting that he needed opioids in order to live with the pain of ankylosing spondylitis. No one wants such a diagnosis. But if you are sick, you would rather have a diagnosis than live without knowing what is making you sick. And so it is for opioids. No one wants to have to take them, but if you are in pain, you would rather take them than live in pain. As Patient Z began to accept opioids and even feel that it gave him some comfort in a life that otherwise would be intolerable, he became aware that the consciousness of the opioid crisis had become a burning social, political, and legal issue. This large-scale change in attitudes and regulatory climate occurred during the same time that Patient Z was coming to the conclusion that his condition was not going to improve and that long-term opioid usage was the only way for him to survive. Like many patients with excruciating systemic pain, Patient Z had contemplated suicide. But in his case, it was an abstract consideration since his pain was controlled. He had bouts of intense pain, bad nights when he could not sleep, and pain during flares that was sometimes at the limit of bearable. The opioids, at least, prevented those bad periods from taking over. By this time, the question on Patient Z's mind was whether it was possible to continue using opioids for decades. He had already completed more than a decade, but would there come a time when the opioids would stop working? He began to read the literature to understand the issue of long-term use.

Most of the studies of high levels of morphine/oxycodone are administered to cancer patients. The justification is normally that it is palliative care, meeting a patient's needs in the home, which can include administration of opioids. It also can include hospice, which is the last refuge where a patient can be comfortable at the end of life. Patient Z thought often about the strange logic that made it acceptable to prescribe high-dose opioids during the final six months of life but not before. The pain is often the same. Then he wondered why cancer was acceptable for opioid treatment and not other painful diseases. Are cancers necessarily more painful compared to autoimmune diseases? Swelling and inflammation are common sources of pain in both, but in many autoimmune diseases, there is systemic attack on tissues, tendons, ligaments, and synovial regions of joints. The pain depends on the severity of the individual case, the type of cancer, and the nature of the autoimmune disease. As he read and talked to people, he came to the conclusion that his pain level is similar to the pain of some cancers. Despite the pain, a patient can live with ankylosing spondylitis for decades. The disease causes progressive damage and discomfort, attacking the neck and shoulders later and then eventually the organs. Ankylosing spondylitis is incurable, and cumulatively, the damage to his tissues will increase the level of pain and decrease function. These are not conversations that one normally has in a pain clinic. Instead, pain clinics regard their responsibility as opioid dose, tapering, compliance, and side effects. Fragmented care combined with the strict regulatory climate forces a focus on the all-important goal of reaching the dose limit set by the clinic. In Patient Z's clinic, that dose was 120 MEDD. The plan for coordination of pain management with treatment of inflammatory or degenerative diseases is not the concern of pain specialists in today's pain clinic.

Pain Clinic Power Games—No Defense and No Argument

Although the doctors and nurses had been as kind as people can be when they are forced to take an action against a patient's will and best interest, Patient Z felt that he needed to question the decision to taper down to 120 MEDD. From what he had read, there should be no forced tapers. He had already tapered down to 180 MEDD. He was distinctly less comfortable after twelve months. He knew his disease and the various pains it would cycle through. Pain is not a constant. It plays tricks on a person's mind. Pain can appear simply as a limitation to movement. The body will refuse to move beyond a certain point because of pain. This is for survival. But the normal reactions are not necessarily helpful when a person's spine has fused and their joints are reforming.

Patient Z summoned his courage and wrote to the director to ask for the clinic policies. He told the director he wanted to understand how the clinic set its dose limit. But the director would not even confirm that the clinic has a dose limit of 120 MEDD per day. He said that it was up to the doctors. He said that they were independent contractors and could make the decisions based on medical considerations. Indeed, the CDC guidelines say that pain clinics should not have hard limits,[468] so apparently, the director of the clinic did not want to go on the record as saying that they have a hard limit. When Patient Z saw the doctor again, the doctor assured Patient Z that the clinic does have a hard limit. If you, the reader, are confused, you should imagine how Patient Z felt.

By this time, Patient Z had advanced-stage ankylosing spondylitis. In the months following the taper, Patient Z realized that the antibody drug, Humira, had stopped working. The human body can develop antibodies to the foreign therapeutic antibody and clear it from the bloodstream. On the lower dose of opioids, Patient Z felt a new combined pain of full-blown systemic inflammation, combined with the bone-on-bone pain from all major articulations and the pain of fused back. By this time, he had been told he needed neck, back, hip, and knee surgery. It felt like torture. Patient Z spoke to an orthopedist who suggested cortisone injections would reduce the pain. Cortisone is known for its anti-inflammatory properties. However, cortisone also suppresses the immune system. Shortly after Patient Z received double cortisone injections, one in each hip, his legs had swollen so much that the skin had split open and formed a large wound. The wound became infected with streptococcus, which spread so rapidly that within hours he was taken to the emergency room and admitted to the hospital. By the time he was seen at the emergency room, he was in the first phase of sepsis. The bacteria had entered his bloodstream but fortunately had not yet begun new infections in his organs. The next step, when the bacteria invade other organs, is often fatal. He spent one week in the hospital on intravenous antibiotics. Afterward, he was so weak that he could barely move. He needed constant help with everything. He went to see a vascular surgeon to discuss the swollen lymph glands in his legs, which had been where the infection began. An ultrasound showed that there was no blockage or obvious cause for the lymphedema.

After the surgeon discussed the events with Patient Z, he advised, "I think you should avoid getting any more cortisone injections. It is likely that they are responsible for the severity of that infection in your leg."

"But without cortisone injections, the pain is too much. I cannot walk," Patient Z replied.

"I would discuss this with the pain clinic," the surgeon responded. "If you tolerate morphine, it is much safer for you than cortisone."

Yet Patient Z knew that the clinic was planning to reduce his morphine even further, and certainly he had no hope of convincing them to increase it. Nonetheless, he had the pain of inflammation because the anti-inflammatory medication, one of the new types of antibody drugs, had stopped working because his immune system had begun to clear it from his system. There are several antibody drugs that bind to the immune messenger, TNF, and Patient Z had started on a new one. However, these drugs take months to become fully active. He had systemic inflammation, which was both painful and irritating. It affected every part of the body from itching in his eyes to a cold feeling in his feet caused by swelling. Meanwhile, he had a large, stinging wound on his leg and skin inflammation caused by the overreaction of his immune system to the infection. He had never experienced so many different types of pain at one time—a stinging large wound, burning inflamed skin, neuropathic pain, joint pain, back pain, swelling in his legs, and a general fatigue from inflammatory pain in his tendons.

Shortly after he was released from the hospital, Patient Z had a routine, monthly appointment with the pain clinic. Because of the COVID pandemic that had swept the United States, Patient Z could not meet with the doctor in person. He was speaking by phone with Dr. Q, whom he did not know well, to discuss his monthly renewal of pain medication. Patient Z understood that the pain clinic was planning to reduce his dose, to taper down his medication. His usual nurse had postponed the taper before the hospitalization, because she had understood that Patient Z had extra pain since his anti-inflammatory medication had ceased to work. However, after hospitalization, Patient Z felt so awful that the thought of adding additional pain of tapering was more than he could bear. After a brief introduction, Patient Z described the series of events that had caused a further deterioration in his health.

"You will always have an excuse," Dr. Q told him. "You have an ungodly high dose, and you have to taper down."

"Ankylosing spondylitis is a progressive disease," Patient Z replied. "I have gotten so much worse in the last few months. But there is some hope. I started on a new anti-inflammatory medication and I believe it is beginning to work, but the doctor says it will take three months. I need an operation for the wound. I had a wound like this one before, and I know that they can use pig bladder cells as a kind of skin graft. It worked well last time I had a wound. In a couple of months I could well be feeling much better. Couldn't we please wait?"

"Many patients have ankylosing spondylitis and they do not need opioids the way you do," Dr. Q shot back.

"I don't understand this statement. Dr. P told me that your clinic has never treated anyone with ankylosing spondylitis before. Where did you get this information?"

"Don't question me," Dr. Q said indignantly. "We are doing this for your own good. On your current dose, you cannot feel anything. You are numb. You are in danger of harming yourself."

"How can I be numb? I am in pain. The harm I worry about is falling down in the shower because the pain is so severe that I cannot hold myself up properly getting in or out," Patient Z said plaintively.

"I do not have time for this endless back and forth. I have already called in the prescription, and it goes down this month. This is all I have time for. Goodbye."

The doctor had revealed a fundamental misunderstanding about the nature of opioid pain relief. Someone who injects heroin may *feel no pain,* in a manner of speaking. But there is a qualitative difference between that emotional lack of a sensation of pain and the experience of a typical pain patient that was discussed in chapter 3. Dr. Q was trained as an anesthesiologist, which perhaps did not give him a good understanding how opioids work in long-term therapy. Moreover, Dr. Q was clearly bluffing concerning his knowledge of ankylosing spondylitis. It was a rehearsed line to bully Patient Z into feeling humiliated and accepting the foregone conclusion of the taper. The pain clinic holds all the cards. Patient Z was devastated after that phone call. He had no recourse.

If a major pain clinic associated with a university hospital cannot treat a patient with an autoimmune disease like ankylosing spondylitis, then where can a patient go? Patient Z was at one of the largest hospitals in the state. Ankylosing spondylitis is a disease with an incidence of one per one thousand of the population. The disease is not *that* rare. And there are many such diseases. There are hundreds of thousands of patients like Z in the United States. If Patient Z, who has insurance and a good PCP, was running into difficulties because how the new regulations have been interpreted, then we must conclude that the system is failing many persistent-pain patients, particularly those without a diagnosis, without insurance, or with other issues such as lack of supportive family or psychological problems.

A persistent-pain patient often feels alone, vulnerable, and scared. But the doctors are also scared. The situation has polarized our society with the relatives of overdose victims claiming that the fault for the death of their loved ones lies with doctors, pharmacists, and pharmaceutical companies. Thousands of lawsuits have overwhelmed the legal system. The threat of a lawsuit weighs heavily on doctors and nurses in the pain clinic. If they make a mistake, they could end up being charged with negligence or a crime, depending on the nature of allegation. The doctors are too worried about their own situation to fight for patients' rights. Moreover, the doctors know how law enforcement works. Patients could become witnesses against them at a trial. The pain clinics are implementing a new legal standard, one that is not necessarily written explicitly, but is enforced by the fact that the DEA can recall their licenses and seize their assets. Without a license to prescribe opioids, a pain clinic must close. Pain clinics insist on patient compliance with a taper. Even the act of questioning the taper could have an unforeseen bad consequence.

Patient Z wrote to the director of the clinic and expressed his grave concern over the taper, the fact that it was so rapid, and the response of the office staff had put him in jeopardy of going without medication at all. He explained that he had spoken with the doctor who had assured him that there was a clinic policy of a hard limit on prescribing. He explained that he wanted to petition to be able to remain on the current dose. He included a short paragraph on the recent hospitalization and what the vascular surgeon had told him. He cited the CDC guidelines, the revised guideline. and a petition in the journal *Pain Medicine* signed by more than one hundred doctors that urged clinics against tapers of patients who are stable, particularly if they have serious diseases.[3,281,282,486] The director sent a return message that said, "Please see the attachment." Attached to the message was a copy of the DEA manual. The DEA manual did not say anything about dosing, but the message was clear.

When Patient Z went to his next appointment, the nurse was friendly and told him that he could wait until summer to continue the taper. The nurse told him that they would taper very slowly. She seemed concerned and compassionate. Then as the nurse was leaving the room, she turned to Patient Z and said, "I have to advise you not to call or write the director again. He is very busy. He told me that if you contact him again, he will have to terminate you. He is very busy. I am sorry about this. I hope you understand."

CHAPTER 9

❦

The War on Drugs Resulted in an Exponential Growth in Overdose Rate

The regulatory reaction to overdose fatalities playing out in pain clinics today is based on a perception that prescription drugs are the root cause of the crisis. This perception is not in accord with the evidence. The evidence, based on CDC data, shows that the prescription rate has been steadily decreasing since 2011, while the overdose rate has been dramatically increasing. The total amount prescribed dropped 35% between 2012 and 2019.[268] For the high-dose patients, there has been a 61% drop over that period.[487] The critics of opioid prescribing point out that the total volume of opioids prescribed was twice as high in 2017 as it was in 1999.[121] Based on the most recent figures from 2020, the overdose rate has risen to 81,000 annually from 17,000 in 1999. The increase is in overdose rate is a factor of five over a period when prescriptions rose by a factor of two. However, this fact masks the true magnitude of PROP's misunderstanding of the origins of the opioid crisis. From 2011 to 2019, when prescribing decreased by nearly a factor of two, the overdose rate increased by a factor of two, from 41,000 in 2011 to more than 81,000 in 2020. Blaming overdose deaths on prescribing ignores the enormous problem of diversion and the even larger role played by illegal drugs. Instead, the net effect of the misguided reasoning is that medications are not reaching those who need them.

The war on prescription drugs has been a war on pain patients and the doctors who treat them. Regardless of the reasons, it is a fact that many pain patients do not receive relief under the current regulatory regime. Please examine figure 3 and consider the question, Why did the overdose rate increase by a factor of two over the same period prescriptions decreased by a factor of two? Why are suicides increasing as well?

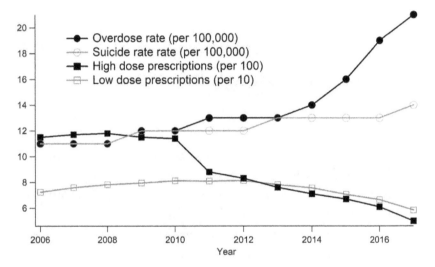

Figure 3. Comparison of opioid overdose deaths, suicide deaths, low dose, and high-dose opioid prescriptions from 2006 to 2017[488]

Citizens hear the news that *overprescribing* has caused the crisis with expert commentary by doctors, law enforcement officials, and politicians. But something is clearly wrong with the storyline. Pain patients report immense suffering, and yet the companies are selling twice as many opioids as they did twenty years ago. Is this all because of increases in the number of pills given out by dentist offices or by hospitals postsurgery? We must recall that awareness of the undertreatment of pain was the impetus for the compassionate care movement. Some pain patients, like Patient Z, did receive high doses, and many of them needed this medication. Even the prescription drug part of this puzzle is complicated by multiple trends. On one hand, there are harmful effects of overprescribing by inexperienced and untrained doctors; the residual attitudes from the marketing blitz of Purdue Pharma and the organized diversion that persists on a smaller scale now that prescription-drug monitoring has been implemented. On the other hand, there is the legitimate need of millions of people for pain relief. In justifying their call for a prescribing cap, PROP focuses on excesses in the treatment of low back pain and osteo-arthritis. There are tens of millions of people in that category who need some level of pain relief, but probably not high-dose opioids in most cases. However, the invisible-patient population of eight million people, with relatively rare diseases, have simply been ignored by PROP, the CDC, HHS, and every other agency, except the FDA. The FDA at least has recognized that there is a diversity of needs and that a one-size-fits-all approach to pain management will bring great harm. We must distinguish different patient populations and determine the severity of the disease before making decisions about how to treat pain. Those who want to portray pain management as a one-dimensional problem that rests on human weakness and drug seeking are misrepresenting the majority of people in society and certainly the vast majority of pain patients. To explain the trends, many observers focus only on the prescription-drug portion of the overdose deaths and ignore the extensive information on the massive drug abuse problem in the US. That focus misses important trends as one narcotic has been substituted for another as the leading cause of death for more than forty years.

According to the CDC, there have been three waves of over-dose fatalities since 2000, the prescription-drug wave (1999–2007), the heroin wave (2007–2013), and the fentanyl wave (2013–present). One of the theses developed by PROP is that pain patients are prone to dependence and addiction caused by their own prescription medi-cation.[11,12] There is a strong tendency in many academic publications to ignore the prevalence of illegal-drug use that has been increasing continuously since the 1970s and has always been a much larger problem compared to prescription-drug misuse. Approximately half of drug overdose deaths arose from illegal hard drugs even in 2011 at the peak of the prescription-drug wave, and even in that year, 90% of all overdoses involved either illegal or diverted prescription drugs, not legitimate prescriptions from a doctor. The detailed analysis is in this chapter and the next. Although the CDC cites the time frame from 1997 to 2007 for the prescription drug wave, the year 2011 is a watershed for prescription drug use because of long overdue implementation of policies that would stop the major diversion by pill mills was completed in 2011.[252,442,462,489] The scale of the diversion is evident in the magnitude of the jump in heroin addiction and overdose that occurred as the prescription drug diversion was slowed down.[49,431]

The Exponential Growth of the Overdose Rate for Forty Years from 1980 to 2020

Although abuse of heroin and cocaine was present at a low level from the time 1900 to 1960, the modern era of drug use in the United States began with the Vietnam War. It came to the attention of Congress in the mid-1960s that heroin addiction rates among soldiers in Vietnam were 10–15%. Heroin was smuggled into the United States on military cargo planes and created a sudden outbreak of heroin addiction and overdose.[490] The reason the first major outbreak was in Washington, DC, had everything to do with the military bases in the vicinity. To understand the trends in opioid overdose deaths today, we should examine the trends starting with the *war on drugs*, which began in 1970 with the passage of the Controlled Substances Act.

Figure 4 shows the data from the CDC database for unintentional overdose fatalities from 1980 to 2018. This figure uses the same public data as those presented by Jalal and coworkers in the journal *Science*.[491] That publication makes the point that regardless of the type of drug, the trend of exponential increase has been robust for nearly forty years. These data include opioids, cocaine, and methamphetamine overdoses. The article also points out that there are significant geographical differences. Methamphetamine is mainly a problem in the southwest; fentanyl, in the northeast; cocaine, in urban areas; and today, heroin is widespread throughout the United States. In the past few years, the majority of deaths are from heroin and fentanyl. For example, in 2017, 47,000 of the 67,700 deaths (70%) involved heroin or fentanyl. The increase in overdose fatalities has been very nearly a single exponential with a doubling time of eleven years while population growth is roughly 10% every ten years.

The war on drugs was worse than a failure; it caused a twentyfold increase in the overdose rate. It catalyzed the growth of an underground drug industry. It increased drug prices, which made the distribution rings and later the cartels wealthy. While cartels and gangs grew in power, purchased sophisticated weapons, and improved their technology, the punitive policies of the DEA and American law enforcement against users and small dealers resulted only in greater misery for those trapped in addiction. An addict who needed to find a new supply of heroin was very vulnerable. The constant pressure of arrests has never eradicated the supply, but it caused disruptions, which increased mortality as users find new suppliers.

Concern for the increase in the overdose rate during the CDC's prescription-drug wave should be put into the context of this forty-year trend. Paulozzi and coworkers examined the same data up to 2002 in a paper published in 2006 and concluded that there was a significant acceleration in overdoses just at the period when the prescribing was also increasing.[492] This was presented in the CDC data, and the same trend has also been presented in the *Annual Review of Public Health* paper by Dr. Kolodny and coworkers that we consider in chapter 11.[12] The short-term view of the data from 1999 to 2010 suggested a direct correlation between prescribing and overdose death increases.[493] From the vantage point of 2020, we can see that overall exponential trend is the crucial feature of overdose fatalities, while the supply side is very complicated because of the rapidly shifting usage patterns.

Drug usage is driven by price and availability. The short-term correlation between prescriptions and prescription drug overdoses was operative for nearly a decade from 2000 to 2010. But that correlation ended abruptly and has not been operative for nearly a decade from 2011 to the present. In 2015, it appeared that overdose deaths were beginning to level off. Perhaps the proponents of restrictive prescribing believed that this was evidence that restrictions on prescribing are effective. However, the CDC guideline implementation in 2016 coincided with the steepest increase in rate of overdose deaths thus far.[50] There are many features and other local shifts that depended on the supply of other drugs. Jalal and coworkers point out how one can account for a spike in fentanyl in 2006 from a lab in Mexico that year. Methadone has been decreasing as state methadone programs have been phased out.[491] Cocaine price and use has been dependent on many factors that influence production in Colombia and the smuggling routes to the US.

There is no simple explanation for what drives people to take drugs so carelessly that they overdose. Jalal and coworkers suggest that the factors are outside of the drugs themselves. This argument implies that the prescription drug crisis is one small phase in a much larger trend and that the hypothesis concerning prescription drugs, diverted or properly prescribed, as a gateway to another drug, fails to take into account the fact that people who are making the decision to take drugs illegally are driven by motives that do not necessarily, and probably do not, depend on the actual drug itself. However, incalculable harm is done to the much larger number of legal and legitimate patients when their supply of medication is reduced or terminated. Based on a great deal of evidence, the reduction in prescriptions is contributing to the desperation in the society at large that has led to record numbers of overdoses in the past few years.[270,437,491]

From 2016 to the present, there has been the greatest pressure on pain patients ever. Patients have been abandoned and tapered suddenly, and there has been an overall 50% reduction in prescriptions. During this time, overdose deaths rose more rapidly than at any time in history. Although there appeared to be a decrease in deaths in 2018,[494] the most recent data on the CDC website shows that the year 2020 set a new record with 81,000 overdose deaths. The introduction of Narcan, a naloxone inhaler to revive overdose victims, has probably prevented the numbers of deaths from increasing even further. Although the number of overdose deaths appeared stable in 2018, the exponential trend has surged to more than 80,000 deaths annually, which is unacceptable for society At what point will decision makers realize that they are actually making the problem worse by cutting off pain patients from their medication?

The overdose problem just gets worse no matter what drug arrives on the scene.[495] The hypothesis that emerges from figure 4 is that greater pressure on drug addicts through more vigorous law enforcement tends to *increase* the overdose rate. A second pressure comes from the lack of affordable, safe, and easily accessible treatment programs. Lacking a treatment option, addicts are often forced to switch from one supplier to another until eventually their luck runs out. A third pressure comes when the general population cannot find a way to relieve the pain of serious disease.

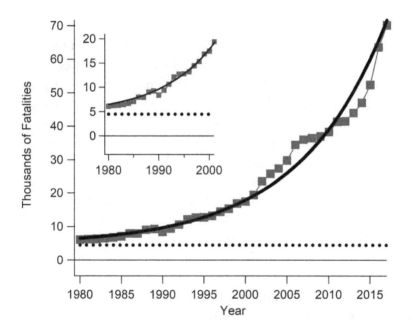

Figure 4. Annual overdose fatalities from 1980 to 2018. The data are presented in raw numbers from the CDC database using the ICD-10 codes for unintentional deaths because of any type of opioid, cocaine, or methamphetamine. Most frequently, multiple drugs were found on autopsy. The blue curve is a fit to the data using an exponential growth model with a baseline. The model suggests that there is a baseline of 4,500 deaths annually, which has not changed significantly since 1970 (data from 1970 to 1980 are not shown). The data from 1980 to 2018 fit to an exponential function with a doubling time of approximately eleven years.

Historically opioid prescribing was seen as a sign of a civilized medical system, and increases in opioid prescribing were indicative of better care because people were not living in pain. Because of some corrupt and inept decisions that permitted a few companies and organized crime to abuse the public trust and divert massive amounts of opioids during the years from 1999 to 2010, we are now paying the price of an overreaction to that excess.

The End of Oxycodone Diversion Leads to the Heroin Wave

Between 2011 and 2017 high-dose opioid prescriptions decreased by a factor of two, while opioid deaths increased by a factor of two.[496,497] According to the Cato Institute study "Overdosing on Regulation: How Government Caused the Opioid Epidemic," after prescriptions began a steep decline in 2010, the deaths from overdose doubled.[270] The prescription rate reported by the CDC was divided into low-dose and high-dose categories. The high-dose category is most relevant for understanding potential relationship between diversion and overdose fatalities. However, a potentially better way to understand drug prescriptions is to track the total volume (measured in morphine milligram equivalents, or MME) for a variety of drugs.[498] Piper and coworkers used the Automation of Reports and Consolidated Orders System (ARCOS) database and track ten different opioids divided into two groups. The group of eight includes morphine, meperidine, hydromorphone, oxymorphone, hydrocodone, oxycodone, codeine, and fentanyl. The two others are methadone and buprenorphine. The study shows that for the group of eight there is an almost symmetric increase up to a maximum at 2011 and then decrease such that both 2008 and 2016 were at approximately 80% of the level of 2011. Buprenorphine prescriptions increased throughout this period from 1% of the total in 2006 to 8% in 2016, while methadone declined from 49% in 2006 to 41% in 2016. These data in aggregate suggest an increasing number of addicts seeking help. Many articles tout the superiority of buprenorphine over methadone for opioid maintenance therapy.[10,295,499–502] The data agree in terms of the trends with the CDC data, but the extent of the decline in prescribing is not as large for the ARCOS data set. We can estimate that the ARCOS data would reach approximately 70% of the 2011 level by 2018, while the CDC shows the high-dose prescriptions at nearly 50% of the 2011 level by 2018. By any measure, prescribing has decreased dramatically since 2011. By any objective assessment, this policy has been a disaster. The overdose and addiction rates have increased dramatically, and the treatment of pain patients has been abysmally bad. The suicide rate has increased, and pain patients have been denied care in record numbers.

In her special series on the Florida pill mills, reporter Pat Beall of *The West Palm Beach Post* showed quantitatively how the drug users who had become addicted to oxycodone during the prescription-drug wave converted within days to heroin addiction when oxycodone was no longer available in 2011.[49,426,427,429–431,444,459,503–505] The Sinaloa cartel predicted the heroin market, had grown the heroin, and had a distribution network in place ready to sell to the new customers. The tragedy extended to pain patients as well as few years later. When the CDC guidelines were implemented in 2016, there was a spate of suicides and new heroin addicts from former pain patients. Patient Z had difficulty believing that pain patients could actually turn to heroin. However, as he read more, he realized that it is not only possible, but it surely has happened to some pain patients who lost their medication and were left with the choice of intolerable pain or heroin. A study of 572 patients in Seattle, Washington, showed a strong correlation between termination from treatment in a clinic and subsequent heroin/fentanyl overdose.[425] Patients with a mean age of fifty-five years were studied in two groups—344 patients who were discontinued and received no further prescriptions and 254 patients who were retained in the clinic after their termination and continued to receive medication. During the study period, seventeen of those from the discontinued group and four of those from the retained group died of an overdose. The terminated patients were four times as a likely to die of an overdose. The conclusion was that the discontinued patients must have resorted to street opioid drugs, which ultimately were responsible for their deaths.[425]

The data from independent sources corroborate the switch from oxycodone to heroin. Although the overall overdose death rate, for prescription drugs and heroin combined, actually dropped from 2010 to 2012 in Florida, nationwide heroin use increased by more than 100% from 2010 to 2012, and the overall drug overdose death rate increased exponentially as shown in figure 4.[496] One study compared Florida to North Carolina, which showed an increase in both oxycodone- and heroin-overdose deaths increased by 20% and 181%, respectively, from 2010 to 2012.[506] There are local variations from the trend in certain states, but the aggregate US numbers show that as oxycodone use decreased, heroin use increased. This agrees with study findings based on information from drug users.[507] According to a specific CDC article, the Florida reports of overdose deaths from the crucial years of 2010 to 2012 showed a decrease of oxycodone overdose deaths of 27% from 13.6 to 9.9 per 100,000.[508] At the same time, heroin-overdose deaths increased from 0.3 to 0.6 per 100,000, which is a 100% increase. The overall decrease in overdose deaths in Florida over from 2010 to 2012 was 18%, while the national overdose rate increased by 8% in those two years. Since Florida was the oxycodone-prescribing center of the US with 90 of 100 top-prescribing pharmacies, there were many local users of oxycodone, and the effect of the crackdown on prescribing in 2011 was a temporary statewide reduction in overdose rate. The general trends in drug use rapidly overtook any gains made. The net effect of the policy was that heroin had been given a large boost by an extremely poorly executed crackdown.[508]

Although the former director of the CDC, Dr. Frieden, made public statements to suggest that heroin use increased proportional to opioid prescribing,[509] the evidence suggests there was a temporary effect that was overwhelmed by larger trends in drug use. One study shows that the proportion of heroin users who started with diverted prescription opioids decreased from more than 90% in 2005 to 67% in 2015.[510] More heroin users are starting directly with heroin or using some other drug first. Rather than general statements about causes of a particular trend, we need real-time assessments of the trends in order to make the correct interventions.[50] The federal and state bureaucracies have given us the opposite of flexible and timely response. Instead, responses are years or even decades too late. One reason is that people see what they want to see. While prescription rates and overdose death rates were both rising in parallel, from 1999 to 2010, the narrative was clearly that prescription drugs were fueling addiction and overdose. To understand the significance of this trend, it is necessary to distinguish between diverted and appropriately prescribed drugs. Since a large majority of overdoses have persistently involved diverted opioids, the statements in the media and political speeches concerning the role of physician prescribing were not on point. When the prescriptions fell and the overdoses continued to rise, Dr. Frieden's explanation was that "a tightly correlated epidemic of addiction, overdose, and death from prescription opioids […] is now further evolving to include increasing use and overdoses of heroin and illicitly produced fentanyl." The spin is evident. Dr. Frieden and members of PROP continue to put the blame on prescription drugs, despite the fact that the vast majority of people are dying from heroin and later fentanyl. PROP's rationale is a dangerous justification for a failed policy to drastically reduce prescribing without a plan for either the patients with legitimate prescriptions who were harmed by reductions or the addicts with diverted opioids who were cut off without a treatment option.

One way to see that there are different routes to heroin addiction is to compare heroin users of Black, White, or Latino heritage. The White population showed an increase in heroin use and declining reliance on prescription drugs from 60% to 20% from 2005 to 2016. The Black population never had high usage of prescription drugs and even showed a tendency not to fill prescriptions for opioids.[511] For Black and Latino populations, the prescription percentage was less than 20% for all years up to the last three years when a slight increase to above 20% was observed.[512] The data reveal that the White population probably used prescription drugs first during the height of prescribing, but that behavior did not extend to other ethnic groups. The recent concern for overdose deaths of the White population reveals one of the biases in the critics of opioid therapy. Dr. Kolodny reports his concern the following way:[168]

> Andrew Kolodny first noticed something was amiss in 2004, when his job as a medical director at New York City's health department was to reduce drug-overdose deaths. An expert in addiction treatment, he opened an evening and weekend clinic with the expectation that his patients would come from New York's rougher neighborhoods, where overdose deaths had been concentrated for decades.
>
> But many of those who turned up came from wealthy areas, like Long Island and Westchester. About a third were elderly; the rest mostly in their twenties and thirties. All were using prescription opioids, whether prescribed by their doctor or bought on the black market. "That's when I recognized we had something awful going on," he says.

The fact that crack, heroin, and methamphetamine had been on a deadly rampage in the city for the past twenty years was in accordance with "expectation," and only when wealthy people from Westchester showed up did Dr. Kolodny recognize that there was "something awful going on." While those wealthy people may well have become hooked on prescription drugs during the *prescription-drug wave* identified by the CDC; the evidence shows that the majority of hard drug users did not get started that way.

The fifty-year trend in heroin use shows the numerous ways that abusers with different backgrounds ended up addicted.[513] There has been a dramatic increase in heroin use over the past ten years and a tendency for heroin use to migrate from inner cities to suburbs and then into rural communities. In the early years, urban use was racially diverse among men averaging seventeen years of age, with approximately equal percentages of Black and White men. More recent heroin use in suburban and rural areas has involved a slightly older demographic (average twenty-three years) of mostly White men and women, in nearly equal numbers. Price was a significant reason for the choice of heroin, although 75% of users in recent years reported that they had started using diverted prescription drugs.[513] The heroin problem was cited as the main reason for the *war on drugs* and formation of the DEA in 1971. Yet today politicians and addiction experts claim that this is a new problem that was brought on because of an "experiment" with prescription drugs. People enter the drug world using the cheapest and easiest route. It is true that while the pill mills were in operation, they provided an access point to drugs. As we discuss in the next chapter, this was well-known to the DEA and state legislatures, yet no one took action for over a decade. To blame this on doctors writing prescriptions to patients like Z is a cynical way to deny the way that government and corporations manipulated the situation while it was advantageous for them.

The drug kingpin, El Chapo, knew about the OxyContin sales in South Florida and saw the opportunity to expand the heroin market in the United States.[503] There was no way for his operation to get directly into the lucrative prescription-drug diversion business, and he could not compete with Colombian cartels effectively in the cocaine and crack trade. But El Chapo could see the handwriting on the wall by 2002. Many states had implemented PDMPs, and Florida had already tried in 2002.[459] It was just a matter of time before Florida would implement the law, and then suddenly, there would be thousands of addicts across the United States looking for an opioid substitute for OxyContin.[49,429–431] El Chapo commanded his minions to sow poppies in the hills of Sinaloa starting in 2002.[503] The new heroin supply was gradually increasing in the US, and heroin-overdose deaths increased by >50% even during the so-called prescription-drug wave.[496] Thus began the CDC's second wave of heroin-overdose deaths. Using court records, internal documents from Purdue, and DEA records, Beall documented how the shift occurred most dramatically in 2011 when Florida finally enacted the PDMP legislation.[506,514] The pill mills were supplying tens of thousands of users in more than thirty states. Heroin distribution networks were set up and ready to go so that literally from one day to the next, the users who could no longer purchase OxyContin legally could purchase heroin at a reasonable price.[496] El Chapo understood the business. People who have become addicted are not able to wait for an alternative if they lose their source. Those people had to be harvested immediately, or they would end up going to a methadone clinic or finding some other way to avoid going into withdrawal. The shift was seen in emergency rooms all over the country within a very short time.[515] A younger, more well-to-do class of people were overdosing on heroin. Heroin is much more lethal than OxyContin, and it was also a new drug for many. The entire situation was exacerbated even further by the arrival of fentanyl, which increased the potency and toxicity of the available powders. The drug kingpin could predict the trend ten years in advance, and our drug experts are still trying to figure out what happened ten years ago.

The real scandal was that the escalation in opioid sales occurred in broad daylight. The massive sales of pills to specific addresses in Florida were tabulated in the DEA database, just like the shipments to Virginia,[505] Tennessee,[516] and California.[517–519] While the state attorney general of California and the DEA were busy prosecuting lone doctors like Frank Fischer, who was completely innocent,[108,303] the pill mills in California were doing a brisk business.[517] While the DEA was making a public spectacle out of the trial of Dr. Hurwitz in Virginia, the Florida and Tennessee pill mills were in their heyday. Both federal and state authorities had ample opportunity to look into these large-scale operations but did nothing for a decade. Once the states finally began to take action using PDMPs and law enforcement actions to close down the clinics, it is inexcusable that no agency, no legislator, or no adviser considered the implications of suddenly stopping the prescribing after permitting it for nearly a decade. This fits a general pattern of complete indifference on the part of authorities to what happens to patients when a pain clinic is shut down. Several thousand have been shut down in the past decade,[303,304,306] and this means that more than one million patients have had to find new sources for their prescriptions on short notice. The disregard for heroin addicts is even worse. The attitude of the society is that they made a choice and they deserve to suffer for it.[485] This cynical attitude appears to extend to pain patients, despite the fact that they did not have a choice in their disease or disability.

Fentanyl Express Delivered Through the US Mail—the Fentanyl Wave

The failure of regulation to adequately deal with the overdose crisis is a tragic blunder whose dimensions are difficult to fathom.[458] By missing the real correlation between heroin- and the drug-overdose rate, the policies focused on prescription drugs rather than on new routes for smuggling such as mail order fentanyl coming from China. The usual smuggling routes were alive and well despite all the talk about building a wall on the southern border.[503] Tunnels, drones, or even hacksaws were enough to get drugs into the United States. Actually, the most common smuggling route has always been trucks that pass through the checkpoints at the border. There was no shortage of drugs before, but as the cartels understood the changing situation, the United States was targeted with drugs by even more creative entry routes. Fentanyl has been responsible for the third wave in fatalities since 2013. While the DEA-mandated pain clinics were being set up, thousands of pain patients were losing their prescriptions, going into withdrawal, committing suicide,[433] or being driven to illicit drugs in desperation; vast quantities of fentanyl were being sent to American households through the US mail.[520] The price of fentanyl relative to income was an important factor in the surge in fentanyl overdoses in eastern and northeastern states.[521] The price of a *fix* dropped to new lows, making it much more convenient to inject fentanyl or heroin laced with fentanyl than any prescription drug. Because of its high potency, then it is likely the main reason for the spike in overdose fatalities in the past six years.[522] In the case of fentanyl distribution, we see that illicit drug distribution is widespread and is the major cause of drug overdose. Given the major role played by illegal drugs in addiction and overdose for more than sixty years, it is clear that the attempt to blame doctors and pain patients for the crisis is misguided. It is sufficiently far from the mark that it begs the question, Who is benefitting from this false narrative?

CHAPTER 10

⤞⤝

The Profit Motive Hijacked the Compassionate Care Movement

The compassionate care movement was primarily intended to reach patients who had undertreated pain, people with serious diseases suffering and an intolerable quality of life.[21,22] Of course, the medical community had an obligation to think about all patients in pain when considering how to expand treatment. It would have been a big step merely to expand palliative care and intractable pain to cover the millions who suffer from incurable diseases. The more ambitious project of extending treatment for pain to the general patient population clearly required better planning to tackle the problem of addiction and a coordinated program of education.[523] Moreover, there were stern warnings at the time of the need to implement controls to prevent diversion.[524] In the aftermath of a movement that Dr. Lembke has called a failed "experiment," [37] we have an ethical responsibility to consider what went wrong and what can be learned. Some might say that the future has already been decided by the CDC guidelines.[281,486] At present, the hard dose limits and forced tapers that PROP has worked to implement are taking away pain medication from hundreds of thousands of patients.[53] People are losing access to medication that they have had for years or even decades.[251,525–527] The mass forced tapering and hard limits currently implemented also constitute an "experiment." The second experiment is crueler than the first and is apparently an even bigger failure, judging from the consistently high overdose death rate since 2016. From a scientific point of view, neither is an experiment. Dr. Lembke should study the scientific method and give more thought to her statements. To accept that PROP's policy is the new standard of care would mean that the medical community accepts an arbitrary and unethical limit on their ability to treat pain. The recent letter from the chief executive officer of the AMA to the CDC director is a strong indication that the medical community has not accepted that these guidelines are the final word.[264]

In 1998, the American Pain Society had endorsed the idea of expanding opioid prescribing to treat chronic noncancer pain.[21,22] In 2000, Congress passed the Pain Relief Promotion Act, which specifically authorizes doctors to treat pain using controlled substances. The bill states that "alleviating pain or discomfort in the usual course of professional practice is a legitimate medical purpose for the dispensing, distributing, or administering of a controlled substance that is consistent with public health and safety, even if it may increase the risk of death." It also has a provision that encourages an expansion of palliative care. In essence, this law is on hold today because of the CDC guideline and DEA influence forged by PROP's lobbying. The guiding concern of the policy makers and government agencies was the rising number of overdose fatalities. The severity of the overdose crisis notwithstanding, we must question the connection between drug overdoses and prescriptions written for persistent-pain patients by examining the evidence. Those who promoted the reasoning that pain prescriptions were fueling the crisis are doing enormous damage to pain management that affects millions of patients and their doctors as well. Even if they were completely accurate in their assessment, great caution would have been needed to avoid a backlash that hurt pain patients. However, media accounts have been sloppy, and many published articles, and even National Public Radio reports,[35] have used experts who have a strong bias. In this chapter, we present evidence that the correlation of overdose deaths is strongest with diverted medications, not medications obtained from legitimate prescriptions.

The inception of the compassionate care movement had a push from the medical community. In the 1990s doctors had been sued by pain patients for undertreating pain.[528] At the same time, the DEA had been investigating and prosecuting doctors for overprescribing with great vigor. The situation had become untenable for the medical community. In 2000, the DEA appeared willing to work with the medical pain community. The DEA met with Dr. David Joransen, director of the Pain and Policy Studies Group at the University of Wisconsin's Comprehensive Cancer Center, and other academic leaders.[419] These conversations led to a consensus document with a joint statement by twenty-one health organizations and the DEA in 2002.[529] This was perhaps a high point for cooperation between the medical community and the agency, but it did not last long. One might suspect that the strongly negative agency review in 2003 by the Office of Management and Budget changed the minds of the DEA director and leadership. The DEA decided to investigate and prosecute doctors with renewed focus to demonstrate their commitment to rooting out diversion in a new *war on prescription drugs*.[303]

This history is a saga of miscommunication and broken promises that has harmed doctors and pain patients the most. The doctors who had taken on the patients with the most challenging conditions during these years were targeted because they were writing prescriptions with the highest doses. Often a fatality that could be attributed to an opioid prescription served as the impetus, but doctors had also been accused of murder for deaths that had no relation to opioids. A doctor treating severe pain is often treating patients with serious diseases, and when pain is severe and the patient requests a very high dose in order to get relief, the doctor has a difficult decision. There had been a recognition of that risk, and there was an agreement not to prosecute doctors for medical decisions made in good faith in 2002, but that agreement did not even last one year. The DEA removed the agreement with the pain societies from its website in order to pursue the prosecution of doctors. The agency did not want lawyers for the defense to prevent them from recommending long sentences for doctors, often much longer than for drug dealers. Many of these prosecutions were overturned on appeal, but some doctors have received thirty years or more in prison merely for prescribing opioids.[247] Of course, some of these convicted doctors worked in pill mills, but the compassionate solitary doctor has always been a target. It is often relatively easy to extract a plea deal by applying the pressure of multiple trumped-up charges based on any bookkeeping irregularity, lapse in record keeping, or by threatening patients to get their cooperation. The DEA's *war on prescription drugs* has institutionalized the need for the agency to become involved in medical decisions in an inappropriate manner. The regulatory fiasco combined with the actions of pharmaceutical companies to make a large profit on the compassionate care movement constitutes a hijacking of that movement by powerful forces in government and the pharmaceutical industry. Doctors have played a role in the crisis, but their role has been greatly exaggerated to direct public anger at overprescribing rather than on the colossal incompetence and corruption that permitted diversion on a massive scale.

Diversion in Broad Daylight—from the Blue Highway to the Oxy Express

Reporter Pat Beall documented how the South Florida pill mills, mainly in Broward and Palm Beach counties, were able to prescribe millions of pills to anyone who wanted to purchase them for more than a decade.[49,426,427,444,459,505] Many of these operations had barely a pretense of being a clinic. Vans from West Virginia, Ohio, Kentucky, Maine, and many other states made the pilgrimage down to South Florida to purchase tens of thousands of pills on each run. The route from West Palm Beach to West Virginia was so commonly traveled by vans full of oxycodone customers that it was called the Blue Highway, owing its name to the color of the thirty-milligram oxycodone tablets made by Mallinckrodt. That company shipped more than five hundred million of the pills to Florida between 2008 and 2012. After 2011, Florida State Troopers intervened to stop that traffic. Why did it take ten years? When highway trafficking became risky a special direct flight, known as the Oxy Express, opened up from Palm

Beach, Florida to Huntington, West Virginia. Transportation Security Agency officials at Palm Beach airport were bribed to let the bags filled with oxycodone tablets go through as carry-on.[49,426,427,444,459,505] The chain pharmacies in the area, CVS and Walmart in Florida, sold millions of pills. Rigg and coworkers described the increase in pill mills from 60 to 150 in 2008 alone in the counties of Broward and West Palm Beach, according to DEA sources.[442]

The diversion of opioids was so well-known to the Florida legislature that talks were held with Purdue Pharma in 2002 to try to convince them to stop selling OxyContin or, at least, not to sell it in South Florida. Purdue Pharma hired former New York mayor Rudi Giuliani's lobbying firm, Giuliani Associates, to influence the DEA and Florida legislature to permit the sales to continue despite the disproportionately large shipments to Broward County.[442,530] In return, Giuliani played a role in private fund-raising for a DEA museum that the agency leadership wanted but could not build with federal funding.[459] In addition, Purdue agreed to pay $2 million to fund a Florida PDMP in 2002.[459] However, there was a catch. The Florida legislature needed to vote to approve the bill prior to 2004. It would not cost Florida anything, but the bill needed approval. When the bill came up for a vote, it was killed by then Florida state senator Marco Rubio. Rubio claimed that he was not opposed to the bill, but the bill was sacrificed in a political feud with Locke Burt.[444] However, with the amount of money flowing from Purdue Pharma into campaign funds, it is hard to know the real reason that a politician had for any decision. The net result was that the pill mills were able to continue operating for another nine years selling OxyContin to half of the United States. Tens of thousands of users had become addicted throughout the US from the Florida pill mills.

Overprescribing vs. Diversion—Which is the Leading Cause of Overdose Fatalities?

In 2011, which was the peak year of the prescription-drug overdoses, half of the overdose deaths involved prescription drugs. Most overdose victims had a cocktail of drugs on autopsy, which made it difficult to determine the cause of death. PROP and federal agencies had seized on the relatively high incidence of prescription drugs to justify extreme reductions in prescribing and hard dose limits. However, 75% of prescription opioids involved in these deaths came from diversion, not from a legitimate doctor's prescription.[374,444,458,459,531–533] The scale of the diversion was only possible because of corporate greed and government corruption that was specific to the opportunity presented by the compassionate care movement. To understand the big picture, we must differentiate between contributions to overdose deaths from diverted prescription drugs that came into circulation through theft, dealers, or blatant pill mills,[532] and those that were prescribed directly by a doctor to a pain patient. Despite a great deal of media attention, internet sales of opioids were found to be a minor component using the research abuse and diversion and addiction-related surveillance (RADARS) system.[534,535] Nonetheless, the total diversion market is estimated to be a $25-billion-a-year market, which is larger than the total legal opioid pharmaceutical market. The size alone indicates the major role diversion played in this tragedy.

To understand the issue, we must precisely define different categories of prescriptions. First, there are legitimate prescriptions to actual pain patients. Second, there are prescriptions from legitimate doctors who are being tricked by a person who is not a legitimate pain patient. Third, there are fake pain clinics, pill mills who sell prescriptions to anyone who walks in the door after a brief consultation. The latter two types of prescription constitute diversion. Evidence from a combined national and South Florida survey of circa 2,700 users revealed that the fraction of the diverted prescription drugs that came from a doctor's prescription was found to be approximately 25% with 13% from a doctor who unknowingly wrote a prescription to a user and 12% from a pill mill.[531] Approximately 50% of pills in the study came from a dealer and 25% from theft or a relative or friend. While it is possible that there is some rerouting of legitimate prescriptions through a dealer, studies on the subject indicate the usual route is from theft or falsified prescriptions. The evidence suggests that doctors who are fooled by their patients represent a relatively small fraction of the total of diverted opioid drugs, about 13%.[531] These data are crucial to understanding the correlation of prescribing to the overdose rate shown in chapter 9.[532] The issue is of vital importance to pain patients since the claim that they abuse their prescriptions threatens their access to needed medications. When an academic medical professional alleges that pain patients are becoming addicted or are addicted, they should pause to contemplate the need for strong evidence given the gravity of what they are alleging.[11,12,18]

The compassionate care movement has been blamed for promoting overprescribing of opioids for minor pain. This may be a valid criticism for some doctors and certain categories of pain patient, such as low back pain, where the range of chronic pain level is very large. Education is needed to ensure that doctors understand to "start low and go slow" and that there is no need to use strong opioids for a number of the minor kinds of pain.[523] However, to confuse legitimate prescribing with diversion is misleading and harmful to every doctor or patient involved in pain management. Care in scholarship is more than an academic good practice when lives are at stake.

Whether from blatantly illegal pill mills, theft, or sale of personal medication, the diversion was on such a massive scale that it could well have exceeded legitimate prescribing at its peak.[444,458,459,531-533] After 2011, diversion became more difficult because of PDMPs.[122,444,458,459] However, heroin and fentanyl overdoses skyrocketed instead of decreasing in parallel with prescribing.[491] PROP made the argument that prescription abuse and overprescribing were the source of the overdose problem.[12] That suited their purpose of supporting the lawsuits that targeted the opioid pharmaceutical companies, but it did not agree with the available evidence.[531] PROP's reasoning led to hard dose limits, forced tapers, and patient abandonment. The implementation of the CDC guidelines has cost many lives. Regardless of the excuse that they make for this failure, it is an enormous misunderstanding of the true situation.

But is this just a misunderstanding? Dr. Kolodny refers to pain patients as *pawns* of the opioid pharmaceutical companies. This is part of a larger attempt to discredit pain patients. Both Dr. Ballantyne and Dr. Kolodny have written articles in medical journals suggesting any pain patient who has a sufficiently high dose is an addict.[11,12,52] In their assessment of the overdose crisis, they ignore strong evidence for diversion that did not involve the typical pain patient. There were certainly patients who received excessive numbers of pills for their level of pain. But there is no direct evidence to support large-scale addiction from this source. On the other hand, the criminal diversion in the pill mills was an industry, and DEA records show the hundreds of millions of pills sent to these various locations. The front operations, the pill mills, were not really doctor's offices in any sense. Since this is all public information, it is difficult to understand how professionals in the field would confuse that abuse with legitimate prescribing. Regarding the treatment of patients and their rights, we should consider pain patients innocent of diversion until proven guilty, not the other way around. There is good reason to believe that the majority of pain patients used their prescriptions as intended.[359] The strong evidence for rates of opioid use disorder of less than 10% among pain patients suggests that the vast majority of pain patients are simply people in need of pain relief.[133,137,138,140–142,144] This description is based on the most conservative estimate from the many studies that have been done. The diversion from legitimate users is correspondingly low.[531]

The causes of continued diversion on a smaller scale after 2011 are still a concern.[531] The criminalization of opioids has created perverse economic incentives that result in a different kind of small-scale diversion. The high cost of prescription drugs, lack of treatment options for opioid-drug addicts, fragmented medical system, lack of insurance, and poverty lead some to the temptation to sell prescription drugs. The market for diverted medication is so distorted that a patient today may pay their rent by selling a few pills a week on the black market. Indeed, diversion is still a problem, but on a much smaller scale than prior to 2011. In any case, diversion should not serve as a justification to punish pain patients in the way that has happened since the implementation of the CDC guidelines.

Follow the Money from Big Pharma to Law Firms—Everyone Got Their Cut

While Purdue Pharma and its allies were thinking about profit during the compassionate care movement, so too are the law firms today who are now suing them for hundreds of billions of dollars.[261] Will these settlements benefit those who became addicted? The leaders of PROP are now among the expert witnesses and consultants who became part of the legal process to sue the opioid manufacturers. The law firms are now lobbying Congress and actively maintaining the narrative that prescription drugs are addictive since this is a central tenet in their court cases. Treating pain patients as though they are on the path to addiction has caused direct great harm to hundreds of thousands of patients.[260] The ethics, motive, and substance of PROP's claims to the detriment of pain patients are highly suspect, given their published statements that pain patients are opioid-dependent, that dependence is addiction and that pain patients are being manipulated by the pharmaceutical companies.

Throughout this process, the people who were supposed to be the primary beneficiaries of the compassionate care movement, the persistent-pain patients, have come last in the power struggle. First, the corporations marketed to the much larger market of low back pain and other such types of pain, pushing the idea that pain should not be just managed but eliminated. Later, pain patients were blamed implicitly because they had been designated as the beneficiaries of the prescribing. In fact, even in the best of times pain patients suffered because of the DEA persecution of doctors. The stigma suffered by pain patients is not washed away in a few years of a movement to treat pain more aggressively.

To win a lawsuit against an opioid manufacturer, it is convenient to make the case that pain patients have been harmed by becoming addicts, just like any other user who had received a prescription that was too large. The lawyers' focus on getting a conviction against the pharmaceutical companies leads them to argue that pain patients have been harmed by the overprescribing. No one appears to care that hundreds of doctors have objected to this reasoning,[1-3] and tens of thousands of pain patients have openly stated that they can no longer get the medications at a level that made their lives tolerable.[283,305] Persistent-pain patients still need opioid medications as a lifeline. PROP's equation of pain patients with addicts increases the stigma and further hardens attitudes that opioid prescriptions should be reduced across the board, regardless of the consequences for those who really need them.[11,12]

It was ironic that blaming pain patients was also the strategy of Richard Sackler, one of the founders of Purdue Pharma. In 2001, the pressure was already beginning because of overdose deaths, and he wrote a confidential email to say, "We have to hammer on the abusers in every way possible. They are the culprits and the problem. They are reckless criminals."[536] By *abusers*, he meant "any customer who used so much of the product that they got the attention of the authorities." In the current legal framework, a patient who has a large prescription for a painful condition may be arrested because of local laws that forbid certain quantities of opioids, irrespective of whether they were prescribed of not. One well-known case is that of Richard Paey, described later. The stigma of the addict is shared by the pain patient. It is not surprising that a disreputable company would try to blame both patients and addicts for the fact that they bring scrutiny to the business practices, but PROP is doing the same thing by writing articles saying that dependence and addiction are the same and patients know that they are drug addicts while their doctors are in denial.

Were Doctors Misled by Purdue Pharma?

Purdue Pharma had been banking on the fact that the intractable pain movement had made an impact and it would be relatively easy for any doctor to write a prescription for opioids once the APS/AAPM statement was published encouraging the treatment of pain as the fifth vital sign.[21,22] However, the persistent-pain population comprised a small share of the total market. Purdue wanted to create new markets to rapidly expand their sales.[505] Rather than a go-slow approach to opioid prescribing, doctors received messages that encouraged them to treat pain aggressively. Purdue held conferences to promote the prescription of OxyContin to thousands of doctors.[299] The marketing of a new opioid drug gave the wrong set of incentives for doctors, including reports that doctors were rewarded financially for prescribing. Doctors were told that addiction poses little risk. As a routine matter, doctors should not obtain their information about medications from advertising by pharmaceutical companies. However, there was a distribution of doctors, some of whom were lazy enough to simply believe that some great new change in research or insight into methods had occurred that would permit them to forget a simple fact that they all once knew, namely, that opioids are addictive. I believe that the majority of doctors are not so susceptible that they would believe something that disagreed with decades of common wisdom. It is an odd position for a doctor to take blaming other doctors. Perhaps Dr. Kolodny should speak for himself rather than claiming that other doctors believed false advertising.

Doctors have years of training and are experts in their field. They are supposed to read the literature and understand the issues, the biochemistry, chemistry, physiology, neurobiology, and more. It is a daunting amount to apprehend, and not all doctors have time to read the literature the way they should. But to admit that Purdue could convince doctors to prescribe in a particular way would say to the world that many doctors get too much of their information from pharmaceutical companies and their sales representatives. What percentage of doctors actually believed statements that were later admitted to be false advertising in a court of law? [458] An interview with Dr. Kolodny was reported as follows[537]:

> Andrew Kolodny, the co-director of the Opioid Policy Research Collaborative, at Brandeis University, has worked with hundreds of patients addicted to opioids. He told me that, though many fatal overdoses have resulted from opioids other than OxyContin, the crisis was initially precipitated by a shift in the culture of prescrib-

ing—a shift carefully engineered by Purdue. "If
you look at the prescribing trends for all the different opioids, it's in 1996 that prescribing really
takes off," Kolodny said. "It's not a coincidence.
That was the year Purdue launched a multifaceted campaign that misinformed the medical community about the risks." When I asked
Kolodny how much of the blame Purdue bears
for the current public-health crisis, he responded,
"The lion's share."

Dr. Kolodny claims, without evidence, that doctors were "misinformed" and "duped" by Purdue Pharma.[18,537] On one hand, doctors may not have received excellent training in pain management,
since that has not been a priority in medical schools. On the other
hand, opioids are not state-of-the-art biologic pharmaceuticals. Some
pharmaceuticals today have completely new principles of action that
did not exist when many doctors studied medicine. An example is
the class of antibody drugs that are used to treat many inflammatory autoimmune diseases. A greater fraction of doctors may rely on
company advertising with regard to these complex drugs, because of
a lack of familiarity and a daunting new literature that would need to
read to formulate an opinion. After all, the FDA approval is normally
the crucial aspect that determines whether doctors should consider a
drug safe or not.

By contrast, opioids are among the oldest-known medicines in
the western world. Doctors did not need to rely on companies for
information on opioids or their side effects since the information is
widely available in the medical literature. Doctors knew that addiction has been the major factor that has prevented opioid use for the
past one hundred years. Dr. Kolodny is claiming that doctors as a
general rule simply put that knowledge aside and believed advertising by a drug company that contradicted the common wisdom. We
need to distinguish between a small minority of doctors who took
kickbacks from the majority who prescribed in good faith. PROP
pretends that the entire problem arose because physicians were

deceived and patients are all prone to addiction without differentiating pain patients or doctors in any way. Was a doctor who took kickbacks deceived? Should we make policy for all doctors based on the consequences of those who took kickbacks? PROP's irresponsible and biased approach to academic articles on public health and clinical studies has led to a policy that effectively punishes those who most need opioid medication for the corruption of some of the opioid manufacturers, the DEA and state, and federal legislatures. Of course, some doctors made mistakes. But the consequences of these mistakes pale in comparison to systematic, high-level diversion, and fraud.

It is a doctor's job to make decisions based on risk. Most medications have some side effects and associated risks. Drugs like aspirin, ibuprofen, and naproxen (so-called NSAIDs, or nonsteroidal anti-inflammatory drugs) cause severe stomach problems for many patients. The annual death rate of patients from NSAIDs was approximately fifteen thousand in 2016.[538] Thus, they are not risk-free. Doctors will tell certain patients to avoid these common drugs if the patient has had an ulcer or requires a very high dose. The idea that doctors were so poorly educated that they could not understand the risks of one of the oldest, most common medicines is disturbing. Yet Dr. Kolodny alleged that doctors were told that there was no risk to prescribing opioids by the pharmaceutical and they simply believed it. That simple story may sound good in a courtroom to people who don't know anything about medicine, but there are numerous other important factors to consider.

For the past one hundred years, doctors have been inhibited with regard to opioid prescribing because of regulatory concerns. After the joint statement by the DEA and twenty-one agencies, the Pain Relief and Promotion Act, and the policy statements by the APS and AAPM, doctors came to the realization that there was a different climate. They could write an opioid prescription without the same fear of legal repercussions. It is believable that doctors were willing to write opioid prescriptions as the professional organizations had told them they could do but were unprepared for the challenge of observing patients for signs of addiction. Identifying aberrant behavior involves more than an awareness of risk. It requires an intervention strategy. Many doctors are unfamiliar with the types of referrals needed for counseling and follow up with patients who do not use their prescription properly. Doctors have little experience with this since they are not permitted to write prescriptions or treat patients for an opioid use disorder under current law unless they have a special waiver, which very few doctors have.

If we accept as a fact that the vast majority of doctors is competent, then they do bear collective responsibility for the significant number of mistakes during the prescription-drug wave. There are many documented cases of doctors prescribing too much and patients becoming addicted. This practice continued after the CDC guidelines were implemented. Although I believe doctors should have been more critical of the changes and used more common sense regarding who should receive a high dose prescription, they were receiving encouragement from pain organizations, the approval of a new federal law, and the strong encouragement of the pharmaceutical industry. But those mistakes pale in comparison to the massive diversion of prescription drugs to pill mills or doctors for hire that was sponsored by Purdue and tolerated by the DEA.

PROP's reasoning completely misunderstood the nature of the criminal diversion that occurred. There is a great deal of evidence that diversion, rather than legitimate prescribing, was the major reason for the prescription-drug overdose wave (1999–2011). Purdue Pharma appeared to have been complicit in diversion right from the start. But diversion on the scale that Purdue wanted to get away with had to involve the DEA. Purdue Pharma urgently needed the support and endorsement of doctors to convince the DEA that it had a legitimate reason for expansion in production and sales. Indeed, once the doctors were on board with Purdue, the DEA signed off on the quotas and watched as the massive shipments were made to various remote counties in Appalachia and particular locations in urban Florida and California.[250,252,253,255] With the doctors apparently agreeing to the need for Purdue's product, the company used Giuliani Associates to then buy cooperation from the DEA,[459,539] the

US Congress,[250] and the Florida legislature.[540] The compassionate care movement was hijacked.

PROP's narrative is that overprescribing is the source of the problem, except that, of course, they claim that doctors are not responsible for overprescribing, because the pharmaceutical companies "duped" them. This convenient allegation defines pain patients as the victims who were harmed by addiction and yet shifts the blame to the pharmaceutical companies because of their false advertising. That argument is perfect for the prosecution of a case against an opioid manufacturer. It also justifies hard limits on opioid medication and tapers for persistent-pain patients. To understand the motivation for making this case, we must bear in mind that certain members of PROP are directly benefitting financially from their role as consultants and expert witnesses in the lawsuits that use these claims as evidence.[260,261] Dr. Kolodny justifies the enormous harm done to pain patients by his machinations by claiming that they are merely *pawns* of the pharmaceutical industry. Dr. Kolodny accuses any doctor who wants to defend patients' rights of being a stooge of the pharmaceutical industry as well. The medical community is powerless to repair the damage as long as there is a policy monopoly promoted by PROP and enforced by the DEA that limits prescribing to fixed levels and forces tapers on patients.

Purdue Pharma's False Advertising—from Addiction to Abuse-Deterrent Formulation

The guilty pleas in court tell us that Purdue Pharma misrepresented the addiction rate in product literature, advertising, and promotional events.[343] Purdue's distortion of the facts had a wider audience than just the doctors. The biggest hurdle to opioid prescribing in the United States is not doctors or pharmacies, but the DEA. Purdue used a sleight of hand—numerous studies that show that the addiction rate is low. Conservative estimates suggest that <3% of pain patients later have opioid use disorder or addiction.[133,137,138,140–142,144] However, Purdue's advertising used the number <1% from the study by Porter and Jick,[137] not only for persistent-pain patients, but for the general patient population. It would be false to state that the addiction rate is that low for a population of healthy individuals. Studies provide numbers ranging from 4% to 8% for addiction rate of the random sample of healthy people who are prescribed opioids.[9,139,141] That is a large difference, not just in total numbers of patients, but also in the attitude a physician will have when considering a prescription. The higher the risk, the greater the need for vigilance.

A second example of Purdue's misinformation was the statement that OxyContin was an abuse-deterrent formation (ADF). Since it was a time-release formulation, it was supposed to prevent users from extracting the active agent, oxycodone, and injecting it or snorting it. One would have to be quite naive to believe this. Abuse-deterrent formulations (ADF) are one proposal to try to curb illicit opioid use, but prior time-release formulations such as Opana had failed to be abuse deterrent. According to a recent expert opinion, "Despite the development of a dozen products with abuse-deterrent features, most of these technologies rely on the same deterrent agent, making it easier for abusers to focus their manipulation efforts and share their experience to defeat the technology."[541] Various strategies from machine learning to postmarketing studies have failed to find a formulation that discourages abuse.[542,543] But more to the point, Purdue's own testing in its FDA application revealed that the ADF did not work (Drug Application to FDA for OxyContin, Pharmacology Review: "Abuse Liability of Oxycodone," Purdue Pharma, Stamford, CN, 1995). There was hard evidence already in 2001 that overdoses in Maine had increased dramatically.[544]

Remarkably, following bankruptcy in 2007, the company continued to produce and market the same OxyContin as before.[343,545] The management changed, but Purdue was shielded from the worst outcome of the lawsuit against it by Giuliani Associates' connections in the DOJ. Purdue created a second version of a supposed abuse-deterrent formulation of OxyContin, which was approved by the FDA in 2010.[458] It is questionable whether the new ADF worked, but it was a moot point.[546] Finally, in 2010, the DEA began significantly lowering production quotas and reining in prescribing.[252] The FDA initiated a restriction of the regulations surrounding prescription and postmarketing of OxyContin in 2013.[547] This was the same year that Purdue Pharma agreed to stop its advertising campaign for OxyContin. Sales fell steadily from 2011 to the present not because of any action that they took voluntarily to comply with the ADF concept, but because limitations on advertising and sales were imposed externally.[548]

Purdue Pharma Tries to Keep the Lid on its Secrets

Although it only had 4% of market share, OxyContin was under patent starting in 1996. Purdue had a much higher profit margin compared to other manufacturers whose formulations were no longer under patent. For example, the widely used time-released morphine, MS Contin, was patented in 1941 so it can be manufactured as a generic. OxyContin was based on a new patent with a significantly greater profit potential. Purdue wanted to maximize their profit advantage by capturing markets quickly using a financial web that extended into Congress, medical professional societies, front business organizations, and the judicial system.[549] However, Purdue was sued by the US government, many states and municipalities, and ultimately, lost in court.[34] Purdue Pharma declared bankruptcy in 2007. According to National Public Radio's report,

> the federal investigation ended on May 10, 2007, when three executives of the pharmaceutical company Purdue Pharma pled guilty in federal court to misleading doctors and patients about the risk of addiction and potential for abuse of OxyContin. Purdue Pharma was ordered to pay over $600 million in fines and other payments to the federal government and the Commonwealth of Virginia.

Given everything Purdue did, the judge's order in the 2007 lawsuit and bankruptcy was a slap on the wrist. Thanks to the extensive lobbying of Giuliani Associates, the judgment was not the end of the line for the Sackler family or for Purdue as a company. However, the company had a lot to hide.[550] When the lawsuits were filed in court, several judges kept documents under seal so that the public would not learn about the tactics used by Purdue Pharma.[33] When the prosecutors wanted to unseal the records in the interest of transparency, Purdue appealed all the way to the Kentucky Supreme Court[551] but lost the case and were required to make public their marketing and promotional records.[552] One relationship that was revealed was a relationship with Abbott Pharmaceuticals, a much larger company than Purdue. Abbott was responsible for the day-to-day marketing operations with a sales force of approximately three hundred sales agents. But this was just the tip of an iceberg of sales and marketing connections, many of them of questionable legality.[246,539,553]

When a company, such as Purdue, makes tens of billions of dollars in a little more than a decade, there is clearly money for many types of "expenses." Many officials received gifts, campaign contributions, or paid vacations from Purdue Pharma.[244] Purdue engaged in bribery, kickbacks, and lobbying to manage their false advertising and shut down enforcement efforts directed against them.[246] Nonetheless, the Sackler family, who owned Purdue Pharma, have escaped criminal prosecution despite the fact that their company and executives have been either indicted or convicted of lying, bribery, and false advertising, while they transferred at least $1 billion from corporate coffers to their own bank account.[244,299] Even as they declared bankruptcy in the US, they constructed a global company, Mundipharma, to replicate the same successful model they had used in the US to market opioids globally. How did Purdue manage to do this in plain sight of the DEA, state law enforcement, the US Congress, and state legislatures?

Purdue Pharma's Marketing Backfires and Creates a Backlash

Purdue Pharma saw an opportunity to get the medical community's implicit approval for their flashy slogans to market the drug

OxyContin. They gave money to medical schools to study pain and thereby promote their product. Like so many corporate-academic partnerships, the company wanted something more than just to help foster research and teaching at a medical school when they initiated the relationship. Dr. Ballantyne clearly regretted having any relationship with Purdue relatively soon after her institution accepted funding from the company in 2000. She was disappointed by Purdue's response to her 2003 publication.[265] Although Dr. Ballantyne described her work as being critical from the beginning, the 2003 publication described opioids as having efficacy but raised concern about side effects in long-term prescribing.[113] Sometime after 2009, Dr. Ballantyne joined others to form PROP, became its president, and began openly opposing Purdue's marketing and advertising as harmful.[8] From around this time, Dr. Ballantyne started on a course to contradict the main conclusions from her early work. She also focused her efforts on writing commentary that pain patients were at risk for addiction. The criticism of Purdue Pharma turned into a criticism of the entire compassionate care movement. For example, the state attorney general of Massachusetts initiated an investigation of funds donated to Tufts Medical School by Purdue Pharma. This might be seen as a natural consequence of the lawsuit filed against Purdue Pharma by the same state attorney general.[265] However, investigating Tufts educational programs for bias is really an investigation of the university. How did the state attorney general come to suspect any bias in the educational program at Tufts? Was it mere coincidence that Dr. Ballantyne worked at Tufts for many years and then later served as a consultant for law firms suing Purdue? [265] It would be easier to assess Dr. Ballantyne's role if it were not for her financial conflicts of interest. One can understand a reaction to the overdose crisis that would lead to a reassessment of prescribing, but Dr. Ballantyne's about-face remains difficult to explain.

After 2007, when Purdue lost in court and declared bankruptcy, it became clear that there would be dozens of lawsuits against pharmaceutical companies.[32,244,245] Drs. Ballantyne and Kolodny became consultants and expert witnesses who can easily make several hundred thousand dollars consulting and testifying in a case.[263] Dr. Kolodny was so deeply embedded with the prosecution of the Johnson & Johnson lawsuit in Oklahoma that the judge was forced to rule on whether he should be barred from testimony as an unbiased expert witness.[35] The judge's bias in the case was evident because he permitted Dr. Kolodny to testify as an expert witness. Dr. Kolodny's writing made it clear that he was a de facto consultant for the prosecution. Persistent-pain patients merely wanted the medical community to take pain as seriously as other symptoms. Yet because Purdue had changed the scope and nature of the pain patient population by their aggressive tactics, PROP came to see reform of the pain patient as part of their agenda. In so doing, they ignored the people with the serious diseases who were the original intended beneficiaries of compassionate care. To establish the principle that overprescribing was a major harm, Drs. Ballantyne, Lembke, and Kolodny have insisted that essentially all patients had been subject to overprescribing and therefore were vulnerable to addiction.[11,12,18,276]

The failure to disclose conflicts of interest raises significant concerns about the true motivations of the leaders of PROP. It is telling that Dr. Kolodny failed to declare these conflicts in several journal articles.[262] In 2019, he published an admission of his failure to follow journal ethics guidelines, because he was caught and called to account.[12,262,554] This is ironic considering how Dr. Kolodny has made it a habit to criticize organizations or individuals that fail to divulge their conflicts of interest.[554] In fact, Dr. Kolodny has used the fact that other doctors have received funding from opioid pharmaceutical companies to attempt to silence their criticism, by claiming that their opinion is compromised by money. Dr. Kolodny has shown that he is acutely aware of the importance of honest reporting. For example, he made sure to report his own conflicts in a crucial publication with the former director of the CDC, Thomas Frieden, that made ten recommendations for policy changes at the federal level with regard to opioid prescribing and addiction.[555] For such a high-profile publication, the failure to report may have had consequences, and Dr. Kolodny did report in that instance. However, elsewhere, such as when he criticized others for failing to disclose their conflicts, Dr.

Kolodny failed to declare his own conflicts.[554] It is scandalous that Dr. Kolodny did not disclose his conflicts of interest at the time that he was playing a major role in drafting the CDC guidelines. It is still not clear whether Dr. Ballantyne disclosed her conflicts of interest at the time of the writing of the CDC guidelines.[260,261]

We will never know the full extent of the role played by PROP behind closed doors in the meetings that led to the CDC guidelines. But many tens or hundreds of thousands of patients are acutely aware of the effect of those guidelines. They are the reason Patient Z has been subjected to his ordeal. Regarding the CDC guidelines, Bob Twillman, executive director of the American Academy of Pain Management, stated,[556]

> Clearly, this is PROP's way of getting what FDA didn't give them when they advocated for an ER/LA opioid label change. I don't think it's a coincidence that this sets a 90 mg MED dose limit, when PROP advocated for a 100 mg MED dose limit in their Citizen Petition to the FDA. That PROP's president and one vice-president are part of the core expert group; their executive director and a board member are part of the stakeholder review group; and another board member is one of the three who will help edit the guidelines after the stakeholders report, all is not a coincidence, and clearly puts their fingerprints all over this guideline. But, of course, no one is supposed to know that."

When they cut ties with the pharmaceutical companies, the members of PROP profited by consulting and expert witness fees, as well as salary and career advancement that followed the new stances that they took, which have been much more lucrative compared to championing patients' rights.

Corruption and Incompetence Prevented the DEA from Taking Action to Stop the Crisis

The DEA's *war on drugs* has resulted in a law-and-order mentality that has skewed medical and regulatory community attitudes toward opioids as pain medications.[421–423,557] Over fifty years, as the failure became glaring, public support for the war on drugs has soured. Most people realize that the drug problem has gotten worse since the "war" began. Two out of three polled believe that possession of drugs should be decriminalized, recognizing that the United States has the highest incarceration rate in the world. In fact, the rate of incarceration has increased by a factor four since 1970 due in large measure to petty drug offenses.[558] Although the total addiction rate for all drugs has been basically flat at 2% of population until recently, the overdose rate in the United States has grown exponentially for the past forty years.[491] Ironically, DEA funding proceeded apace.[489] As the overdose rate grew year after year, a procession of different drugs have been the leading cause of death—heroin, crack cocaine, methamphetamine, prescription drugs, heroin again, and finally fentanyl. However, often overdoses involve mixtures of drugs, making it difficult to identify the precise cause of death. When politicians or government officials state that the heroin-addiction problem started in the 2000s, after opioid prescribing increased, they are misleading the public. Heroin addiction has been a problem in the United States since World War II and has waxed and waned depending on the availability of alternative drugs. In 2000, heroin addiction was at a lower rate (0.2%) than it had been for many years because of the easy access to cocaine and crack, but there were still approximately six hundred thousand heroin addicts during this period. Access is everything in the drug world. Each of these drugs—heroin, crack, cocaine, fentanyl, and diverted prescription drugs—has contributed to the exponentially increasing drug overdose death rate. Of all the drugs, heroin has been the most consistent cause of death over the past forty years. Those who blame prescription drugs for "causing" the problem are confused by recent trends. Heroin addiction increased significantly after 2011, spurred on by the availability of a cheap supply of heroin from Mexico. The history of how politicians and government agencies ignored the problem while receiving donations from opioid manufacturers reveals a sad state of affairs in our society, described in the following sections of the chapter. The facts show that it is disingenuous of anyone to blame the continuing drug crisis on doctors' opioid prescribing.

The DEA Avoids a War on Pill Mills

DEA officials, lawmakers and the media knew from 2002 that the scale of the diversion in south Florida alone was staggering.[426,427,444] Despite declaring *war on prescription drugs* in 2004, the DEA did not take any action against one of the largest opioid diversion schemes in US history. We will have to make do with the information that is in the public domain in our discussion of DEA actions. Requests by journalists for additional documentation under the Freedom of Information Act (FOIA) have been denied by the DEA. There were also other centers of diversion in Virginia,[505] Tennessee,[516] and California[517–519] that were well documented.

Late in 2003, the DEA had received the results of a congressional review of the DEA's war on drugs. The Office of Management and Budget had given the DEA a score of 0 out of 100 for its thirty-year-long *war on drugs*. Journalists, academics, and think tanks have been writing articles documenting the failure of the strategy and implementation of the DEA's war on drugs in Latin America, Laos, and Afghanistan, as well as on the streets of America for more than twenty-five years,[421–423] but when the congressional financial watchdog declared an agency to be total failure, swift action was required. To justify their continued funding in the congressional committees, the DEA announced its new mission of a *war on prescription drugs* as a justification for expanded agency funding.

The DEA controls opium imports, opioid production quotas, and licensing of doctors and pharmacies.[252,255] Given the obvious diversion that was ongoing in Florida and elsewhere, there were plenty of targets for the DEA. Given their total control of manufacture, all licensing for distribution or prescription, it would appear to be impossible for the DEA to lose a war on prescription drugs. However, the DEA had been hamstrung by Congress, the revolving door with the opioid industry and lobbying by Giuliani Associates at the state and federal levels.[530] Purdue's strategy did not leave out any angle in nailing down the DEA's support.[459] They bought the medical community's support,[299] Florida lawmakers' support,[459] and US Congress's support[250] and paid lobbying and technology firms to make the case to the DEA that their product was a legitimate abuse-deterrent pharmaceutical,[246] which was in high demand. The DEA never made a move against Purdue Pharma or its major suppliers or pharmacies or the major pharmacies despite inside information that upper management was fully aware of illegal sales.

The DEA Was Constrained Not to Wage War Against Purdue Pharma

The DEA never took action against obvious diversion by Purdue, its distributors, or the large pharmacies, despite evidence of employees who alerted the corporate offices of suspicious activity. The 2019 Office of Inspector General Report states,

> We found that DEA was slow to respond to the significant increase in the use and diversion of opioids since 2000. We also found that DEA did not use its available resources, including its data systems and strongest administrative enforcement tools, to detect and regulate diversion effectively. Further, we found that DEA policies and regulations did not adequately hold registrants accountable or prevent the diversion of pharmaceutical opioids.

There was evidence from many quarters that diversion was occurring on a massive scale during this entire time. Ex-DEA agent Rannazzisi's revelations made him a whistleblower who exposed the extent of agency inaction and protection of the corporate executives for many years.[559] In an interview on *60 Minutes*, Rannazzisi made the explosive allegation that the three largest distributors—Cardinal Health, McKesson, and AmerisourceBergen—all knew that opioids were being sent to disreputable "pill mills." Rannazzisi painted a picture of an agency that was overwhelmed at first by the sheer magnitude of the diversion, but when he and others began to focus on the fact that they needed to target the distributors, suddenly their process was slowed down by the upper management of the DEA. The distributors had been found to be in violation and had paid fines in the tens of millions of dollars but continued to ship millions of pills to remote areas.

Early in the process, Giuliani Associates was directly lobbying the DEA but later successfully lobbied a campaign that led to the passage of House Resolution 4709.[250] An expose in *The Washington Post* revealed that

> ["t]he drug industry, the manufacturers, wholesalers, distributors and chain drugstores, have an influence over Congress that has never been seen before," said Joseph T. Rannazzisi, who ran the DEA's division responsible for regulating the drug industry and led a decade-long campaign of aggressive enforcement until he was forced out of the agency in 2015. "I mean, to get Congress to pass a bill to protect their interests in the height of an opioid epidemic just shows me how much influence they have."

The legislation was passed in 2015, so this set of facts cannot explain the fact that for fifteen years prior to its passage, the action by the DEA was so ineffective. The fact that lobbying and campaign contributions to Dan Marino (R, Pennsylvania) and Orrin Hatch (R, Utah) were successful suggests that there may have been other backroom manipulations to prevent the agencies from taking action.[250] Ironically, Congressman Marino stated that "the DEA was too aggressive and needed to work more collaboratively with drug companies." According to the *Post*,

> [p]olitical action committees representing the industry contributed at least $1.5 million to the 23 lawmakers who sponsored or co-sponsored four versions of the bill, including nearly $100,000 to Marino and $177,000 to Hatch. Overall, the drug industry spent $102 million lobbying Congress on the bill and other legislation between 2014 and 2016, according to lobbying reports.

The crucial point is that this parallel diversion directly by the manufacturer and largest distributors means that there is a need to examine the myth of PCP overprescribing as the cause of the crisis. During the peak of the crisis, medical examiners who investigated opioid-overdose deaths suggested that most involved drug diversion and abuse.[560] In the crucial years prior to 2011, the DEA could have had the most significant impact if it had intervened to shut down some of the largest diversion schemes. A study in West Virginia at the peak of the prescription-drug wave showed a large role for prescription drug abuse. The 63% of people who died from pharmaceutical overdoses had taken one or more drugs for which they did not have a prescription. The 21% had prescriptions for controlled substances from five or more physicians in the year prior to death. The 16% also had illicit drugs, such as heroin and cocaine, contributing to their deaths.[561]

The *Los Angeles Times* documented a similar operation in California, which was nothing more than an organized drug ring that hired a retired doctor as a front.[517] According to the *Times*, which published numerous emails as evidence, Purdue Pharma was aware of the criminal nature of the orders they were receiving. *The Washington Post* article continues with a statement by DEA director Mulrooney[250]:

> "At a time when, by all accounts, opioid abuse, addiction and deaths were increasing markedly"

the new law "imposed a dramatic diminution of the agency's authority," Mulrooney wrote in a draft 115-page article provided by the Marquette Law Review editorial board. He wrote that it is now "all but logically impossible" for the DEA to suspend a drug company's operations for failing to comply with federal law. The agency declined to make Mulrooney available for an interview.

Lindsey Barber played a key role in writing the legislation and advocating for its passage by his testimony before Congress. In April 2006, Barber was the top lawyer for the DEA's Office of Diversion Control. After the legislation was passed, in July 2017 Barber became the senior vice president in charge of regulatory affairs at Cardinal Health. He had intimate knowledge of the DEA's strategy for interdicting drug shipments. The legislation essentially put that activity on hold. Although Lindsey Barber had been tough on the companies along with Rannazzisi, he went through the revolving door and helped them later. *The Washington Post* estimated that up to fifty-six DEA officers and lawyers ended up leaving the agency and working for the health industry. The revolving door and lobbying protected Purdue Pharma from federal prosecution and from being closed down after their admission of guilt and bankruptcy in 2007. After that judgment against Purdue, Giuliani's influence permitted the company to continue to do business with the federal government and gave it immunity from further prosecution, which was unheard of after a conviction of that type.[539,545] These contacts combined with the hundreds of millions spent in lobbying Congress, which helped to keep the companies in business selling high volumes of opioids.[250] Two democratic senators initiated a probe to examine Giuliani's contacts with the DOJ's political appointees, who overruled career prosecutors. Giuliani had effectively stopped any further investigation of Purdue.[562]

The DEA's Shameful War on Doctors

Despite this poor record of enforcement against the major diversion during the years 1999–2011, the DEA and state law enforcement agencies unjustly prosecuted dozens of doctors who were treating legitimate persistent-pain patients.[303] There is practically an industry in trying to get a conviction when a doctor is accused of diversion in opioid prescribing or Medicaid fraud. As Dr. Libby describes in his book *The Criminalization of Medicine*, the DEA and Office of Inspector General of the Department of Health and Human Services (DHHS) have a history of making cases out of the weakest of evidence.[108] But their success with Congress and taxpayer rests on making convictions. If a doctor is targeted for suspected opioid violations, the agents search records looking for any discrepancy, incorrectly coded billing, or possible infraction to add as many additional charges as possible. They interview patients and try to turn them against the doctor. They look through death records and see if there is any possible way to blame the doctor for a patient death. The goal of the strategy is to put so much pressure on the doctor so that a plea bargain will seem like the best strategy. This maximizes the conviction rate. Never mind what it does to the doctor or his patients.

Watchdog agencies can function to prevent fraud and abuse. The pill mills and their diversion were (and are) a major source of the corruption of a well-intentioned movement to prescribe opioids to people who have genuine pain. To the extent that the DEA and state law enforcement have prosecuted those illegal activities, they have acted in the interest of pain patients and society at large. However, when an agency decides to prosecute a doctor in order to meet law enforcement targets or to prove itself to Congress and the public, there is a great danger of wrongful prosecution. Just as pain patients suffer the stigma of opioid use and are often suspected of abuse, particularly when their pain is severe and the dose needed for relief is high, doctors who treat these patients also suffer from the stigma of the pill mills. Doctors who prescribe opioids to very ill patients are the most vulnerable to the kind of pressure that the DEA uses to force doctors to admit to some crime in order to avoid the threat of a long jail sentence. The patients who seek out doctors willing to prescribe higher doses are often the very ill patients like Patient Z. There are patients whose pain is so intense that they need high-dose opioids for treatment in order to function. It is crucially important that we understand that many of the doctors who have been prosecuted or harassed by the DEA are caring and talented physicians who have treated people whose pain was so severe that the patient had thought there was no hope. These cases have shown that some individuals with severe pain from Ehlers-Danlos syndrome or adhesive arachnoiditis can live a somewhat normal life if they have a very high dose of opioids. Some have criticized the doctors for prescribing what have been called "lethal" doses. Indeed, if a pain-naive person who had no prior exposure were to take a dose of one gram of morphine (1,000 MEDD), it would be lethal. Yet many patients have shown that they can live for long periods on such a dose after they have gradually increased their tolerance. However, these patients are highly vulnerable to a rapid worsening of their health if they are suddenly cut off from their prescription. It turns out that it is not the dose that is lethal, but the actions by the DEA that are often lethal for such patients. Many patients have died when the DEA closed down a doctor who prescribed these large doses. The DEA agents felt justified because they reasoned it was harming the patients to take such large doses. DEA agents are not doctors, and it is absolutely chilling when they make statements about what a particular dose means. The agency appears oblivious to the dozens of documented deaths it has caused. Patient Z has mentioned how frightening this prospect is and how it prevents him from seeking doctors who might be more understanding than the pain clinic. There are still a few left, but they are threatened with extinction. It is a patient's nightmare to have a doctor who has understood their pain suddenly unable to write a prescription.

Because of the chilling effect of these arrests and perhaps even following Libby's testimony before Congress in 2005,[303] several studies were conducted to assess whether the arrests of doctors were improper.[563] Jung and Reidenberg investigated the cases of forty-three of the doctors prosecuted in 2005. They concluded that any doctor who keeps good records has nothing to fear. The article also cited previous work by state medical board investigators who maintain that the prosecution rate against doctors who are honestly treating patients for pain is "non-existent." It is difficult to reconcile these conclusions with the dozen cases that are in the public domain with ample press coverage. As with so many aspects of this controversy, various authors give diametrically opposing views. Most of the cases are complex. As I have studied them, it is often the case that the doctor's practice or behavior could be improved. However, the penalties are outrageously disproportionate to any wrongdoing or lack of adherence to regulations in any of the cases that have been documented in newspaper accounts[239,305-307,564-567] or Dr. Libby's book.[108,303]

There is a fundamental problem with law enforcement making judgments about medical matters. State medical boards are in a much better position to make informed decisions about the propriety of a doctor's prescription. They can also mete out a punishment that is appropriate by simply taking away a doctor's license to practice medicine.

There were a total of 726 doctors charged associated with writing opioid prescriptions between 1998 and 2006.[304] This represents 0.1% of the practicing patient care physicians in the United States. It is interesting that Dr. Goldenbaum refers to this as a low rate, given that 80% of US physicians no longer prescribe opioids. Thus, among the set of prescribing doctors, that is an incidence of 0.5%. Of these, approximately 70% were sentenced to prison. Most of the cases ended in plea bargains because the doctors could not afford a lawyer when their assets were seized and they were told that unless they accepted a plea bargain, the DOJ would prosecute them with the full force of criminal justice system in order to get a conviction for a twenty-to-thirty-year sentence.[239,303,305,306,564,565]

The DEA has prosecuted doctors with the help of many unscrupulous people who made their living testifying against doctors on behalf of the DEA.[248] A common strategy is to pit patient against doctor. The DEA agent will tell the patient that they are going to prison for a narcotics violation unless they join the government and testify against the doctor. The DEA's own inspector general has found millions of dollars misspent on informants who lied or abused the confidence of the agency.[248] Expert witnesses make significant sums of money in trial testimony or giving advice to the DEA to investigate doctors. This entire industry is a disgrace to law enforcement.

One of famous cases of a doctor prosecuted for prescribing high-dose opioids was that of Dr. William Hurwitz. This case was discussed in the documentary "Dr. Feelgood," which presented the ethical dilemma of patients who turned to Hurwitz in terrible pain and having given up hope. Hurwitz's pain clinic was located in McLean, Virginia, and patients came from thirty-eight states to see him. Because of the high doses he was willing to prescribe, he had disagreements with the Virginia Medical Board. Although the board had sanctioned Dr. Hurwitz, the board wrote that his prescriptions had all been made "in good faith." Dr. Hurwitz had some flaws. He was aware that some of his patients sold their medications, but he had the attitude that he was not a law enforcement officer and there was nothing he could do about his patient's behavior. Unfortunately, that was a naive position to take in a country where the DEA can decide to prosecute. Eventually law enforcement approached those patients who were dealing and gave them a reduced sentence in return for testimony against Hurwitz. In 2004, Hurwitz was convicted of drug-trafficking charges and sentenced to twenty-five years in prison. Several members of the jury were outraged by the sentence since they felt that on the technical merits he was guilty but that he had acted in good faith to help people in pain. Ironically, the patients who were actual traffickers were given very light sentences in return for their testimony against Hurwitz. In 2007, he won an appeal and his sentence was reduced to four years and nine months.[247]

The case of Frank Fischer was one that was more clearly a case of prosecutorial overreach from start to finish. It is surprising that it did not end up a case of prosecutorial misconduct. Fischer practiced pain medicine in Redding, California, for a few years before he was arrested and charged with murder. The Harvard-trained doctor had a practice with three thousand patients. Approximately 5% had chronic pain. A Medi-Cal insurance office noticed a number of high-dose opioid prescriptions coming from Redding, and they were traced to Dr. Fischer's office. Fischer said that he prescribed pain medication at high doses only when it was warranted. The state sent undercover agents to his office seven times to try to get him to write a prescription for a made-up reason. Fischer never wrote a prescription to the undercover agents. Then state investigators decided that there must have been someone who died under his care because of the opioids. They began searching death records. They found two patients who had died and charged Dr. Fischer with murder, drug trafficking, and Medi-Cal fraud. His assets were seized, and the process against him was started. After an unnecessarily lengthy investigation, it was revealed that neither of the individuals had died of opioids. Quite obviously, the murder charge was not going to stick. It took nearly four years for three court cases to clear his name. He was found innocent in three jury trials. By that time, his career was destroyed, and he could no longer practice medicine.[307]

Even the leaders of the community of pain physicians have been targeted by the DEA. In 2010, the DEA opened an investigation into manslaughter charges against Dr. Lynn Webster of Salt Lake City, Utah, past president of American Academy of Pain Medicine (AAPM).[239] After a four-year investigation, the district attorney dropped the charges, and Dr. Webster was never prosecuted. However, his medical practice was severely damaged by the investigation.

Dr. Webster had been an expert witness in a trial against a pain doctor in Des Moines, Iowa. Dr. Daniel Baldi had been charged with manslaughter charges when a patient under his care died. One has to keep in mind that the people treated in pain clinics are often quite sick to begin with. It is rare for patients to die of an overdose when following the doctor's advice, but it can happen, and it is not necessarily negligence. Patients sometimes die from the complications of their disease or because they take illegal drugs. There are many reasons including possible physician error, but none of those should be called manslaughter. Dr. Baldi was found innocent by a jury.

In 2018, the DEA raided the office of Dr. Forrest Tennant in Los Angeles, California, for suspected narcotics trafficking [305] Dr. Tennant was one of the pioneers in the field of intractable pain and had a fifty-year practice helping severely ill patients with persistent pain. He returned from a brief trip serving as an expert witness in a trial against a Montana doctor for prescribing opioids to find that the DEA had kicked down the door to his house in an effort to find evidence that he had profited illegally from prescribing opiates. Dr. Tennant was seventy-seven years old at the time. He simply shut down his practice rather than deal with the legal issues.[305]

The website and organization Doctors of Courage started by Linda Cheek keeps a database of one thousand doctors who are currently or have been targeted by the DEA and DOJ for alleged opioid prescribing abuses. It is remarkable how many doctors have been prosecuted without a clear crime having been committed. The prosecution looks into every death that occurred during the doctor's practice and attempts to find some involvement of opioids that can be used to blame the doctor. These doctors are tried for years in the court of public opinion before their actual trial. It is noteworthy that there is a disproportionate number of African American or foreign-born doctors on the list. A recurrent theme in statements by prosecutors is to infer that when doctors receive Medicaid payment for opioids, then they must have done something wrong. Of course, doctors who practice in poor areas will need to accept Medicaid. Moreover, many patients who lack insurance have poor records. Neither of those facts is the fault of the doctor. The point is not that all doctors are innocent, but the tactics used are unfair and the DEA does not understand medicine.

The case of Dr. Harvey Jenkins in Oklahoma City is one example from Dr. Cheek's collection of more than one thousand doctors who have been charged. There was no evidence of diversion. The allegations against him were based solely on the amount he prescribed. Comments made by a representative of the attorney general's office, Ms. Fry, were reported in a local news source[566]:

> I would say that operation was dangerous to our society. There's not an abundance of doctors specializing in pain management who see mostly Medicaid patients. Though Jenkins may have been seeing patients that other doctors would

not, that fact makes Jenkins' alleged conduct all the more egregious. It put him at a higher standard, because he knew what kind of patients he was getting. These are the ones who had very difficult cases.

Ms. Fry appears to be saying that a doctor should be held to a higher standard because he took on difficult cases that other doctors turned away. Such statements exemplify the issue of poverty that is not receiving appropriate attention in the debate over opioid therapy. The implication is that poorer patients are more likely to abuse their prescriptions and Dr. Jenkins should have somehow taken this into account. The authorities always pay lip service to the need to ensure that all citizens have access to pain medicine. Yet when they closed down Dr. Jenkins's pain clinic, hundreds of patients were left without anywhere to turn. Dr. Harvey's case with twenty-nine charges of drug trafficking was remanded for trial in 2017, but there is no record that it is has been heard. This information strongly suggests a plea bargain, which is the usual outcome.

The War on Pain Patients

It sounds like an exaggeration at first, but as the facts are clarified, it becomes clear that the consequences of anti-opioid zealotry have negatively impacted pain patients in an increasingly direct manner. Elderly and sick patients who have relied on a doctor for years or live in a remote area have few options for continuing their medication when their physician is suddenly arrested or a clinic is shut down. It is astounding that state medical boards have no contingency plan for the patient abandonment that occurs in such cases. *Patient abandonment* is not the correct phrase since the doctors do not willingly leave their patients but are prohibited from writing prescriptions. Although not a victim of prosecution, Sean Greenwood was a patient of Dr. Hurwitz who lost access to his pain medication when Dr. Hurwitz was arrested. Greenwood died in 2003, only a few years after he lost access to the dosage of medication he needed to alleviate the pain of Ehlers-Danlos syndrome. He died of a brain hemorrhage probably caused by the high blood pressure he experienced from the painful condition he had. His wife, Siobhan Reynolds, made a documentary called "The Chilling Effect" about his life and Mr. Paey's experience. In addition, Dr. Tennant's patient Trini Yaeger, who suffered from adhesive arachnoiditis, was put on life support after her opioid dose was cut. The governor of California finally interceded as an act of mercy to request that she receive medical help—the opioids—she needed.[565]

When the DEA and state law enforcement close down a clinic, the DEA cannot possibly have considered the health status of the patients. Every doctor who prescribes opioids has to live in fear that if a patient of theirs dies for any reason, even one that has nothing to do with the opioid prescription, they may be blamed for the fatality. Yet when the DEA prosecutes a doctor and patients die as a result, it is not even noticed by the authorities. When Dr. Hurwitz was arrested, two of his patients committed suicide shortly thereafter. One of Dr. Tennant's patients committed suicide shortly after his practice was closed.[305] Patients who die of complications from pain or a combination of pain and withdrawal are rarely counted.[268]

No one could argue that the federal agencies are showing compassion for pain patients, but has the *war on prescription drugs* become a *war on pain patients*? Dr. Humphries, one of the proponents of strict limitations on opioid prescribing, denied that there is a *war on pain patients* in an interview on National Public Radio.[35] Later I will discuss the inaccuracies in Mr. Mann's report, but here I will provide information that describes the plight of pain patients denied by Dr. Humphries. Dr. Kline's practice in Raleigh, North Carolina, was shut down by DEA agents apparently because of complaint by a heroin addict in New York State who did not like his YouTube videos on pain management. Dr. Kline had practiced for forty years at the time he was forced to close. Dr. Kline has stressed that his patients were all people who had serious, rare diseases. Dr. Kline found a doctor in Virginia who took on the thirty-four patients remaining in his practice. Subsequently, the doctor in Virginia received notification that Medicare would not reimburse him if he continued to write opioid prescriptions for the patients. If this is not a war on pain patients, then someone needs to explain why the federal government is so determined to make these people suffer. Dr. Kline is still under investigation, but it is unclear what the allegations are. None of his patients died, and no one has accused any of his patients of selling their prescriptions.

The case of Richard Paey was an example of how the size of a prescription alone became incriminating evidence against a patient. Richard Paey was severely injured in a car crash in 1995. He was paraplegic and in severe pain. After a surgery gone wrong, he also began to develop symptoms of multiple sclerosis. He moved from New Jersey to Florida with a large number of prescriptions from his previous doctor to last him until he could find a new pain specialist. He did find a new specialist, but in the meantime, the large doses he was prescribed came to the attention of local law enforcement when he filled his prescription at a Florida pharmacy. They followed him and attempted to find evidence of diversion. When they could not find any evidence of diversion, they approached his Florida pain specialist and lied to him, saying that Paey had admitted that the prescriptions were forged. The doctor agreed to testify against Paey. After three attempts at jury trial, Paey received a twenty-five-year sentence. Ironically, he was given the higher doses of morphine that he needed while in prison because of the fear that he would die in prison without sufficient pain medication. Ultimately, the governor of Florida pardoned Mr. Paey.[567] It is truly a perverse policy that gives better treatment to pain patients in prison than under a doctor's care.

Prescription Fentanyl Spray for Breakthrough Cancer Pain or Whatever Ails You

There is yet another scheme for illegal distribution of prescription drugs that was revealed in court in the past few years. Although Purdue Pharma has been convicted of false advertising, it is still not clear how their various distributors sent such large shipments of pills to the pill mills. We do not know the extent to which the sale of opioids to specific large volume pill mills was initiated by the distributors or, alternatively, the result of criminal organizations that realized an opportunity and negotiated with the distributor. However, the smaller company, Insys, provides an even more direct insight how a company can facilitate the sale of a large quantity of opioids for a purpose that they were not intended. Insys's major product was a sublingual fentanyl spray known as Subsys. The fentanyl spray delivered intense short-term relief and was FDA approved for breakthrough pain in cancer patients. The company's founder, John Kapoor, realized that his company was initially having financial difficulty because the market for breakthrough pain in cancer is relatively small. Kapoor hired a sales team who had relatively little knowledge of pharmaceuticals to implement a corrupt strategy of directly rewarding doctors with bribes and sexual favors, admitted by employee John Burlakoff, who entered a plea deal with federal prosecutors. According to the allegations, bribes including money paid as a "speakers' program" fee for their supposed participation in speaking events, which were often little more than a business dinner. The system of rewards or bribes for the doctors was based on prescribing Subsys, but also on increasing each patient's dose of Subsys. For a drug as a strong as fentanyl combined with the rapid delivery of a sublingual spray, this was a prescription for addiction.

More than seven thousand people have died of Subsys overdoses.[568] Less than 10% of them were cancer patients. The deaths comprise more than 3% of all drug overdoses during the past three years. The scheme used to sell Subsys ultimately led to prosecution of the Dr. Kapoor and several members of the sales team for racketeering.[569] This is a well-documented specific example of an illegal use of opioids that must be separated from appropriate use for cancer pain. The narrative that the origin of the crisis is legitimate doctors prescribing opioids for pain developed by PROP totally ignores the diversion by Purdue and bribing of doctors by Insys, both of whom engaged in pushing sales of opioids irrespective of any medical need. After the conviction of Insys president and several company officers, prosecutors have begun to investigate whether other companies engaged in similar practices. There are pending investigations of Amerisource Bergen, Amneal Pharmaceuticals, Johnson & Johnson, McKesson, Mallinckrodt, and Teva Pharmaceutical Industries.[570] PROP and others are blaming the major portion of the problem on doctors and their prescribing, not on criminal diversion. Yet in the case of Subsys, the problem is apparently 90% one of criminal diversion. It is important to distinguish these carefully because blaming legitimate prescribing is a major reason for the current war on pain patients. While doctors have acted badly in these instances, there has been systemic mismanagement and criminal intent from outside the medical community behind much of the harmful prescribing.

Blaming the Heroin and Fentanyl Overdose Waves on Prescription Drugs

By 2010, a drumbeat of media reports, public policy debates, government agency actions, and political speeches focused on the narrative that prescription drugs are responsible for addiction and drug overdose. Up to 2011, the trends in the data supported that view. But that was a temporary correlation. A longer-term view, even then, would have given a different perspective of a larger problem. For the past forty years, one drug has been substituted for another as drug use has increased steadily. Price and availability have largely been the determining factors of which particular drug is most prevalent. The narrative used by the authorities to explain the failed policy is the *gateway drug* concept. In the 1970s, marijuana was called a gateway drug. Today studies show that states that have legalized marijuana have lower rates of heroin addiction, which contradicts that particular gateway drug theory. Because many of the people dying of overdose today once tried OxyContin, the proponents of the current version of the theory claim that Oxy is a *gateway drug*.[571] This narrative is a way to deflect responsibility for failure to take any action for ten years, the lack of planning once prescriptions were restricted, and the extremely poor state of services for addicts that result in fatalities. The gateway drug narrative implies that if a particular drug were missing, the addiction rate would decrease, ignoring the fact that there are parallel pathways to addiction.

Neither the addiction nor overdose rate has decreased in any of the past forty years. Every time one drug was in short supply, another drug took its place. It was a poor practice to overprescribe OxyContin, but that did not mean that Oxy *caused the epidemic*. A Rand Corporation study placed the blame on Medicare Part D, which expanded access to opioids in people sixty-five and older.[572] Medicare Part D, which expanded coverage to outpatient prescriptions, was fully implemented in 2006. The Rand study suggested a 10% increase in medical access to opioids led to a 7.4% increase in opioid deaths. This is a small fraction of the total drug overdose deaths. The report purports to provide a causal explanation, but it ignores the major role played by diversion in opioid overdoses. Given the sources and magnitude of diversion that we have considered up to this point, there is no evidence to support the notion that elderly individuals would be a more likely source of diverted opioids than pill mills and an extensive black market.

Pat Beall's articles showed quantitatively that rapidly terminating prescriptions of prescription drugs resulted in significant number of users making a switch to heroin in 2011.[507] Instead of saving thousands of people who had been affected by the diversion schemes tolerated by the DEA and state legislatures, the policies introduced to crack down on prescribing pushed those people to take a much more dangerous drug and dramatically increased the overdose rate. This mistake has been repeated numerous times in other locations during the crackdown on prescription medications. To add to tragedy, none of this justified taking medication away from legitimate pain patients, as is happening today.

As the crisis evolved, the nature of overdose deaths changed. It is important to understand that heroin was present and responsible for many of the deaths even during the prescription-drug wave. Because of its much higher potency, a kilogram of fentanyl has nearly twenty-five times monetary value higher than a kilogram of heroin. It is also at least one hundred times as dangerous. Heroin and *synthetic opioids* fentanyl and carfentanyl caused 80% of the opioid deaths in

2018 and 2019.[270,573] The addiction problem has taken on a whole new dimension because of these very powerful drugs. There is no doubt that fentanyl used by addicts is not derived from a prescription source. Fentanyl prescriptions are dwarfed by the amount of illegal fentanyl that makes it to market in the United States. Despite these facts, the link between prescription drugs and drug overdoses has been forged in the mind of the public by politicians and media. The media continues to develop this narrative despite the fact that prescription drugs were involved in less than 20% of overdose deaths in 2019. When we consider that the 20% is composed of 75% diverted and 25% directly prescribed, the percentage of overdose deaths from directly prescribed prescription drugs is 5% of the total.[513]

Thus, the overdose deaths from pain patients who obtained a legitimate opioid prescription from their doctor is small fraction of the total. Many of the 5% of overdose deaths can be attributed directly to prescription of benzodiazepines with opioids. Benzodiazepines are an antianxiety medication and sedative that should never be combined with opioids because they dramatically increase the risk of respiratory suppression. The rate of accidental overdose by patients with their own prescriptions is very low and mainly because of mistakes in prescribing. Pushing for hard limits and tapering patients is harmful to patients, and it only exacerbates the overdose crisis.

In a recent study, Gallagher and coworkers wrote the following[574]:

> The narrative of the opioid crisis is that ill-informed and careless prescribing by physicians has led to increases in opioid-related harms including overdose deaths. Focusing on reducing the access to prescribed opioids without treating substance use disorder has led to increases in use of heroin and illicitly produced fentanyl. Overall prescribing of opioids has declined causing collateral damage to those who use opioids appropriately to reduce pain and improve function. The complexity of this issue requires a change in focus and

broad changes in society's approach to substance abuse and mental health.

This is a response to PROP's arguments that pain patients are in danger of addiction because of their own prescriptions.[11,12,52] We should be concerned about what happens to patients when they lose their prescriptions or when their doses are drastically reduced. When pain becomes unbearable, people will consider things that they never would have thought to do under normal circumstances.

Nowhere to Turn—a Paucity of Opioid Treatment Programs Exacerbates the Crisis

Receiving treatment for addiction in the US has always been difficult.[499] There has been a common attitude that maintenance therapy should not be provided to help heroin addicts recover. However, abstinence is not possible for majority of addicts.[485] The private insurance system of the US makes treatment expensive or simply not accessible for most addicts. Wealthy families can pay for rehabilitation, but others would have to apply for Medicaid. Given the legal ramifications and stigma, there is great fear among addicts to reveal their identity.[575]

Rather than treating people, the legal system has been putting them in jail for possession charges or even minor infractions. Incarceration tends to increase the overdose rate. People who have been incarcerated and are released are twice as likely to die of a fentanyl overdose compared to the general population. The greater the duration of their imprisonment is, the greater the likelihood of them overdosing. When people get out of prison, they are at their most vulnerable and they do not know what trends have affected the society. For example, the change from heroin to fentanyl happened relatively quickly, and some users may have no warning about the potency of the new drug.

There is a need for greater access to treatment programs with methadone/buprenorphine, syringe services programs (SSPs), and psychological counseling services.[576] Many members of local communities had moral objections to SSPs, and even users are often discouraged despite the increases in HIV and hepatitis C that occurred without such services in rural parts of the United States.[577] These negative community attitudes toward syringe service programs (SSPs) and opioid-treatment programs (OTPs) mean that they are underfunded and are often intimidating to the intended participants.[578]

Methadone clinics are the lowest-cost option for those who want to recover. As an example of the obstacles, *The West Palm Beach Post* series described how the Florida Department of Children and Families (DCF) failed to approve new methadone clinics for years, forcing those addicts who wanted to find a way out to drive up to one hundred miles per day to pay the twenty dollars to receive a dose of methadone.[429] In fact, by 2011, when the need was greatest there was such a shortage of methadone clinics in the state that many addicts were giving up. Pat Beall documented the story of one woman's struggle for survival. She had been beaten beyond recognition as a young woman and had an abusive husband, who died when he eventually turned to heroin. Then she decided she would go to a methadone clinic to quit heroin. She knew that people were dying of fentanyl added to the heroin powder. However, a person in rehabilitation must get a dose of methadone every day. The state does not permit a person to consume the methadone outside the dispensary. One day, she drove to her dispensary, only to find that it had closed down because of state negligence in approving the renewal. The next day she was found dead of a fentanyl overdose.[429]

Patients who can pay more are often steered to buprenorphine.[10,295,499–502] Buprenorphine is a partial MOR agonist, which explains its analgesic effect, but it is also a KOR antagonist, which helps to reduce anxiety and other adverse side effects of withdrawal.[181] While buprenorphine appears to be the most recommended alternative to methadone today, in a study of more than five thousand patients who were being given methadone or buprenorphine, the study found that the buprenorphine patients were 2.8 times more likely to quit the program and the methadone patients were 1.8 times more likely to be discharged on recommendation of the provider.[579]

Comments made by former addicts suggest that buprenorphine is unpleasant, while methadone is tolerable. Neither is considered pleasant, but they both satisfy the craving that addicts have and prevent withdrawal symptom. It appears that even wanting to feel comfortable is seen as a weakness or moral failing. Despite this fact, many drug users are switching because they realize that it is a matter of life and death.

If addicts could be seen in private by a medical doctor, it could greatly increase their willingness to seek treatment.[580] However, addiction is still not formally treated as a disease, despite some progress over the years. The separation of pain medicine from addiction can present a problem of how to treat a pain patient who shows signs of addiction. A doctor can receive a diplomate of board certification in pain management or addiction medicine, but not both. Thus, pain patients can be terminated for any suspicion that they have misused their medication, and after that, they are unlikely to be seen by a pain-management specialist. Instead, they are stigmatized with an opioid use disorder. Each case is different, of course, but what often happens is that a patient who is an outcast from a pain clinic or primary care doctor for violation of an agreement or any irregularity is on the path to being classified as an addict. Addicts have pain too. How do people with addiction receive treatment for pain? Historically, it was always possible for a doctor to write a prescription for methadone for pain, even for a patient known to be an addict. But today, because the issue has become so charged, very few doctors would consider even meeting such a patient, let alone writing a prescription. As one doctor put it to me, "Those conversations just don't happen anymore."

Starting in 2000 with the Drug Addiction Treatment Act, it has been possible for medical doctors to prescribe certain opioids, today mainly buprenorphine, to opioid-drug addicts. This is known as medication-assisted treatment (MAT). MAT is the first step toward treating opioid use disorder as a disease.[581] However, there are still many obstacles to widespread use of MAT in the treatment of opioid addiction. A physician who wishes to prescribe using MAT must attend training and obtain a waiver, which is basically a special permit from the DEA, a so-called "X" permit. While MAT is preferable to state-run methadone clinics and cheaper than rehabilitation,[582] there are many barriers to convincing physicians to take on the added risk,[583] and fewer than 5% of doctors have elected to obtain a MAT waiver.[584] Doctors are reluctant to prescribe buprenorphine because of the challenge of insurance reimbursement, and also because some of them do not want recovering drug users in their clinics.[502] Some fear diversion of buprenorphine.[585] While buprenorphine is potentially a promising opioid for pain management,[586] it is incompatible with morphine in the sense that a patient on heroin or fentanyl (or any other drug in that class) must taper down to zero before starting to take buprenorphine. A second aspect of buprenorphine is its long half-life, which means that administration requires a completely different routine than other drugs.[587-589] A third aspect is the fact that buprenorphine tends to become less effective at higher doses, unlike other opioids such as morphine, oxycodone, or hydromorphone. We say that those opioids have no ceiling.

Many areas in the United States are opioid-treatment deserts with no options for heroin addicts.[590] The government could improve the situation simply by making the waivers easier to obtain, reducing the fear of prosecution by establishing clear and reasonable guidelines, and helping ensure the medical coding is appropriate for insurance reimbursement.[295,296] On the other hand, some lawmakers have indicated that they would prefer abstinence to giving any kind of relief for the craving of withdrawal, despite the failure of abstinence program in producing results.[485,591] In reaction to these inhumane policies, some doctors are beginning to call for deregulation of buprenorphine, which would permit them to treat persons with opioid use disorder without the barriers that exist today.[592]

There is both a shortage of facilities and an unwillingness of drug addicts to seek out treatment. While the treatment facilities are operating at 80% capacity, only 60% of addicts are being treated. Significant gaps between treatment need and capacity exist at the national level.[593] There is good evidence showing that people are not seeking treatment. Despite a sixfold increase in heroin addiction rates from 2000 to 2014, drug detoxification treatment rates were essentially constant.[594,595]

The Failed War on Prescription Drugs

It is hard to imagine how the DEA, an agency that controls every aspect of import, production, prescription, and sales, permitted as large a scandal as the prescription drug phase of opioid crisis to occur. The explanation of the three waves presented by the CDC is worse than an embarrassment for law enforcement, including the DEA and politicians in the Florida legislature and in Congress in Washington, DC. However, it is a scandal that the American public will not know about as long as their anger is directed at *Big Pharma, the pharmacies,* and even *the doctors* for producing, selling, and prescribing drugs. While PROP is trying to portray the pharmaceutical companies and the American Pain Society as the guilty parties, they are leaving out the larger context. The corruption that permitted the movement to be coopted extends to the highest levels of government and involves numerous examples of influence peddling and lobbying to prevent the DEA from taking action against the large companies. Some people's addictions have started in doctors' offices. That was a preventable tragedy, and people have a right to be angry. However, the image of this type of prescribing as the cause of a major epidemic distracts from much larger forces at work. Illegal drug use, in aggregate, has been increasing for the past fifty years. The only reason that the heroin addiction rate was lower in the 2000s compared to previous decades was because cocaine and crack had taken the dominant position. Focusing on prescription drugs, pill mills were selling millions of pills in a blatant manner that was recorded in the DEA database. Shipments of huge volumes of opioids from the pharmaceutical companies were sent to sparsely populated counties in Appalachia and to Broward and Palm Beach counties in Florida.[250,252,253,255,459] Each one of these operations affected thousands or even tens of thousands. The lawsuits against the Big Pharma and the pharmacies keep the media focused on prescription drugs, but the public has not been given the information in a way that clarifies the true criminal nature of what happened. The media reports need to spell out clearly the cause and effect that led to the current heroin and fentanyl epidemic to prevent further confusion. That is not happening because law firms are now the ones driving the politics by making campaign contributions and keeping the narrative of the prescription drug epidemic foremost in the minds of the public.[261] Their campaign contributions and influence with Congress benefits their multibillion-dollar legal strategy to sue every opioid manufacturer and pharmacy.

CHAPTER 11

꧂

Succumbing to the Fear of Addiction

Opium has been used to treat pain in the Western world for hundreds of years. After 1680 opium was used in an alcohol solution known as laudanum as a sedative and as pain medicine.[17] In 1803, Friedrich Saturner first extracted morphine from opium, and in 1855, Alexander Wood developed the hypodermic syringe used mainly for the injection of morphine into patients in pain. By the middle of the nineteenth century, it was common to use morphine to treat terminally ill cancer patients. In 1874, John Kent Spender, a doctor in Bath, England, wrote the following[17]:

> Seldom does it afford more pride and pleasure to be a physician. One of the chief blessings of opium is to help us in granting the boon of a comparatively painless death. The medical man who (from ignorance or timidity) withholds hypodermic medication from a patient afflicted with cancer is totally without excuse.

It was recognized that morphine is addictive, but it was not considered a major public health issue in the nineteenth century. The change in attitude began in 1874 when the diacetyl derivative of morphine known as heroin was synthesized by Dr. C. Alder Wright. Ironically, Wright had been searching for a less addictive form of morphine. Initially, heroin was sold in a formulation with aspirin as a remedy for headache. However, in 1900 users in the United States discovered that the heroin could be extracted from the headache pills and taken in a variety of ways as a potent euphoric drug. This led to a new phase in the history of addiction and ultimately to new laws that would criminalize all opioids. The punitive policies toward addiction have been creating misery for addicts, pain patients, and the society at large ever since.[485]

During the 1960s, Dr. Cecily Saunders of Saint Christopher's hospice in London gave terminal cancer patients sufficient doses of morphine and heroin to alleviate their suffering during their final days and weeks of life.[64] The philosophy was not vastly different from that of Dr. Spender in 1874, except that by 1960, there was fifty years of history of criminal prosecutions and a campaign against addiction that added to the barriers to use in hospice. Dr. Saunders pointed out the absurdity of worrying about whether someone who is dying of cancer is going to become addicted to opioids. But beyond palliative care of terminal cancer patients, it would take decades before the general use of opioids to alleviate suffering of patients with other painful diseases, such as sickle cell disease, multiple sclerosis, lupus, ankylosing spondylitis, psoriatic arthritis, and so on. Now PROP has effectively put a stop to those efforts to treat persistent pain. PROP has made it a mission to redefine the epidemiology, public policy, and clinical study by raising the specter of addiction as the necessary consequence of the treatment of chronic pain patients.

Clinical Ethics—Individualized Care Is Required When Definitive Evidence Is Lacking

A brief discussion of medical ethics is warranted prior to examining the arguments advanced by PROP. In a 2010 article in the journal *Pain*, Dr. Ballantyne gave an ethical justification for refusal of treatment with opioids as a responsibility of a physician who has reason to doubt the benefit of treatment or can predict a sufficiently high risk.[130] The ethical review is a reaction to ideas of patient satisfaction, which had gained sway in medical practice. She argued that physicians must use their own judgment and should not feel compelled to provide opioid therapy simply because patients demand them. While she was speaking of the need to be firm, her publication shows significant sensitivity to the needs of individual pain patients. However, in light of the formation of PROP in 2011 and the subsequent effort to lobby for restrictions on all pain patients, the ethical arguments in the letter appear to justify not just an individual or case-by-case consideration of whether to deny care, but rather a decision to deny care to all pain patients. Her ethical argument was criticized in 2015 by Cohen and Jangro, who pointed out that in such a *data-thin* field as opioid therapy, with such a long history of consensus, clinical ethics should apply.[5] That is to say, individual needs and conditions are paramount and general policies that apply to all patients are not ethically justified. Clinical ethics require consideration of individual patient needs in the absence of good evidence regarding the efficacy; it is unethical to deny therapy that might be efficacious for some patients.

PROP's Case That Pain Patients Are Intrinsically at Risk of Addiction

In an article entitled "The Prescription Opioid and Heroin Crisis: A Public Health Approach to an Epidemic of Addiction," in the *Annual Review of Public Health*, Dr. Kolodny and coworkers explain their viewpoint that prescription opioids are harmful to *all* patients, even the patients who take them as directed.[12] The hypothesis of the *Annual Review*[12] is that opioid prescription will lead to addiction of any patient, even pain patients. Dr. Kolodny equates this inherent propensity toward addiction with *iatrogenic addiction*. Iatrogenic refers to "a disease or condition that is caused by the medical procedure." The *Annual Review*[12] has some suggestions for how to treat addiction, but the perfunctory section on prevention of addiction lacks originality and could easily be replaced by standard language from the National Institute on Drug Abuse website. The point of this article is clearly to make the case that pain patients are intrinsically at risk for addiction.

PROP is reacting to the failure of the compassionate care movement to consider addiction as a significant risk when prescriptions increased in 1996. Many observers agree that doctors who prescribed large doses of opioids should have been more vigilant in checking whether patients showed signs of succumbing to addiction. However, our medical and legal system separate pain management from addiction treatment in a manner that makes it all but impossible for a doctor to treat both. Treating addiction is only possible with a waiver or other special circumstances.[295,296] Addiction treatment has been neglected for a long time. Nonetheless, the failure to include referral for counseling and treatment for addiction as one of the agenda items in a multifaceted program to treat persistent pain is a major failing. It is crucial to consider the issue of addiction as the medical community assesses what has been learned from the compassionate care movement.

Rather than consider how the medical system could expand care to treat both pain patients and drug addicts with compassion, specialists in addiction medicine, like Drs. Kolodny and Lembke, claim that addiction is inevitable and persistent-pain patients are especially vulnerable. Dr. Kolodny is trying to prove that addiction is inherent in opioid prescribing and that the drug companies knew this harm existed. Is it coincidence that this argument strengthens the case against Big Pharma in the courtroom? Dr. Kolodny attempts to discredit his critics in the medical community, and even pain patients, by claiming that they are paid by pharmaceutical companies. Meanwhile, he is being paid by the law firms who are suing the pharmaceutical companies. I have no connection to the companies, and I am as outraged as Dr. Kolodny about Purdue Pharma's false advertising. However, I strenuously disagree with Dr. Kolodny's methods and his goals, because I can see the enormous harm his advocacy has done to pain patients. The objection I am raising to the *Annual Review*'s case for "iatrogenic addiction" is not a defense of Purdue Pharma. It is a defense of pain patients. Dr. Kolodny's callous disregard for the welfare of hundreds of thousands of pain patients is a breach of clinical ethics. Clinical ethics require that patients should be treated as individuals in the absence of definitive evidence of a specific harm that would argue against prescription of a medication.[5]

The fear of "iatrogenic addiction" is raised in the *Annual Review* as the justification to limit prescribing. However, the evidence is weak or misattributed. In the section entitled "Opioid Addiction Is a Key Driver for Morbidity and Mortality," a number of publications are cited showing that people with a history of substance abuse are more likely to die from an overdose.[561,596] The authors of the *Annual Review* wrote,

> The sharp increase in the prevalence of opioid addiction is a key driver of opioid-related morbidity and mortality. The misattribution of the opioid crisis to nonmedical use or abuse rather than to addiction has stymied efforts to address this crisis because it has led to a focus on policies to prevent such nonmedical use at the expense of greater resources committed to preventing and treating opioid addiction in both medical and nonmedical users.

The articles cited in the *Annual Review* publication are particularly poorly chosen because they provide no information on the relationship between medical use and addiction. In fact, the limited evidence the references provide supports the hypothesis that the nonmedical use is associated with opioid use disorders, precisely the point that Dr. Kolodny wishes to dispute.

The reference by Hser and coworkers was a follow-up with heroin addicts from the 1960s each decade up to the 1990s.[596] In this thirty-three-year retrospective study, approximately 60% of the heroin addicts had passed away and most of the others still had substance abuse problems. This observational study had nothing to do with prescription opioids. The study by Hall and coworkers[561] showed that 84.5% of decedents from drug overdoses in West Virginia in 2006 obtained prescription opioid drugs either by diversion or doctor shopping. There was no evidence that these individuals were pain patients. The third reference was a study in Utah on victims of unintentional overdose. The study found 80% of the overdose victims were substance abusers.[597] There was no evidence presented that there is any intersection of the population of heroin addicts and prescription opioid abusers with legitimate pain patients in any of these studies. Therefore, these studies did not offer any evidence regarding the addiction of pain patients.

The Weak, Weak, Weak Evidence for Iatrogenic Addiction

Generalizing for all pain patients, Dr. Kolodny and co-authors wrote,[12]

> The incidence of iatrogenic opioid addiction in patients treated with long-term [opioid pain relievers] is unknown because adequately designed prospective studies have not been conducted. However, opioid-use disorders appear to be highly prevalent in chronic pain patients treated with [opioid pain relievers].

The *Annual Review* article[12] further made the claim that doctors are causing addiction and overdose in their patients by providing the opioid medications. The article uses a non-standard acronym OPR for opioid pain reliever, which we have spelled out in the excerpt below, for clarity.

> Over the past decade, federal and state policy makers have attempted to reduce [opioid pain reliever] abuse and [opioid pain reliever]-related overdose deaths. Despite these efforts, morbidity and mortality associated with [opioid pain relievers] have continued to worsen in almost every state. Thus far, these efforts have focused primar-

ily on preserving access to [opioid pain relievers] for chronic pain patients while reducing non-medical [opioid pain reliever] use, defined as the use of a medication without a prescription, in a way other than as prescribed, or for the experience or feeling it causes. However, policy makers who focus solely on reducing nonmedical use are failing to appreciate the high opioid-related morbidity and mortality in pain patients receiving [opioid pain reliever] prescriptions for medical purposes.

First, it was not clear why the *Annual Review* article[12] made this argument in 2015 since by that time the trend was already evident that mortality associated with opioid pain relievers had decreased since 2010 while the overall overdose rate due mainly to heroin and fentanyl had increased dramatically. The figure used in the publication showing a parallel increase in prescribing and overdose between 2000 and 2010 was already outdated by the time the paper was published. Second, the evidence cited to support the contention that pain patients have a high mortality, because their own medications consisted of two isolated data sets that are not obviously related. Based on 2011 data, the greatest nonmedical use of prescription medications was by the fifteen-to-twenty-four-year-old age group and decreases steadily with age. The interpretation was that older users tend to use legitimate prescriptions, while diversion was greater for younger people. The data also showed that the forty-five-to-fifty-four-year-old age group had the highest prescription drug overdose mortality in 2011.[12] Since people in the older age group tended to be legitimate pain patients rather than drug users, the authors concluded that "opioid overdoses appear to occur more frequently in medical OPR [opioid pain reliever] users [pain patients] than in young nonmedical users." This conclusion ignored the larger context of drug use. As the *Annual Review* article[12] showed, heroin overdose fatalities in the younger age group were growing rapidly throughout this period. The fact that relatively few younger users died of diverted prescription medications in 2011 was directly related to the shut-down of the pill mills, and massive diversion schemes in 2010, as we have already discussed. Finally, after many years of corruption and incompetence, PDMPs, as imperfect as they are, were put in place, and the diversion market had become prohibitively difficult. This disproportionately affected the younger age group. Evidence suggests that the younger age group of drug users turned to heroin as sources of OxyContin were closed down.[507] The younger group was dying mainly of heroin overdoses. Prior to 2007, the overdose rate of all age groups increased in parallel, but after 2007, the heroin death of younger users skyrocketed and prescription overdose rates fell for that group.[598] According to CDC death rate statistics, prescription drugs were involved in 39% of drug overdoses in 2011, the peak year for prescription drug overdoses.[598] There has been a substantial increase in heroin overdoses in the older age groups as well in recent years, although they are still far less than the younger age groups.[599] The analysis of the death statistics must also account for the fact that multiple drugs are present in most of the deceased. The comparison between the age groups does not tell us percentage who died in total from each type of drug, which complicates the comparison.

Dr. Kolodny claims that the abuse potential of prescription opi-oids is as great as that of heroin. Causality is difficult to determine. One can understand the trends by examining the overdose fatality data for all drugs to have an estimate of how many people died from prescription drugs relative to illegal drugs. This is a point missed by Kolodny and coworkers, who make a relative comparison of age groups to try to determine the risk of prescription drug overdose. In aggregate, prescription drugs are found on autopsy on 39% of over-dose fatalities, the cause of death is likely to be heroin for the 19% of overdoses where both heroin and prescription drugs are found. Thus, approximately 20% of overdoses in 2011 were due solely to prescription drugs. Several sources agree that approximately 75% of those who died using prescription drugs obtained them illegally.[600,601] If we assume that 25% of all prescription drug users who died of an overdose had a legitimate prescription, one can conclude that at most

10% (i.e., 25% of 39%) of total overdoses were caused by prescription pain relievers from legitimate prescriptions in 2011.

What can we say about the relative risk of overdose from use of prescription drugs compared to heroin? According to the *Annual Review* article,[12] there were 10 million persistent-pain patients receiving opioid prescriptions. According to the Substance Abuse and Mental Health Services Administration (SAMHSA), in 2012, there were 2.1 million Americans addicted to prescription opioids and 669,000 addicted to heroin.[601] Using 10 million as the total population of pain patients receiving an opioid prescription, the overdose rate *among prescription drug patients* is 41.4 per 100,000. We can compare this to the overdose rate *among heroin users*, which was 692 per 100,000. Contrary to Dr. Kolodny's assertion, the data show that heroin is seventeen times deadlier than prescription drugs.

The authors of the *Annual Review* article[12] state that "[opioid pain relievers] have an abuse liability similar to that of heroin." The implication is that the "abuse" is from legitimate pain patients who receive a prescription. According to the *Annual Review* article,[12] 25% of pain patients who used prescription opioids had opioid use disorders. The value of 25% is rather high compared to any of the published studies on use disorders.[4,9,133,137–139,141,142,300] The official statistic that there 2.1 million people with opioid-use disorder and 10 million pain patients with prescriptions sets the maximum for abuse at 21%. However, there is no evidence that these groups overlap and percentage of actual pain patients who have opioid-use disorder is estimated by many studies to be significantly lower. Diversion of prescription drugs is responsible for 75% of the 2.1 million who abuse those drugs according to the sources chosen by Dr. Kolodny and coworkers.[143,600,601] One can conclude that the percentage of legitimate pain patients who develop opioid use disorders is circa 5% (i.e., 25% of 21%), which is in a range that agrees with other estimates cited above. Dr. Kolodny's main contention appears to be that addiction caused by legitimate prescriptions has been ignored, but the publications he cites show that diverted prescription drugs are responsible for the majority of overdose deaths. His own evidence refutes his contention.

The *Annual Review* article creates the fear that opioid prescribing is causing addiction. The concept of *iatrogenic addiction* is based on a conjecture about how two distinct data sets may be correlated. There are many trends in drug abuse that are larger than prescription drug abuse: heroin/fentanyl, crack cocaine, cocaine, methamphetamine, MDMA, and many others.[495] Taken together, these other trends are many times greater than true prescription drug abuse of the type that Dr. Kolodny and coworkers are considering with their hypothesis of iatrogenic addiction.

Who Is a Pain Patient, and Who Is a Substance Abuser?

Our medical and legal system has created a situation in which the line between legitimate pain patient and substance abuser is so crucial and yet simultaneously poorly defined. That line is blurred repeatedly in the *Annual Review*, where the question is supposed to be whether legitimate pain patients are in danger of being led into addiction by their prescriptions. There is evidence that pain patients tend to follow their prescription. For one thing, in the current system, any patient who deviates even slightly from the contract is dismissed from the pain clinic. Most often one infraction is sufficient. The patient may subsequently be labeled with a substance-use-disorder diagnosis. By constantly doubting pain patients, by failing to support them when they are most vulnerable, and by not taking their pain seriously, our society and medical system are both pushing pain patients toward aberrant behaviors. While there is good evidence that pain patients respond differently to opioids than pain-naive people, the assumption is that pain is controlled. When pain is not controlled, the psychological consequences can be devastating. A medical system that does not recognize that fact is cruel.

Another important issue is to understand the origin of substance abuse. Depression and psychiatric problems are two common reasons for substance abuse. Patients can abuse prescription drugs, but that does not mean that denying access to prescription drugs will end the tendency of the patients to seek opioids or other drugs. There are other trends buried in the comparisons discussed above. For example, older people tend to have a cumulative balance of health conditions and psychiatric issues that may lead to use disorders and to thoughts of suicide. A study of 1,149 overdose deaths nationwide primarily arising from prescription drugs found that there was a significant component of the older population who committed suicide using their prescriptions.[602] Deaths from prescription drug overdose also increased by nearly twofold in Sweden from 2006 to 2014. Sweden is a useful point of reference since it has drug statistics more like the United States compared to any other European country. Using the national database, the results of patients who received opioid medication for pain and those who had known substance use disorder (SUD) were tracked to discover that most of the overdose deaths were attributable to the SUD population.[603] The Swedish paper drew the conclusion that there were two separate populations, those who use the opioids for pain relief and those who have a psychological disturbance or SUD that leads to either suicide or unintended overdose. We cannot deny treatment to all patients because some of them are at risk for suicide. Rather, we must understand the conditions that give rise to the at-risk population and find ways to help them.

The Evidence Refutes the Concept of Iatrogenic Addiction

The *Annual Review* article[12] admitted there were no adequate studies to support the claim of *iatrogenic opioid addiction*. The authors cited an article by Boscarino and coworkers in the journal *Addiction Research Reports* to address dependence in pain patients and how that might lead to addiction.[143] A collection of 705 patients who had received more than four prescriptions for opioids per year compared to a control group he found that approximately 22% of patients exhibited signs of "opioid dependence." The precise meaning of the term *dependence* is not defined anywhere in the article, except that it refers to the *Diagnostic and Statistical Manual of Mental Disorder, 4th edition (DSM-IV)*.[13] That source gives the following definitions.

Substance Dependence: A maladaptive pattern of substance use leading to clinically significant impairment or distress is manifested by three or more of the following, occurring at any time in the same 12-month period:

- Tolerance, as defined by either of the following:
    - A need for markedly increased amounts of the substance to achieve intoxication or desired effect
    - Markedly diminished effect with continued use of the same amount of the substance
- Withdrawal, as manifested by either of the following:
    - The characteristic withdrawal syndrome for the substance
    - Taking the same (or a closely related) substance to relieve or avoid withdrawal symptoms
- Taking the substance often in larger amounts or over a longer period than was intended
- Having a persistent desire or unsuccessful efforts to cut down or control substance us

Boscarino and coworkers did not report asking patients about opioid tolerance or withdrawal. Thus, they could only have determined "dependence" based on the prescriptions written. The criterion is often "taking the substance often in larger amounts or over a longer period than was intended." The patients were queried regarding prior substance abuse, depression, anxiety, mental disorders, use of psychotropic drugs, and childhood trauma. Based on these questions, it was concluded that risk factors for "dependence" include age (being less than 65), pain level, depression, use of psychotropic drugs, and previous substance abuse. For example, 33% of the patients acknowledged previous opioid abuse, which could be seen a bias in the study if the goal is to determine whether a legitimate prescription tends to cause iatrogenic addiction. The study was looking for correlations with mental disorders and, not surprisingly, found that those patients who had a previous history of opioid abuse were eight times as likely to be "dependent." The diseases of the patients were not mentioned, so we have no idea why this patient population was prescribed the opioids to begin with. In the conclusion, the authors wrote, "Our study suggests that opioid dependence may be higher than expected among chronic pain patients," which tells us nothing since the authors did not state what the expected value was. Finally, Boscarino and coworkers show that chronic pain is less likely to lead to dependence than risk factors such as psychotropic drugs or previous substance abuse. It is important to bear in mind, however, that a pain patient may be accused of an opioid-use disorder for a minor "infraction," such as accepting a prescription from a dentist following oral surgery. While the *Annual Review* does not present any actual evidence to support its claim of iatrogenic addiction, it does create more suspicion and fear of pain patients by doctors who may be considering whether to continue to prescribe.

Stigmatizing Pain Patients Does Not Show Compassion

The *Annual Review* article[12] stresses the dangers to pain patients who are following their prescriptions. However, the evidence suggests that the true accidental overdose rate is very low.[257,604] Dr. Kolodny's own source suggests that the at least 75% of pain patients use the medications appropriately,[143] and other sources suggest that 80% or more use their prescriptions as indicated.[600,601] The evidence for addiction in the *Annual Review*[12] relies heavily on the overdose rate. The percentage of the total overdose rate resulting from abuse of nondiverted prescription drugs is less than 10% (see above). Some studies indicate that the overdose probability increases with increasing dose. However, attempts to interpret such studies as evidence for dose dependence[381,605] are flawed because the definition of the equivalent dose is poorly defined and dosing itself is unscientific.[126] The body surface area, possible metabolic issues in individual patients, and diseases-related specific considerations are not part of the dose strategy.

For legitimate pain patients, there is an accidental overdose rate, and sadly a significant portion of that may be because of poor prescribing practices combined with mental health issues.[606] The co-prescribing of inappropriate medications or, in some cases, needed medications that have an inherently higher risk is a factor in a great many of the prescription overdose deaths. Many studies on overdose rates make a disclaimer that they do not consider effects of secondary drugs such as benzodiazepines (such as Valium, Xanax and other commercial brands) in their statistics. This is a major oversight and likely source of systematic error since it has been estimated that between 25 and 50% of all overdose deaths involve synergistic effects of benzodiazepines.[607,608] But there are also antidepressants, barbiturate, antipsychotic, and other psychotropic prescription drugs found on autopsy of more than 70% of prescription drug overdoses. Patients need appropriate consultation to ensure that they know about the dangers of using sleep medication, alcohol, or other potentially lethal drug combinations with opioids.[609] Even nonprescription sleep medication can be dangerous for patients taking opioids. A proper study should always record the presence of sedatives or alcohol in the death statistics since these clearly have a major effect on the statistics.[126,610] Overdoses can occur even at low opioid doses, especially when secondary medications are involved.

Aside from the fact that the supporting evidence for a pain-patient prescription overdose epidemic is extremely weak in the *Annual Review*, the AMA has addressed the harm in the stigma created by these arguments for pain patients and addicts alike.[575] It is one thing to warn clinicians of the danger signs and help them to work with patients who may have inner conflicts, depression, or untreated pain. But the *Annual Review* does not address those issues and refers instead to enforcement of narcotics contracts and the reluctance of patients to discuss their *drug-seeking* behaviors because they fear being terminated. Pain patients frequently have a shame-guilt complex that accompanies obtaining opioid medications. Patients will question themselves even when they should not. The mind game proposed by the *Annual Review* paper is that the physician should ask the patient to conduct a self-examination to determine whether he or she has become *dependent* on the pain medication. Pain patients frequently ask themselves whether they are addicted, even when they have pain and the medication is being taken for that reason. This is most often caused by internal pressures, not because of any self-destructive tendencies or craving. Every pain patient feels the need for opioids when the pain comes on, but that is a valid reason for taking the medication and has nothing to do with addiction. American society is so obsessed with the possibility that someone might be feigning the pain that even the patient who has a legitimate need has the fear of being seen as a pretender. The first fear is the patient's own self-doubt, which arises from societal pressure. The second fear is that someone will decide that the patient is feigning pain and take away medication. Patients live in constant fear in this society, and sometimes they do exactly the wrong thing in response to a situation because they are so afraid. These comments are based on observations on Patient Z and others like him who do not have a prior history of substance abuse. There is good reason to believe that Patient Z is showing normal pain patient behavior. One can misinterpret behavior rather easily in such situations, particularly when a bias exists that any request for more pain medication is driven by "iatrogenic addiction," rather than a legitimate need for pain relief. The *Annual Review* fails to present evidence that iatrogenic addiction is *prevalent* in the pain patient population.[12] No one can deny that there are pain patients who have psychological problems and physicians need to be vigilant,[606] but the evidence tells us that it is relatively rare among the population of pain patients.[133,137,138,140–142,144]

The treatment recommendations in the article are for rehabilitation of addicts, not for a medical solution to addiction. One can contrast the *Annual Review*'s[12] public health statements with the more balanced approach in the article by Saloner and coworkers.[360] The concern for destigmatization of both addicts and pain patients, sensible prescribing combined with services for addiction are commonsense public policy proposals. In their final section Saloner and co-workers write as follows[360]:

> Deregulation of medication-assisted treatment and targeted decriminalization approaches are incremental steps toward a reevaluation of the federal controlled substances regulatory system. Under the federal Controlled Substances Act, the US Drug Enforcement Agency has broad purview over health care and pharmacy practices as they relate to controlled substances. The US Drug Enforcement Agency has been driven by criminal justice metrics that bear little relation to public health and lack the scientific expertise to appropriately calibrate patient care. Better public health outcomes could result if the regulatory system were reevaluated based on the likely balance of risks and benefits to public health.

Finally, there is a valid concern that some people who come to a pain clinic are not actually in pain. There are compelling physiological reasons for the difference in addiction statistics between a genuine pain patient and a pretender. A person in pain has a different body chemistry and an actual need for pain relief. Nonetheless, many physicians are frustrated with the burden that the current system places on them. They are expected to be practically clairvoyant in detecting the role-play of a fake patient. Perhaps one reason why it became acceptable to prescribe opioids to cancer patients is that it is difficult to fake cancer. Nonetheless, there are many diseases that have clear diagnoses and severe symptoms that make a claim of being in pain highly believable. While it is more challenging to treat pain of patients who do not have such compelling evidence, a good doctor-patient relationship is by far the best way to do this. The pressure that doctors feel in making treatment decisions would greatly relieved if addiction were treated as a disease rather than a crime.

PROP's Concern for the Overdose Rate vs. the Reality of Pain Patient Suicide

Aside from the repeated statements alleging that pain patients are at great risk for addiction, the reasoning for wanting draconian limits on prescribing is based largely on the claim that the overprescribing of opioids is responsible for the increase in overdose deaths that began in the late 2000s. Yet the evidence shows that the rapid reductions in prescribing after 2011 have had the largest unintended effect of increasing the overdose death rate in the history of public policy.[49,426,427,503] At the same time, it forced persistent-pain patients to reduce or stop taking medications that they had relied on for years. The result was misery and even suicide.[611] Although there is a concern that pain patients may commit suicide by ingesting opioids, the findings of several studies indicate that firearms are a more frequent cause of death.[612] The study by Petrosky and coworkers of the death records in eighteen states that participation in the National Violent Death Reporting System showed that less than 20% of suicides among pain patients involved opioid poisoning.[613] A pain patient who has a good relationship with their doctor knows how much trouble the doctor will get into if the patient overdoses. Often the suicide note makes this clear. Not surprisingly, many pain patients have formed a strong bond with their prescribing physician, because the doctor who understands and treats the patient's pain is a truly special human being. Patients are keenly aware of how tenuous the entire medical relationship is given the constant interference of the DEA in doctor's practices and the potential for the doctor to end up under investigation or prosecuted. The suicide rate by opioid poisoning remained constant from 2003 to 2014 at 1.5% of total suicides, during which time the percentage of suicides involving all chronic pain patients increased from 7.5% to 10% of total suicides. The overall suicide rate in the United States has increased by 30% since 2011, the largest rate of increase in history. There is no real escape from persistent pain, which makes treating it even more difficult than addiction.

Suicide as the Ultimate Pain Control

In an era when there are already many preconditions for suicide because of a rapidly changing economy and loss of earning potential, even livelihood, arising from mechanization, automation, and globalization, the pressures leading to suicide are great.[437] The dire situation and its relationship to pain medication have been documented in the recent book *Deaths of Despair and the Future of Capitalism*.[614] In this regard, opioid prescribing overlaps with social realities. Poor people have a much more difficult time obtaining treatment for their pain. People who live alone often have a more difficult time because of *safety concerns*. Today, doctors ask patients about depression as a routine part of an office visit. Depression may also be seen as a risk factor. These may all be connected since there is evidence that greater pain is associated with poverty arising from poor medical care, poor diet, and poor environment, which has led to broken homes and depression. However, there is evidence that denying pain treatment for any of these reasons pushes a person toward greater risk of suicide.

The Painful Truth of a Utah Doctor's Career

Dr. Lynn Webster, former president of the American Academy of Pain Medicine, wrote an editorial in 2014 describing the dilemma a pain specialist can face.[615] He described how a pain patient of his who had three failed back surgeries suffered excruciating pain. Dr. Webster had installed an intrathecal morphine pump and felt that the dose should be sufficiently high that he was compelled to significantly reduce the patient's dose of oral opioids. Dr. Webster was concerned he would be in legal jeopardy if his patient died of any opioid-related condition. His patient told him three times that he could not bear the pain, but Dr. Webster had confidence that the pump would take care of the pain and the patient just needed to stabilize. However, Dr. Webster learned that he was wrong when the patient shot himself and left a note saying that the pain was too much.

Dr. Webster had been one of the doctors who prescribed high doses of opioids to treat some of the most serious cases of pain. He wrote about how his patients spoke to him when he reduced their dose as he had done for the patient who committed suicide. Patients told him that without pain medication sufficient to relieve an intolerable condition, they had no reason to live. But Dr. Webster had no choice. After 2010, he was investigated by the DEA in connection with charges for manslaughter because some of his patients had died of opioid overdoses over a number of years.[37] Dr. Webster's career exemplifies the debate over treatment of pain in all aspects. Dr. Webster only accepted patients by referral, patients who had tried other pain clinics and whose pain was intractable. Some of the patients wanted to escalate their doses. They claimed it was because of pain. Dr. Webster listened to them and increased their doses as they had wanted. Some of them died. The *Annual Review* is precisely directed at this issue. In fact, one of Dr. Webster's theories was that patients who dose-escalated because of pain had an apparent addiction, a pseudo-addiction. This notion was attacked by PROP. Whether one calls it *pseudo-addiction* or *iatrogenic addiction*, addiction is a real possibility when patients dose-escalate. However, the available evidence suggest that these few cases are exceptions.

Dr. Webster's book *The Painful Truth* describes how he wanted to take on the most difficult intractable pain cases. Pain often comes from disease, and such a practice is by its nature high risk. The critique that patients die or that their pain is not completely controlled are failures of opioids is often off the mark. Patients with serious diseases have a higher mortality compared to the general population. The cause of death of a person with an incurable disease is often difficult to determine, but when opioids are involved, they are usually considered the cause. An article in the *Deseret News* describes some of the personal stories of the patients who died of overdoses. These tragic stories pose the dilemma: What does a doctor do when the patient claims the pain is intolerable at any dose? Telling the patient that there is nothing more you can do may lead to a suicide, but increasing the dose may result in an overdose. Dr. Webster was exonerated of all charges in the manslaughter case brought against him,[37] but his willingness to prescribe high doses during his career has put him at the center of controversy.

Dr. Webster had treated thousands of patients in his clinic and provided relief from pain for many. He had been sought after by many pain patients who wanted relief, but he only accepted patients by referral. There are not many doctors who will take on the challenge and risk of treating someone who has persistent pain; Dr. Webster considered this his life's mission. However, since he has conducted research supported by pharmaceutical companies to develop new pain medications, he is on the list of people that Dr. Kolodny has testified against in court, either directly or indirectly. Dr. Webster faces at least eighty lawsuits for his role as president of the American Academy of Pain Medicine, which received funding from numerous pharmaceutical companies. Dr. Kolodny has made allegations against anyone who had any financial ties with pharmaceutical companies, even for research, suggesting that they have conflicts and they are biased. Indeed, they may have conflicts, and that is why they should disclose them. Why then didn't Dr. Kolodny disclose his conflicts of interest from hundreds of thousands he earned from his expert testimony against Johnson & Johnson in the Oklahoma lawsuit? Dr. Kolodny has impugned the professional organizations, but these exist mainly for conferences, professional contacts, and outreach to the public. These relationships exist in all fields of research. Most corporate funding to these professional organizations supports conferences and legitimate scientific organizational activities. The attacks on the professional organizations show the extent to which these lawsuits are about money rather than corporate or medical ethics.

Prescription Drug Overdose Is Not Primarily a Problem of Pain Patients

Aside from the *created* debate over efficacy of opioids discussed in chapter 6, there is a debate over the origin of the increase in overdose rate that occurred from 1999 to the present. We should not have to debate this point, since the official statistics are available on the

CDC website, but so many reporters in the media have stated or insinuated the overdose crisis arose because of a *prescription drug crisis* that two terms have practically become synonymous in the public mind. The CDC data show the dramatic divergence of numbers of prescriptions, which went down by a factor of two from 2011 to 2018 and overdose deaths, which went up by a factor of two during the same period. As of the writing of the book, the CDC has posted a headline on its vital statistics page, stating that opioid-overdose deaths decreased by 4.7% in 2018. However, they failed to mention that suicide deaths increased by even greater margins in 2019 and 2020. Opioid- overdose deaths increased by 5.4% to 72,000 in 2019 by 12.5% to at least 81,000 in 2020 (the number was report as of mid-December 2020). The agency is looking for something good to say about its failed policy, but the sad truth is that the best option for the agency is to leave dated information on the site and ignore what is currently happening. Many doctors understand the reality of patient death caused by government policy. That is the meaning of the title of Dr. Kertesz's article, "It's Time to Start Counting."[268]

It is disheartening to hear inaccurate reporting on National Public Radio. Reporter Brian Mann has repeatedly portrayed an epidemic of overprescribing that is leading to addiction. Aside from the vast amount of evidence of diversion, government corruption, and the already existing drug problem that his journalism ignores, it is an example of extremely sloppy journalism even in the reported facts. For example, the reporter, Mr. Brian Mann, claims,[35]

> In 2016, the CDC issued strongly-worded guide-lines, urging doctors to avoid opioids or to minimize their use whenever possible. Roughly half the states have implemented some form of regulation designed to curtail prescribing. But scientists, government officials and front-line medical workers interviewed by NPR say those efforts have fallen dangerously short.

The characterization of the CDC guidelines is seriously in error. As we have discussed, the actual wording is not severely restrictive, although there is a statement that first-time prescriptions by a PCP should not exceed 90 MEDD unless a valid medical reason can be provided.[281] This is precisely the clause that hundreds of doctors and the AMA have asked be removed or amended to give doctors the liberty to treat pain without fear of sanction. Mr. Mann's final statement that doctors believe that the guidelines "have fallen dangerously short" focuses narrowly on the issue of excessive prescribing by dentists or surgeons and ignores the major problem that millions of people in pain have had their prescriptions reduced or terminated without medical justification.[121] Hundreds of doctors have petitioned for changes in the guidelines to eliminate the limits on prescribing and leave those decisions up to doctors.[1,282] The AMA sent a letter to the CDC on June 16, 2020, describing harm caused by the CDC guidelines to patients.[264] The CDC itself issued a clarification in 2019 after hundreds of doctors had petitioned the agency.[486] In a balanced report, Mr. Mann would have pointed out that many pain patients are harmed by the rigid interpretation of the CDC guidelines and that the overprescribing by dentists and surgeons that persist is a matter for physician education, not a government-mandated limit on dose for all patients. By ignoring the larger issue of the suffering of millions of pain patients and making the incorrect connection between prescribing and the overdose rate, the article is an advocacy piece for government interference in medicine to reduce prescriptions to an arbitrary level irrespective of the disease a patient suffers from. Sadly, NPR has refused to acknowledge or answer e-mails, letters, phone calls, or texts regarding this inaccurate and biased reporting.

Rather than recognize the deadly trend that they have set in motion, the designers of this new "experiment" in mass tapering and arbitrary dose limits have decided to explain the failure of their proposal to rein in overdoses by blaming persistent-pain patients themselves for the increases in overdose deaths. Aside from equating pain patients with addicts, Dr. Kolodny has stated that he believes that "[t]he PR firms working for opioid makers…are very good at manipulating opioid-dependent pain patients."[616] How exactly do pharmaceutical companies manipulate people who are sick and disabled and can often barely leave their homes? In reality, it is Dr. Kolodny who uses pain patients as his proxies to make the case against the pharmaceutical companies as strong as possible in his expert witness testimony. Making the case that the product is harming the intended recipient is a crucial step in the chain of evidence. The most convincing way to make the case for the guilt of the pharmaceutical companies is to present evidence that pain patients themselves are becoming addicts. For this reason, Dr. Kolodny argues that overdose deaths are primarily a consequence of those who obtained drugs legally from their doctor, contrary to abundant evidence that illegal drugs and diverted prescription drugs account for over 90% of overdose deaths. The *iatrogenic addiction* argument gives this destructive and cynical narrative a veneer of respectability.

The *Annual Review* article focuses on a minority of patients with concerns of abuse and ignores the issues of seriously ill patients with chronic diseases and persistent pain. Not all patients have low back pain or osteoarthritis pain. This demographic is the most studied and considered most likely to be overmedicated. What happened to individualized care and concern for the patient? PROP has implemented hard limits that make a mockery of their claim that doctors are using opioids as "shortcuts." Having one policy for all patients is the ultimate shortcut. This policy is cruel when applied to Patient Z and others like him. People whose bodies have been damaged by disease, who are living with systemic inflammation, and who have exhausted all medical treatments are being denied care by the tens of thousands. In examining the dynamic of the situation today, one has to consider the consequences for a patient who has been tapered or terminated and still has intolerable pain. When Dr. Kline's practice was shut down by the DEA and the North Carolina State Board of Health, he responsibly found a doctor one hundred miles away who would take the thirty-four elderly patients with rare diseases and continue their care. Subsequently, pharmacies refused to fill their opioid prescriptions, and ultimately Medicare Part D refused to reimburse the new doctor until he dropped the patients. The doctor was not permitted to taper the patients gradually but was forced to let elderly people who had depended on opioids for survival to fend for themselves. To the deniers I ask, How is this not a war on pain patients? Indeed, if such patients turned to street drugs in desperation, Dr. Kolodny could count them as an iatrogenic-addiction statistic. By what twisted reasoning is the action of putting elderly sick people through the pain of sudden total withdrawal protecting them from harm?

Who Is the Real Persistent-Pain Patient?

Will the real persistent-pain patient please stand up? This is the problem in a nutshell. Every doctor who prescribes opioids is confronted with the fact that there are people who want to obtain a prescription to abuse it or divert it. Such pretenders create a problem for both doctors and legitimate pain patients. Doctors must worry that being fooled puts them in jeopardy since a doctor may be held liable for any abuse by the pretender. Pain patients are harmed, quite obviously, because they must constantly fear being mistaken for a pretender. The accepted solution appears to be to treat every patient as a suspect and to use enforcement mechanisms to test patients' honesty. Although narcotics contracts, PDMP, and urine testing are flawed methods, I believe it is best to accept them as necessary to garner public support for the treatment of pain. The tragedy is that even with the implementation of these methods, patients are still being denied treatment in record numbers. The best method would be to return to multidisciplinary pain clinics or at the very least give doctors and nurses enough time to know their patients. Of course, addiction is always a danger. Even if the risk is 1%, it is still something that a doctor must watch for. The tragedy in America is that we have such poor ways of dealing with addiction that the fear of addiction makes this problem worse than it should be. Many pain patients would regard being classified as an addict to be a death sentence, and they are basically correct. The treatment of addicts in the society is so terrible that a persistent-pain patient would probably not be able to continue under the strain. Then there is the problem that these commonsense ways of delivering health care cost more money, and every aspect of health care is designed to cut costs. In the end, our current policy is one of disregarding the needs of a large segment of the population, and it is not managing to reduce the large number of overdose fatalities.

CHAPTER 12

⤫

The Not-So-Many Alternatives to Opioid Therapy

Can pain clinics offer persistent-pain patients any alternative to opioid therapy? There is a *range of pain therapies* that the staff of a pain clinic will mention. But when it comes to the time for actual discussion about those possibilities, the reality is that there are few options other than opioids, and those that exist work only in certain specific and limited cases. Some alternatives include acupuncture, cognitive behavioral therapy, aromatherapy, music therapy, hypnotherapy, and herbs. These types of suggestions may be appropriate for the pain of lumbago, a recurring mild headache, a sprained ankle, or mild osteoarthritis. Such alternative therapies are not a good way to relieve serious autoimmune or mechanical pain from inflammatory or degenerative diseases. These alternatives are based on distraction from the pain. A sensory input can close the gate and inhibit pain (see chapter 3). This approach can work for relatively minor pain that may plague a person at work or while driving. However, distraction is not going to supersede the grinding, burning, or piercing pain of inflammation, tumor, or pinched nerve. When these methods are insufficient, pain medication should be used as recommended by the WHO in a three-rung ladder of medication: (1) acetaminophen, NSAIDs; (2) tramadol; and (3) morphine. The rule is to proceed slowly and stop when pain is controlled.

Comparison of the Toxicity and Mortality of Acetaminophen, Aspirin, and Ibuprofen

The nonsteroidal anti-inflammatory drugs (NSAIDs) include aspirin, ibuprofen, naproxen, and the cyclooxygenase-2 (COX-2) inhibitors (e.g., diclofenac). Acetaminophen is not an NSAID, but it has a similar profile of pain relief and similar severity of side effects. The NSAIDs work by blocking the biosynthesis of prostaglandin, both in the brain and in tissues. NSAIDs, beginning with aspirin, the first pharmaceutical, bind to the active site of cyclooxygenase-1 (COX-1) and cyclooxygenase-2 (COX-2). Acetaminophen blocks the action of the same enzyme by preventing the oxidation step. It is a weaker drug on a per-weight basis than NSAIDs.[618] The ulcers and gastric bleeding caused by continuous use of NSAIDs result from their binding to COX-1 in the gastrointestinal tract (GI). COX-2 enzymes are found elsewhere in the body. If it were convenient to inject NSAIDs, the effects on the GI could be avoided. But this is rarely done for practical reasons. A number of pharmaceuticals have been developed that bind to COX-2 and thereby lack the toxicity and unpleasantness of the NSAIDs. However, COX-2 inhibitors are associated with an elevated risk of heart attack. The latter is a rare effect, but usually fatal. The difficulty with COX-2 cardiotoxicity is that it is difficult to predict. Diclofenac can be administered as a gel and applied topically. It is a remarkably effective painkiller for certain arthritis conditions where the penetration depth of the drug is sufficient to reach the target tissue. It appears to be much safer than oral diclofenac. The gel is known as Voltaren in Europe, and it is sold as a nonprescription drug. In the US, it is still only available by prescription. However, diclofenac gels do not alleviate the pain of many conditions, inflammatory arthritis, cancer, or sickle cell disease, to name a few.

The NSAIDs and acetaminophen both have potentially life-threatening side effects. One side effect that they have in common is irritation of the gastrointestinal tract that can lead to bleeding (except the COX-2 inhibitors). More people die every year from intestinal bleeding caused by NSAIDs and acetaminophen than die from prescription opioid overdoses. To clarify, this comparison refers to legitimate prescription opioids, not diverted opioids. There are serious concerns about the hepatotoxicity (liver toxicity) of acetaminophen as well,[619] which are exacerbated by alcohol consumption.[620] Comparison of patients admitted to hospitals who took either ibuprofen or acetaminophen found that they both had similar mortality (circa 12%) and similar types of problems, GI bleeding or ulcers. Those who took acetaminophen spent an average of fourteen days in the hospital compared to eleven days for the ibuprofen patients.[621] In-depth studies of the side effects of acetaminophen include elevated blood pressure, cardiovascular disease, asthma, and renal injury, and the effects of in-utero exposure.[622] The estimate of 16,500 deaths from GI bleeding caused by acetaminophen was based on an extrapolation from a small sample.[623] More accurate estimates are considerably lower.[624] A high-quality estimate for the year 1999 is 3,200 deaths.[625] Acetaminophen is widely used in Europe, and a number of studies suggest that it is safer than the NSAIDs, although weaker as a painkiller and lacking in anti-inflammatory action.[618] The annual death rate of patients from NSAIDs was approximately 15,000 in 2016, which is five times greater than the estimate for acetaminophen fatalities. Putting those numbers together, the total deaths from all causes including both acetaminophen and NSAIDs is higher than the opioid overdose deaths, for patients who used opioids as directed. I base this statement on the number of opioid overdose deaths in 2016, which is 47,000, and then removing heroin, fentanyl, and methadone, which leaves about 20% that could possibly be because of prescription drugs, giving 9,700 patients compared to more than 18,000 for NSAIDs and acetaminophen. A study that directly compared the annual mortality of opioids and NSAIDs found all-cause mortality for patients taking nonselective NSAIDs compared with all opioids was 48 per 1,000 compared to 75 per 1,000, respectively.[411] Thus, this estimate indicates that opioids have a 50% higher mortality than NSAIDs and acetaminophen. It is more difficult to obtain aggregate numbers for acetaminophen or the NSAIDs because they are not tabulated by the CDC in the same way that opioids are. While this comparison looks, at first, like it means that opioids have a greater risk than the NSAIDs and acetaminophen, it must be borne in mind that the fatality rate for opioids in this comparison includes street drugs, heroin, and fentanyl, which is anywhere from 50% to 80% of the total overdose rate. By both estimate, NSAIDs and acetaminophen are more dangerous than opioids and may even have a greater risk of mortality when used for medical reasons.

What Is the Evidence for Efficacy of NSAIDs and Acetaminophen Compared to Opioids?

A Cochrane review of 4,449 articles found two high-quality studies with a total of 1,785 patients with low back pain.[626] They found high-quality evidence that there is no difference between acetaminophen (four grams per day) and placebo from one to twelve weeks. They found further that acetaminophen has no effect on quality of life, function, global impression of recovery, or sleep quality. This is more definitive and higher quality than any of the studies on opioids, and the result is negative for efficacy of acetaminophen. Studies on NSAIDs have shown lack of efficacy for more painful conditions, such as rheumatoid arthritis, while simultaneously producing significant gastric distress.[627] A meta-analysis of opioid therapy for rheumatoid arthritis concludes that there is fair evidence for efficacy of low-dose opioids and insufficient evidence to comment on high-dose opioids. NSAIDs are found to have no efficacy.[628] In one early study, the pain relief amounted to approximately one-point reduction in the pain scale compared to placebo for 3 MEDD of the opioid dextropropoxyphene, which is currently banned because of adverse side effects.[408,629] Several German authors have recommended that opioids should be considered for serious osteoarthritis pain since they are more effective and have fewer long-term side effects than NSAIDs.[630,631] In fact, an observational study of 63,101 patients found that 19% used opioids for long-term pain relief.[632] Most studies of opioid treatment discussed in chapter 6 included osteoarthritis, and many of those studies found some efficacy with fair or poor quality of evidence. As discussed in the appendix, recent high-quality studies in Germany support the use of opioids for these conditions.[40-46,312,352] However, in North America, there is great controversy over any such statement as can be seen in media reports concerning the Canadian study by Busse and coworkers.[38,39] This is still being studied and opioids are used for osteoarthritis in Europe. In the United States, it is becoming increasingly difficult for osteoarthritis patients to obtain opioid medications.

Nerve Blocks and Radiofrequency Neural Ablation

For more than one hundred years, the significant alternative therapy to opioids has been a "nerve block." The permanent version of this intervention is a radiofrequency neural ablation. The idea is to eliminate a specific nerve that is transmitting the pain. The block can be temporary as is usually suggested for surgery or some short-lived pain.[633,634] Clinicians recommend a temporary block using a steroid or a lidocaine injection near the nerve of interest. One must make sure that there are no side effects, no motor control or other bodily functions that would be damaged by ablating the nerve. An epidural is an extreme type of temporary nerve block, most often used during childbirth. Temporary nerve blocks are used for surgery.[635] If a temporary nerve block works, then the permanent ablation may be proposed. However, getting a nerve block that works is difficult at best.

Physically, the technique used is to chemically or physically interrupt a pain signal, usually in the extremities, so that a particular nerve or joint is targeted. The majority of successful nerve blocks are associated with surgery, such as hip or knee total arthroplasty.[636,637] Approximately 10–15% of patients receive a temporary nerve block, which is deemed a success if it reduces the number of days in the hospital from eight to seven.[633] For more complicated types of pain, a nerve block is not practical. For systemic diseases, one would need many nerve ablations to provide real relief.[633,634] Radiofrequency neurotomy of nerves in the sacroiliac joints did not show effective reduction in pain.[638] Patient Z was tested twice in different clinics, but they gave up rather quickly when the initial nerve block failed. The doctors did not seem surprised.

Spinal Cord Stimulation as an Alternative Pain Treatment

Spinal cord stimulation by implanted electrical circuitry has been known since 1967, but until recently, it has lacked the feedback control needed to make it effective.[639] The concept is related to deep-brain stimulation referred to in chapter 3; however, the device is placed in the spine to stimulate nerve cells electrically and disrupt the pain signal. A device has recently been tested that continually reads the electrical activity induced in the target nerve. The output is automatically adjusted to keep nerve stimulation within the therapeutic range.[640] For specific pain in the spine and leg, a new high-frequency theory has been shown to give superior results and reduce side effects.[641,642]

And Then We Are Back to Opioids

Years ago, Patient Z's friend Brad mentioned that his brother-in-law had failed back surgery that had left him permanently disabled and in persistent pain. Brad explained that for years, his brother-in-law had suffered because he could not get adequate pain relief. Finally, Brad's brother-in-law found a good doctor and "got the right medicine." The way that Brad related this story, Patient Z had assumed that the problem was that opioids were not taking care of his pain and that he needed to find a doctor who could give him a suitable alternative. A few years later, after Patient Z had struggled with pain clinics, he asked Brad about his brother-in-law. Patient Z finally worked up the courage to ask.

"So what medication did they finally use to take care of his pain?"

"Oh," Brad replied sheepishly, "they gave him morphine."

Patient Z was puzzled. "I don't understand. Morphine is the first opioid any doctor would try. Why did it take him several years to get the right medicine?"

"You know how restrictive things have become," Brad responded. "He had to find a doctor who trusted him enough to write a prescription that would take care of his pain."

Doctors are scrutinized when they write a prescription for more than 100 MEDD for any patient.[643] If a patient is irresponsible in any way or dies for any reason, the doctor may lose his or her practice or be prosecuted.[304] It is a lot of risk to assume for one patient's comfort. Many doctors refuse to take that risk. It stands to reason that doctors would screen their patients carefully, and the process of finding a doctor would take time. The climate has become much more restrictive in recent years because of the opioid-overdose crisis. Finding a doctor who will take the risk just to make a patient's life bearable is more difficult than ever. How can any doctor act differently when a dose above 120 MEDD is considered "poor care" according to the national quality standard?[48]

Methadone and Buprenorphine for Treatment of Pain

The remaining suggestions for alternatives to opioids are other opioids. Recently, there has been a suggestion that pain patients should be treated as opioid dependents and switched to buprenorphine.[10,51,124] Both methadone and buprenorphine are considered less addictive than morphine. They both have significantly longer half-life in the bloodstream, fifteen to -fifty-five hours and sixteen to twenty-four hours, respectively, compared to the morphine half-life from four to seven hours. However, methadone and buprenorphine are so different in their properties that they really have nothing in common except for their historical use as maintenance therapy for former heroin users.

Methadone is much less common than morphine for pain management.[644] The risk of overdose is at least 50% times higher than using morphine.[385] The nonstandard dose-response of methadone makes it difficult to properly dose. The long half-life is also potentially a problem since methadone can build up in a person's body. Switching between morphine/oxycodone and methadone requires skill to get the dose and timing right. Methadone-maintained populations can be treated with morphine for breakthrough pain following surgery. There are reports methadone by itself can have good efficacy as an analgesic in cancer[645] and for neuropathic pain.[340] A survey comparing treatment options for pain in geriatric concluded that levorphanol is a good substitute for methadone with fewer disadvantages.[646]

Buprenorphine is a partial agonist of the MOR and an antagonist for the KOR, which is a significantly different mechanism of action from morphine. Despite being a partial agonist, it binds very tightly to the MOR. The partial agonist property refers to how the drug affects the signaling in the nerve cell rather than how tightly it binds. In recent years, buprenorphine has become the first-line drug recommended for opioid maintenance therapy.[499] It has also been recommended as an alternative to morphine and oxycodone for pain patients.[10,588] Recent studies suggest that buprenorphine may be a reasonable alternative for treatment of pain.[586,647] It is considered to be less addictive.[648,649] A buprenorphine patch has been shown to be adequate for long-term pain relief.[587] Buprenorphine is like methadone in that it has a long half-life, which makes rotation more difficult. Given the significant push to prescribe buprenorphine for pain, one would hope that it will be classified so that it is not seen primarily as a maintenance drug for addiction. Pain patients struggle with being seen as addicts because there is such a pervasive stigma associated with opioid use.

Opioid Rotation—the Need for a Scientific Approach

Opioids are ligands that bind to a receptor with a binding affinity. In chapter 3, we have shown a simple equation for the equilibrium binding: MOR + O = MOR(O). MOR is the mu-opioid receptor, O is the opioid, and MOR(O) is the complex formed when the opioid binds to the receptor. There are two types of receptor binding—agonist (activator) and antagonist (blocker). An agonist binds to a receptor and triggers a response. On the other hand, an antagonist binds but inhibits the transduction of the message; it blocks the receptor.

Opioid rotation is based on the idea that different opioids have slightly different effects. While they all bind to the MOR, some also have some binding affinity for KOR or DOR. The exact mode of binding may affect the nature of the signaling in the nerve cell. Therefore, to the extent that a patient's body has developed a tolerance, the replacement of one opioid for another may reset the interactions and give more relief for the same equivalent dose. In a feedback response, nerve cells decrease the number of MORs or desensitize the MORs in response to morphine in the system as a feedback response to the presence of high concentrations of the agonist (active agent).[650] However, the scientific understanding of the relative potency of opioid drugs is still poor. Use of MEDD as an equivalent unit follows a common practice in pain medicine. However, this practice is not based on rigorous scientific comparisons of the effects of the drugs.[126,127] Different studies have significant differences in their equivalencies. In the US oxycodone is usually considered to correspond to 1.5 milligrams of morphine, but in the recent EU standard, that value is 2.0 milligrams. Fudin and coworkers have been outspoken in their criticism of the lack of scientific rigor, which impedes a good understanding of how well one drug will substitute for another, and there were enough variations of morphine-like drugs with tables showing the relative potency of the substitutes so that one can calculate a substitution and substitute one medication for another while keeping the overall potency roughly the same.

Since the basis of opioid rotation is differences in mode of action, the more the drugs differ, the greater the effect. For example, it is standard practice to prescribe morphine and oxycodone together to give slightly different types of pain relief.[651] Hydromorphone, hydrocodone, and weaker forms such as codeine can give more relief if the body has not been exposed to them for a time. Opioid rotation is a rational calculated substitution of one opioid for another to give a patient's system a chance to lose the tolerance for specific aspects of a painkiller. Since all of them bind the MOR as a main mode of action, opioid rotation is not perfect.

Tapentadol and tramadol are both mu-opioid receptor (MOR) agonists and serotonin/norepinephrine reuptake inhibitors (SNRI). The WHO recommends one of these medications as the second line of treatment for cancer patients, beyond NSAIDs and acetaminophen, but prior to morphine. Because of the SNRI mechanism, tapentadol and tramadol have a dose limitation unlike the morphine class of opioids. The reason for the dose restriction is that the SNRI mechanism can lead to seizures at very high doses. Of course, this case be dangerous for people who abuse tramadol or tapentadol. Ironically, PROP has claimed that tramadol and tapentadol are dangerous for treatment of persistent-pain patients because of the abuse profile. This is like saying that you should not buy a sports car because there are people who drive sports cars too fast. Any of these drugs can be abused. But, unlike other opioids, these two drugs do have an upper safe limit. Tramadol should not be prescribed at a dose higher than four hundred milligrams per day (40 MEDD). These two medications are safe when used as directed, and they have a significantly different mechanism, which means that they can be used to complement morphine or in an opioid rotation.

Tapentadol is three times weaker than morphine. Therefore, a substitution of three times as much tapentadol for morphine could potentially give greater relief for a period of weeks or months as the nerve cells stop producing quite as many mu-opioid receptors. Tapentadol has some similarity with tramadol, but unlike tramadol, it does not require activation in the liver.[652] Tramadol is a pro-drug, which means that it requires activation within the body and specifically in the liver. This both slows down its activation and increases its potency because of action of cytochrome P450 oxidation enzymes. Since not all patients can activate tramadol, tapentadol is potentially useful as a secondary drug that could complement morphine, with relatively low abuse potential.[653]

> There is a recognized treatment pathway for persistent pain based upon the World Health Organization (WHO) cancer pain ladder, whereby patients progress from non-opioids such

as paracetamol and non-steroidal anti-inflammatory drugs (NSAIDs) to weak opioids and finally
strong opioids. Tapentadol is a centrally acting
analgesic which has two mechanisms of action,
namely mu-opioid receptor agonist (MOR) and
(serotonin)-noradrenaline reuptake inhibition
(SNRI).[24,654]

American medicine often skips the weak opioid step. Certainly
this was the case when Purdue got involved with the marketing of
OxyContin. They were marketing a form of oxycodone, which we
should remember was first synthesized as a substitute for heroin.
Oxycodone is a powerful painkiller, but it is not a first-line therapeutic, unless there is an acute situation that calls for extreme medication
quickly—a serious accident, a burn, or a major surgery postoperative treatment. These examples indicate the difficulty of comparisons based on equivalent dose tables.[645,655–660] Opioid rotation entails
some risk and therefore requires experience and personal attention.
Rotation is not an alternative to opioids but could be a way to use
them at lower doses and greater effect for their desired effect to control pain. Unfortunately, the current climate has made clinicians concerned about how opioid rotation appears to regulators rather than
focusing on delivering maximum pain relief with a minimum dose.

Intrathecal Delivery—Surgically Implanted Opioid Pumps

The intrathecal delivery method can be quite effective for long-term
opioid therapy. The intrathecal method consists of implanting a delivery pump that provides a constant supply of opioid to the patient.
Intrathecal pumps were pioneered by Onofrio in 1980, and since then,
there have been over three hundred thousand implanted pumps.[661]
Fentanyl transdermal patches (skin patches) are a similar but less invasive approach for long-term delivery in a modality that is not easy to
abuse.[662–665] Transdermal patches have been shown to give high rates
of pain relief with relatively few side effects compared to oral delivery.

Intrathecal pumps and transdermal patches are two of the methods that can be classified as abuse-deterrent formulations (ADFs).[666]

The reasons for trying pumps can range from problems with opioid metabolism to deterrence against abuse. Some patients do not tolerate or cannot metabolize oral opioids.[667] Others need high doses and would prefer not to have to manage so many pills. Intrathecal therapy is most often based on a morphine pump, but hydromorphone has also been used with success.[668] One of the downsides of intrathecal morphine delivery is pruritus, the extremely unpleasant itching side effect that appears to be particularly common for morphine pumps. But a pump can also be used for hydromorphone, or the two can be alternated on a schedule to permit side effects to be mitigated and to reduce tolerance. This approach is combination drug rotation and intrathecal delivery approach. It is perhaps because of expense[669] that when the intractable-pain-patient movement began to gain traction, this option was not recommended over a time-release formulation.[670]

An intrathecal pump is considered by many to be the method of last resort.[666,671] Yet other studies suggest that a high percentage of patients get good pain relief with tolerable side effects.[672] A recent innovation has been developed to reduce the potential for abuse using the channel blocker ziconotide and morphine in an intrathecal pump.[673] This pump is analogous to the idea of combining different medications into one pill, such as Vicodin, which consists of acetaminophen and hydrocodone as a deterrent to abuse.

Opioid Adjuvants for the Treatment of Neuropathic Pain

There are many types of pain, nociceptive, inflammatory, neuropathic, and others. Combination therapy has been proposed for complex cases with multiple types of pain.[674] This approach must be implemented with appropriate caution. Many sedatives, such as the benzodiazepines and barbiturates, are dangerous in combination with opioids. Sedatives are involved in nearly half of all prescription drug-overdose deaths. While the sedatives may help to relieve anxiety, they are not analgesics. On the other hand, the tricyclic antidepressants, such as amitriptyline, appear to play a dual role in ameliorating depression but also managing neuropathic pain.[675-677] Neuropathy is not necessarily caused by mechanical or physical damage, but rather from a chemical change in state of the nerve cell. Neuropathic pain can result from medical treatment, such as chemotherapy, stimulants and opioids, but also from diseases, such as diabetes and even infections. Opioids tend to relieve nociceptive pain, but they are significantly less effective for inflammatory pain or neuropathic pain. Amitriptyline has efficacy in treatment of neuropathies associated with chemotherapy or other drugs, but not tumor pain.[678] An antidepressant from a different class, duloxetine, is both a serotonin and norepinephrine uptake inhibitor and suppressor of TNF, which can provide relief for both neuropathic and inflammatory pain. These drugs can be used in combination with opioids, which may help to treat multimodal pain.[679-682]

Amitriptyline may also help to address the role of opioid-induced hyperalgesia (OIH) in humans.[683] Experiments in laboratory rats have shown that amitriptyline can ameliorate OIH induced by common opioids[684] but does not alleviate OIH from remifentanil.[685] This suggests that amitriptyline and other tricyclics may be useful to determine whether pain has a neuropathic origin. In an era when there is such a great discussion about minimizing the opioid dose, it is important to consider drug combinations, such as opioid and amitriptyline, that may provide greater relief at a lower-opioid dose, particularly when neuropathic pain is a component of a disease. The risk of respiratory suppression is significantly less than for sedatives.

Patient Z developed neuropathies over time from severe immunological irritation of tissues in his legs. However, amitriptyline was prescribed only later, when he entered palliative care. A low dose of amitriptyline alleviated the neuropathic pain, specifically to an extent that would have been difficult to achieve with opioids alone. Yet no one mentioned this possibility during five years in three different pain clinics. This experience further confirmed Patient Z's observation that pain clinic's primary function was to control opioid dose rather than to treat pain. The focus on opioid dose was such an obsession that the doctors never took the time to understand the various origins of Patient Z's pain. Ironically, based on his later experience, he came to the realization that they could have helped his pain significantly without increasing the opioid dose. The information provided here is not medical advice or a recommendation for treatment, but general information based on the medical literature and one patient's case study.

The Recurring Claim That There Are Many Alternatives to Opioid Therapy

In the media and academic articles, authors frequently state that there are many alternatives to opioid therapy. While there is some promising research, the reality today is that there are no good options for most patients with severe, persistent pain. For all the options that doctors discuss in the pain clinic, opioids are still the basis of most of them. For most patients who have intractable chronic pain, opioid drugs are the only option that provides long-term relief. In fact, opioids manage 90% of cancer pain.[686] In a setting where the medical community apparently takes pain seriously, such as cancer patients in hospice, opioids are routinely administered. It is understandable that terminal patients are given relief from pain in the last few months of their lives, and no one questions this use of opioids. Therefore, alternatives to standard opioids, morphine and oxycodone, are recommended for cancer patients only when the standard treatment fails to provide relief.[24] What are the reasons for not doing this to other patients who are sick and suffering with bad pain? The objection that "we don't have good data" on long-term use is based on biased arguments used to reject existing studies discussed in chapter 6. The critics ignore the fact that opioids have been shown to be effective for severe cancer pain in hospice for the past sixty years. They reject the observational studies, knowing that there are ethical concerns that prevent long-term RCT studies of severe, persistent pain because of the suffering it would cause. Our medical system only permits that degree of suffering in real life.

CHAPTER 13

❧

Adverse Effects of Opioid Drugs Compared to Untreated Persistent Pain

There are three main objections to the use of opioids to treat people with incurable chronic diseases. First, there is concern that opioids cease to be effective because of tolerance. Second, there are unpleasant side effects. Third, opioids can lead to addiction and associated risk of respiratory suppression. To be objective, studies of the side effects of opioids should be compared with studies of the side effects of other analgesics, such as the NSAIDs and acetaminophen, which are more dangerous than most people are aware. These should both be compared to the side effects of untreated pain. The latter is the most difficult to study, but the great medical and ethical failing of the current reaction to the *prescription opioid epidemic* is a narrow focus on dose to the exclusion of the important issues people confront living in pain. Instead of asking what the risks of opioid therapy are, we should ask, What are the risks of living in persistent pain? These considerations apply to all types of pain, but few of the studies or commentaries make a distinction between minor pain and persistent pain, particularly the pain of autoimmune or degenerative diseases.

To Taper or Not to Taper—Is That a Question?

A return to common sense in prescribing does not mean that every patient should have a dose limit. Rather, it means that pain should be titrated until it is controlled, and the dose should be increased until the point where the patient can at least tolerate daily living. Pain medication should not be doled out freely, but it should be prescribed appropriately to those who need it. The argument for drastically restricting or eliminating opioid pain medications is that many people are overmedicated. However, not everyone is overmedicated! Having examined how the compassionate care movement was taken over by outside forces, one can propose that pain management could be done correctly if the proper safeguards were in place, a required educational component is introduced, and addiction is treated as a medical problem.[535] Surely some kind of rational plan is better than ignoring disease entirely, which is the plan of the pain clinics today. The current CDC guidelines result in the same criteria for treatment of a patient with osteoarthritis and ankylosing spondylitis. The current policy even ignores cancer pain, except in hospice when the patient is clearly at the end of life.

The current dose restrictions and forced tapers have been nothing short of disastrous for many persistent-pain patients. The doctors in PROP have made some statements in the literature to indicate that doctors should show compassion and that tapers should not be too rapid.[10] But the fear of addiction prevalent in their writing outweighs these statements, and the legal force behind the guidelines leads to a pressure to force patients to taper. The paper entitled "Rethinking Opioid Dose Tapering, Prescription Opioid Dependence, and Indications for Buprenorphine" by Chou, Ballantyne, and Lembke suggests that pain patients who initiate a taper and then have pain or other symptoms could be diagnosed with *prescription opioid dependence* as a distinct condition.[10] The authors do not say whether they are discussing a voluntary taper or not. A patient who is convinced by the doctor's claim that they will feel better if they taper may agree only to learn that the pain is much worse. Then following Chou and coauthors, the doctor will claim that the pain is a withdrawal symptom and evidence of dependence. Further, the authors suggest that patients should *voluntarily* change their diagnosis to include the term *dependence*. Once a patient agrees to change the diagnosis, the patient is on a slippery slope because *dependence* has been equated with *addiction* by these same authors.[11] The authors claim that the benefit of this diagnosis comes from the fact that the patient *may* be on the path to opioid use disorder and this diagnosis will help the patient avoid that danger. The patient is in a vicious cycle since the suspicion of opioid use disorder suggests that the patient should taper, but then any complication in the taper becomes more evidence of opioid use disorder. The similarity of the reasoning with the methods of Spanish Inquisition are disturbing. The authors wrote the following[10]:

> As tapering experience accrues, clinicians have observed that many patients with chronic pain receiving long-term opioid therapy struggle to reduce doses. Why are tapers a challenge in some patients? An important reason is dependence, characterized by withdrawal symptoms when opioid doses are decreased or discontinued. In addition to somatic symptoms, withdrawal may manifest as psychological symptoms. Even with stable doses, patients can experience continuous subthreshold withdrawal between doses, dysphoria, and hyperalgesia, all which can be exacerbated by tapering.

In their etiology, they consider only the possibility that the patient is undergoing withdrawal, not that the patient's pain may have become unbearable at the lower dose. The authors in PROP write as though pain is not real. There is an enigmatic statement in the introduction that says, "Quality of life may be adversely affected despite perceived pain benefits." In Patient Z's case, it is impossible to separate *quality of life* from *pain benefits*. The opioids improve quality of life because they control the pain. If someone is actually in pain, this is the only logical way to describe their reaction.

The significant therapeutic recommendation of the publication is that persistent-pain patients who encounter difficulty tapering should consider switching to buprenorphine. Of course, today buprenorphine is primarily used in maintenance therapy for opioid use disorder, for recovering drug addicts. This suggestion could make sense if buprenorphine efficacy for pain relief had been established, and it did not also carry the connotation that the pain patient was recovering from addiction. Both psychologically and in terms of the social stigma, it is harmful to patients to suggest that they are addicts. It is particularly insidious for the greater than 96% of pain patients who are not addicts. Since many people, including the leaders of PROP, consider pain patients to be addicts, every pain patient worries about anything they might do or say that could be used as evidence of addiction. This creates a climate of fear and anxiety that is not healthy for a patient population already suffering from serious disease. It would be another matter entirely if the focus of this publication were the merits of buprenorphine for relieving pain. If the drug has a benefit, why not change the designation of buprenorphine as a drug to a pain medication rather than change the pain patient's diagnosis? Rather than an emphasis on patient welfare and destigmatizing a potential medication, the focus is on the question, Is the pain patient really an addict? In a humane world, it should not even matter.

Patient Z has repeatedly asked his pain clinic for an explanation when they discussed the risks of opioids. He has been on opioids for more than ten years including at doses much higher than his current dose. Why is his risk greater now than at any time in the past ten years? There are many indications that tapers can destabilize patients. Since Patient Z is really quite ill, why should he change any medication that appears to be working? No one at the pain clinic has been able to define the risk. They speak about hyperalgesia and the risk of overdose. Hyperalgesia would mean that Patient Z has some new serious pain that has been caused by the opioids. However, in his case, there is a strong correlation of opioid dose and pain relief. Even after ten years he gets more pain relief at a higher dose. There is simply no reason to discuss hyperalgesia when a patient is stable and responding to the medication the way Patient Z is. The risk of overdose is always a concern. Patient Z has naloxone present on his bedside table, and the family knows what to do if he stops breathing. But in more than ten years, he has never had such an episode. What is the major risk that justifies suffering more pain and changing the equilibrium that he has established?

When a pain specialist writes a publication to suggest that any difficulty with tapering is evidence of a withdrawal symptom, the patient is doomed from the start. A patient who has genuine pain is bound to experience some kind of issues when the medication is reduced. Perhaps there are other medications or interventions that could help, but the patient needs to be seen as a pain patient and not primarily in terms of their relation to dependence or addiction, which are actually subjective terms. The pain medicine literature seldom focuses on function. Ability to stand, walk, and carry out basic tasks is the test of whether pain management is working. The difficulty a person has standing or walking is something that can be measured, unlike *quality of life*, which is discussed in subjective questions on a form.

At a time when there is extreme pressure to taper all patients, doctors are searching for easy ways to justify the taper. This behavior is evident in the way that doctors talk about the side effects of opioids. On a visit to the pain clinic, side effects are continuously reintroduced into the conversation in order to convince patients that the harm of opioids is greater than any benefit.[477] Telling the patient that the side effects are worse than the relief that they feel from the opioids is not particularly convincing to most persistent-pain patients. A persistent-pain patient is someone whose quality of life has already been greatly impaired by disease and pain. Most patients are aware of the side effects if they are taking opioids already. Those patients who have bad reactions to opioids self-select and opt not to continue. However, many patients feel that the worst side effect is the internal conflict about using opioids because of the stigma. Some decide that they would like to taper merely because of a sense of morality.[675] A person with significant pain who has such an internal conflict may end up with a larger problem caused by the experience of living in persistent pain. However, today most pain specialists would welcome any reason to taper a patient who is higher than the limit. In the words of one medical-legal specialist, "The regulatory climate now appears to favor underprescribing." [26] Living in pain has become more acceptable, and according to some specialists, pain is good for patients.[18] Patient Z could explain the harms of persistent pain if the experts would take the time to listen.

Overview of Side Effects of Opioid Medication vs. Side Effects of Untreated Pain

The major negative effects of opioid medications are constipation, nausea, pruritus, sedation or cognitive impairment, loss of sex drive, and hyperalgesia. Respiratory suppression is more than just a side effect since it can be lethal, and will be discussed separately. As we examine the physical origins of each of the opioid side effects, we also consider ways that they can be managed.[688] While these side effects sound serious, Labianca and coworkers also noted that[689]

> balanced against the adverse effects of pain man-
> agement medications, there is a need to be mind-
> ful of the widespread, often serious, adverse con-
> sequences of poorly managed pain itself.

As a contrast to opioid side effects, the side effects of untreated pain are high blood pressure, stress, and overactivation of the pituitary gland, which secretes adrenocorticotropin.[422] There is a risk of falls, and nausea is also possible when pain is extreme. Pain can lead to loss of sleep, which has many secondary effects—loss of mental acuity, a lowered immune response, and a general inability to function. When Patient Z was in extreme pain, he was at risk of falling, mainly because he was so tired that he could fall asleep standing up. One of the most difficult things for painful conditions is finding a comfortable position that one can stay in for a long period. Many pain patients cannot lie down, but they also cannot sit for long. In a recliner chair they must constantly change the position because of pain. That fact makes it very difficult to sleep. There are few things more miserable than being unable to sleep for days on end.

Misplaced Fears of Opioid Toxicity

The lack of pain management training in medical schools has given some doctors exaggerated and ill-informed ideas about the meaning of tolerance and its relationship to the systemic effects of opioids.[691] Opioids can suppress the immune system, but this can actually be an advantage for patients with autoimmune diseases.[690] While there are dose-dependent risks, toxicity is not high among them. The exception to this is patients who already have kidney[692] or liver damage. In those cases, antioxidants and other protective drugs may be needed. At an early stage in his disease, Patient Z once was on a flight sitting next to a surgeon. Patient Z mentioned about some of his medical issues, which were mainly manifesting themselves in his back at the early stage of the disease. When he mentioned that he was taking morphine, the surgeon proclaimed that he needed back surgery for his back pain and that morphine would kill him. Not only would he need an ever-increasing dose, the surgeon said, but the morphine would destroy his liver. Anyone hearing such a dire prediction is bound to be upset. Patient Z stayed calm throughout the flight, but once the plane landed, he went straight to his hotel room, connected to the internet, logged in to the Web of Science, and downloaded every article he could find on the liver toxicity of morphine. He stayed up much of the night reading. Contrary to the pronouncements of the surgeon on the plane, opioids have low-liver toxicity unless the liver is already damaged by some other conditions. Consistent with this information, Patient Z always had normal liver function, even after taking high-dose opioids for more than ten years. One study suggested that the oxidation of DNA was significantly higher in morphine-treated mice compared to the control. However, the study found that the effects could be counteracted quantitatively by taking antioxidants, principally vitamin C.[693] Despite the fact that the person whom Patient Z met on the plane claimed to be a famous surgeon, and did seem knowledgeable about anatomy and physiology, he did not know anything about the safety or efficacy of morphine. In the current division of labor in a hospital, sedation would be managed by an anesthesiologist. Most pain specialists know that morphine can be used in a reproducible and stable way to treat pain. They test for liver function as a precaution, but problems of that type are seldom the reason for recommending a different course of treatment. A patient with compromised liver function may have problems, but usually, the liver damage preceded opioid use. Clearly, anyone who takes opioids long-term should consult a doctor and regularly test for liver enzyme function. Vitamin C is a naturally occurring antioxidant that prevents a number of harmful oxidative processes that are associated with aging. It has no known harmful side effects. Likewise, vitamin E is a fat-soluble antioxidant that can complement vitamin C.

Opioid-Induced Constipation and Nausea

Of the common opioid side effects, constipation is the one that has the greatest general impact on the day-to-day life of a new patient. The effects of opioid-induced constipation may be related MORs present on a number of non-neuronal cells and specifically on the lining of the gastrointestinal tract.[694] The effects on the gastrointestinal tract have been confirmed using MOR-knockout mice.[695] The presence of MOR in the intestine is therefore thought to be the physical origin of constipation and nausea. Most of the studies of the burden of constipation for patients have been conducted on cancer patients, which may be a confounding factor.[696]

These side effects appear to depend on the binding of cytoplasmic beta-arrestin-2 to the MOR following drug binding to the MOR.[696] This understanding is leading to research on inhibitors of beta-arrestin-2 binding that may prevent the side effects.[193,698] The various opioid receptors and cellular signaling pathways that reduce peristalsis and motility in the intestine have been thoroughly studied.[697] While injection of opioids caused less constipation than oral ingestion, a meta-analysis of ten studies found that epidural administration (injection directly into the lower back) resulted in greater nausea and pruritus than either of the more common routes of administration.

Ileus, or blockage of the intestine, is a relatively common consequence of constipation and is one of the most common reasons for trips to the emergency room. One relevant statistic is that severe constipation is a major cause of emergency-room visits, which increased from 440,000 to 700,000 cases from 2006 to 2011.[699] While constipation is a generally acknowledged side effect of opioid treatment, for many patients the severity can be mitigated using laxatives.[700] In some cases, common laxatives are not effective, and then the strong laxatives prucalopride or lubiprostone may be more effective.[688,701] In more extreme cases, MOR antagonists can be used provided these do not cross the blood-brain barrier.[701] Naloxone is an antidote for opioids, most important for respiratory depression, but it works for other symptoms as well. Some pain clinics cite constipation as a serious side effect that should lead patients to consider tapering.[477] However, for many patients, overcoming constipation in long-term use of opioids is a matter of modulating diet, careful monitoring and using laxatives.

While nausea is a side effect of opioids, many diseases also bring on nausea—cancer, lupus,[702] multiple sclerosis,[703] and others. This may be caused by attack of an imbalance in the immune system or the changes in physiology caused by tumors. The extreme stress response that is brought on by persistent pain can cause nausea. There are drugs that can overcome nausea or mitigate it. If the opioids are bringing relief, nausea is not necessarily a reason to stop treatment. Of course, the patient should be the one to decide, in consultation with a doctor.

Morphine as a Sedative—Cognitive Effects of Opioid Use

The idea that morphine is a sedative that makes a person unable to reason, stay awake, or be a danger when driving a car is anecdotal. The few observational studies that have been conducted are inconclusive, in part because it is nearly impossible to accurately define the patient populations. Perhaps cognitive effects are applicable to patients in hospice.[704] When morphine is used in end-of-life palliative care, it does have more of a tendency to exacerbate patients' delirium, perhaps because doses in hospice are often higher than other settings[705] Oxycodone was found to be a good substitute.[704] Anesthetic doses of morphine given for surgery can put a patient to sleep. But at normal therapeutic doses taken in a routine manner, patients can be alert and capable of driving a car without being impaired.[366,706]

Pain patients who have direct experience will point out that pain is the greater danger when driving a car. The sudden onset of severe pain can cause a person to become distracted to the point where it is not possible to focus on the road or the traffic. When a person is in constant pain, it is not possible to get a good night's sleep, and one is much more likely to fall asleep at the wheel or suffer from lack of attention due simply to exhaustion. This is not to say that one should ignore the sedative properties of opioids. One must be mindful that motor and cognitive impairment by prescription opioids can be problematic for older adults, particularly at higher doses or for severe diseases.[695] Older patients in hospice will sometimes ask for lower doses to remain alert in order to be able to relate to loved ones. This is consistent with what was stated above since doses in hospice can be very high. However, many long-term pain patients, who have routine prescriptions, are attentive and careful drivers and are alert, such that an observer would not be able to tell that the patient is taking opioids.

Pain can prevent sleep. In this way a person can become so compromised that it is not possible to carry on a conversation or take care of the most basic function. Patient Z went through a phase when his pain was so debilitating that he could hardly sleep for days even weeks at a time. He was so tired that he clearly could not drive a car, but in fact he could not safely make tea. Opioid medications were not an immediate cure for this condition since he also went through an initial period of adjustment to the medication as he initially began to escalate the dose to manage his pain. However, within a month of starting opioid therapy, his sleep improved markedly and he no longer was at risk of falling or spilling hot liquids. With time he became habituated and was as lucid as he had been prior to taking the opioids. As he came to regard opioids as another medicine that he needed, he began to mention to others in conversation what he was taking. Watching people's reaction was always interesting because many people have the notion that opioids stupefy a person. Since Patient Z was always extremely alert and cogent in his conversation, he felt that it was appropriate to let people understand the reality of living with persistent pain. It was pain rather than the opioid medications that was the greater threat to his mental well-being and acuity.

Pruritus—Opioid-Induced Itching

The itching condition known as pruritus can be excruciating. Some say worse than the pain that opioids are used to treat. Pruritus can also be brought on by fabrics or certain materials that cause skin irritation. Conditions such as eczema or dermatitis herpetiformis can cause it. Tumors or vascular problems can also give rise to an itch. In opioid therapy, pruritus is a condition that most often arises from intrathecal delivery of opioids—that is, opioid pumps. It may be one of the most serious disadvantages of the technology that sounds promising in many respects. Clearly, an opioid pump would not lend itself to diversion. Treating pruritus becomes a priority for use of the pump technology. One solution is to give the patient MOR antagonists that cannot cross the blood-brain barrier. An antagonist is an interesting way to solve the problem with the MOR antagonist that basically undoes the action of the MOR agonist in the lining of the stomach. However, as I have emphasized, opioids relieve pain not only by their effect on the brain, but also by their effect on the MORs along the dorsal horn of the spine. Introducing an antagonist could change the nature of pain relief even if the antagonist could not enter the brain.[708]

Effects on Libido and Bone Density— Testosterone Replacement Therapy

Treatment with opioids can reduce levels of testosterone in men. This occurs by a mechanism known as opioid-induced androgen deficiency.[709] The reduction in testosterone has effects on sex drive, but also other health factors, such as muscle mass and bone density.[710] In general, a patient's mood is negatively affected. The decrease in sex drive is perceived as a great disadvantage by many men and has been discussed in doctor conversations about tapering.[477] However, testosterone replacement therapy is a reasonable solution in cases where the opioid is effective and reduction would cause significant pain.[92,710] The effect of loss of sex drive also occurs in women, but is even less well studied.

Hypogonadism is a common occurrence in older men even without opioid usage. The health risks are cardiovascular disease, type 2 diabetes, Alzheimer's disease, and premature death. Given the severity of these symptoms, particularly the last one, it is advisable to seek treatment. Fortunately, hypogonadism can be treated even if it is caused by opioid use. One common treatment is the drug clomiphene, which stimulates the synthesis of testosterone within a week or two if taken daily. Testosterone injections are also possible, but a somewhat harsher way to make up for the deficiency.

The Symptoms of the Disease Called Persistent Pain

Pain does significant damage to the human body. In the field of geriatric medicine, this is described as the *allostatic load*.[711] This fact is ignored in most of the discussion of opioids and their effects. What are the risks of untreated pain, and how many of the risk factors that are identified associated with opioid use are also risk factors for pain itself? High blood pressure (hypertension) is common in diseases such as osteoarthritis[89,712,713]; but even more so in more painful inflammatory diseases such as rheumatoid arthritis (RA), psoriatic arthritis (PsA), ankylosing spondylitis (AS), and spondylytic arthritis

(SA), to name a few. Hypertension may be a primary result of the disease, which has caused some dysregulation on the vasculature because of autoimmune attack. However, there is also a secondary effect of pain, which is general for any painful condition. The harmful health effects of hypertension can be life threatening. It increases the risk of stroke and heart attack.[89] Indeed, sometimes the hypertension can be treated using standard *blood pressure medications*. The most common of these medications (lisinopril) blocks the processing of angiotensin peptide, the protein responsible for causing constriction of blood vessels. A second common medication (losartan) binds to the angiotensin receptor, which has a similar physiological effect. Analgesics and antihypertensives (painkillers and blood pressure control medication) are often prescribed together to mitigate the pain. But nonsteroidal anti-inflammatory drugs (NSAIDs) such as ibuprofen often increase blood pressure and reduce the efficacy of blood pressure medications aside from the toxicity discussed previously.[714] Opioids of various types from the weaker tapentadol in doses of 100 to 250 milligrams[715] to stronger morphine have been shown to relieve these symptoms and contribute to a lowering of blood pressure. Opioids can both relieve pain and reduce blood pressure at the same time.

Insomnia is also a symptom of untreated pain. Insomnia caused by pain is poorly managed by benzodiazepine (Valium), which is effective for reduction of anxiety.[716] The consequences of extreme insomnia can be life threatening. The risk of falls or other actions that might cause self-inflicted burns or wounds are a real danger if a person is sufficiently sleep-starved. Normally, it is nearly impossible to reach such a state, but a person in pain can be unable to sleep for days on end. Relieving the pain with an adequate dose of opioid medication can cure insomnia brought on by pain. Extreme caution is advised if sedatives or sleep aids prescribed with opioids. It is generally best to avoid these combinations and to attempt to treat the pain.

Pain brings on stress. Abnormal levels of adenocorticotropin hormone (ACTH)[93] and overworking of the adrenal system that result from the constant assault of intense pain cause long-term damage that may even be fatal.[91] The effects of pain on the neuroendocrine system can impair immune function.[113] The imposition of stress disrupts the homeostasis (balance) of the immune system, which is essential to its function in combating disease.[717]

Finally, pain can bring on depression. Studies suggest that there is a negative synergy between pain and depression.[718] Aging populations have a very high incidence of multimorbidities (patients with three or more common diagnoses),[719] but the comorbidity of pain and depression with one or more of the above complications can be treated only if the pain can be alleviated.

Pain biomarkers have been discovered in recent research. There is hope on the horizon that it will be possible not only to determine that a patient has pain but even to pinpoint the physiological harms and mitigate them with greater specificity. MicroRNAs in blood can be measured to identify fibromyalgia,[720,721] spinal cord injury,[722–724] complex regional pain complex,[725] and osteoarthritis.[726] These conditions are often difficult to assess by other methods, which has led some in the medical community to dismiss them.[18] Having biomarkers will hopefully provide objective information that can be used to identify pain. Circulating inflammatory factors, such as cytokines and tumor necrosis factor, can be measured to provide evidence of inflammatory pain.[76] Other proteins and metabolic intermediates have also been identified as biomarkers of pain.[75] We will also be able to predict variable reactivity of opioids and other drugs in the body using pharmacogenomics.[727] The decision to use opioids is highly individual but can be aided significantly by a knowledge of individual genetic differences. For those who have severe pain and would be unable to function without opioids, the ethical imperative for treatment is clear.

Those in the medical community who want to significantly curtail opioid therapy for all patients appear to ignore the harm of letting a person live in pain. This harm is not mentioned in their articles. The harm and the misery that many patients feel while waiting for premature death is nowhere to be found in the consideration of these doctors. They see the potential for addiction as a dominant consideration. With the current state of knowledge, there are many facts about a pain patient that could be discovered in order to assess the risks. Aside from the genetics, which account for 50% of the risk, a strong doctor-patient relationship would permit an understanding of the motivations and disease indicators of the individual. When evaluating the dangers of opioid use, doctors should also ask patients about the health consequences they have experienced because of persistent pain.

CHAPTER 14

⤌⥥⤍

Allergic Reactions vs. Tolerance—Two Extremes Confused for Hyperalgesia

The strongest sensitivity that a person can have to a drug is an allergic reaction, but these are extremely rare for opioid drugs. True allergic reactions to opioid medications affects <2% of patients.[728,729] Anaphylactic shock is extremely rare for opioid treatment. However, some patients experience symptoms that have the appearance of an allergic reaction because of the release of histidine from mast cells. This type of reaction is called a pseudoallergy.[730] To separate a true allergy from a pseudoallergy, one can use a skin prick test or a test for a specific type of antibodies (IgE-type), although true documented cases of IgE antibodies are rare.[731] Allergic or pseudoallergic reactions that involve histidine release can be serious and may also appear as hyperalgesia, a hypersensitivity of nerve cells to certain stimuli.[728,732–736] Even when individuals show an allergic reaction to an opioid, it is almost unheard of for an individual to be allergic to all three chemical classes of opioids: phenanthrenes, phenyl-piperidines, and phenylheptanes. One of the classes of opioids is likely to be effective in pain management. The various different opioids have very different effects on hyperalgesia, a type of neuropathic pain, but this is far from understood. The fact that it is not well understood does not appear to inhibit the doctors in typical pain clinics from bringing hyperalgesia up at every convenient stage of the conversation.

Hyperalgesia is a form of neuropathic pain. Opioids are not alone in causing hyperalgesia. Chemotherapy agents and many other drugs can also cause neuropathic pain in mice. Back pain can be excruciating because of the high density of neurons along the spine. Pinched nerves can lead to sensitization or neuropathic pain, which is a major concern for lower back pain and is an indicator of poor outcomes.[737] Chemical modifications of morphine in the body have been studied as the potential cause for hyperalgesia[738] There are many kinds of neuropathic pain that may arise from disease or treatment history with other drugs that can be mistaken for opioid-induced hyperalgesia (OIH).

Some have argued that tolerance has been misidentified as hyperalgesia.[739] Logically, both tolerance and hyperalgesia may show up in a similar way—namely, that the opioids no longer control a patient's pain.[740] However, the course of action should be exactly opposite in these two cases. To overcome tolerance to a given dose, the doctor should increase the dose within reasonable limits; while for hyperalgesia, the doctor should lower the dose. The hyperalgesia narrative is the more popular one with doctors since it fits with the administrative and regulatory environment today when pain clinics invariably are looking for reasons to reduce the dose. In practice, the pressure to reduce patient's dose or to taper will almost inevitably result in greater pain. The pain specialist can hope that the condition is temporary and that the patient will adjust to the lower dose. But how often is the patient's request to return to the higher dose respected? The reaction of doctors today exposes the pressure they feel.

Mechanisms of Hyperalgesia—Potential Causes of Neuropathic Damage

One can only study the molecular mechanism of OIH in an animal model.[741-751] These data may be useful because of the similarity in the fundamental neural transmission mechanisms in both mice and humans. However, there are important differences. Mouse studies of pain involve a surgery in the mouse to create an inflammatory or pain state followed by observation. Invasive biological tools are used to determine the neural pathways, receptors, and cellular effects of pain and its mitigation in a mouse model. There are obvious physiological differences that make the interpretation of data from mice problematic for humans. Inflammation may cause sensitization of neurons, and the preparation of mouse models often involve neuropathic damage, which leads to hyperalgesia.[752] Any study in this field must recognize that hyperalgesia is caused by many diseases, chemicals, wounds, and burns separate from any opioid treatments. A patient who suffers from neuropathic pain may find that it is impossible to distinguish their usual pain from a suspected OIH. For years the conventional wisdom said that opioids could not treat neuropathic pain.[40,45,113,753-755] Recent research suggests that adjuvant opioid therapy with amitriptyline may be a valid approach to neuropathic pain, and perhaps even to hyperalgesia.[674,677,678]

The body has a natural system for reducing inflammation in nerve cells involving the noradrenaline (also called norepinephrine) neural pathways descending from the locus coeruleus in the brain to the dorsal horn (back corner) of the spine. Binding of noradrenaline to its receptor has an anti-inflammatory effect that prevents neuropathy.[756] When these neural pathways are damaged or interrupted, hyperalgesia can ensue.[757] There is evidence that involvement of calcium channel receptors in OIH may cause further hypersensitization of neural signals and exacerbate inflammatory pain in a mouse model.[758] Ketamine has been used as an antidote to this type of inflammation. Ketamine acts as a noncompetitive inhibitor of the calcium channel receptor and thereby reduces nerve cell sensitization by morphine or even by strong opioids such as remifentanil used in surgery.[759,760] Ketamine may amplify the effect of morphine and simultaneously reduce inflammation. Magnesium ion also blocks the calcium channel receptors. Surgeons have found that adding magnesium sulfate to a wound during surgery prevented OIH.[761,762] Despite the vast number of studies of opioid-induced hyperalgesia in rodent models, complete with molecular mechanisms, the significance of OIH for human health is uncertain.[763,764] For this reason, pain specialists should use caution when interpreting animal studies as a justification for reduction of dose.

Opioid-Induced Hyperalgesia—the Infallible Justification for a Taper

More than one pain specialist has told Patient Z, "The opioids you are taking are causing you more pain. You should cut back, and you would feel better." They were not mentioning this because Patient Z had complained about excess pain. They were volunteering the information in order to convince Patient Z to taper down his medication. The excess pain that the doctors were referring to is OIH.[287,765] While OIH is well-documented in laboratory mice and rats,[744,766] experimental conditions are typically high-dose exposure followed by cessation or significant reduction of the opioid treatment.[751] In humans a similar phenomenon was observed in surgery following administration of extremely strong opioids such as remifentanil or in heroin addicts who had habituated to high doses because of tolerance.[767–770] However, quite a number of studies have failed to observe hyperalgesia resulting from routine prescribing[771–773] or indicated the controversial nature of the observations.[761] Several studies suggest that OIH may be associated with withdrawal from heroin addiction.[774-776] This may explain the difference between methadone patients who are opioid-naive (and have no hyperalgesia) and recovering addicts on methadone, some of whom suffer from hyperalgesia. The effect of the opioid medications is not a mechanical damage to nerves but arises from neuroplastic changes in nerve cells that can occur upon intense activation of the MOR. The distribution of channels or receptors or their communication may be altered by a sufficiently large unnatural chemically triggered set of events in the neuron after binding of strong opioids, such as remifentanil and heroin.[775] In such cases, the pain, once provoked, is considered to be neuropathic since it arises in the nerve cell itself.[777] Since there are many potential causes of neuropathic pain, one should be careful about jumping to the conclusion that their patients have OIH, even if they are in fact showing symptoms of hyperalgesia.

When studies have been carried out in humans—that is, by asking them to reduce their dose and then report their pain—the evidence is far from conclusive. A meta-analysis by Fishbain and coworkers that searched all studies of hyperalgesia on humans conducted prior to 2007 was summarized by the Centre for Reviews and Dissemination, an international center engaged exclusively in evidence synthesis in the health field at the National Center for Biotechnology. Their summary is as follows[778]:

> This well-conducted review concluded that there was insufficient evidence to determine the existence of opioid-induced hyperalgesia in humans, except for normal volunteers receiving opioid infusions, but these data were inconsistent. The strength, quality, and consistency of the data appear to have been poor and the authors' cautious findings appear to be reliable, but there was a risk of publication bias.

Studies of OIH are receiving a great deal of emphasis, which begs the question whether physicians have a bias in the direction of justifying the hyperalgesia narrative since it gives them one of their best justifications for reducing a patient's dose. For those who take umbrage at the allegation of bias, I ask, in which other context do doctors tell patients what they are feeling? One doctor even went as far as to tell Patient Z, "You are feeling more pain from the opioids, but you just don't realize that are feeling it." Doctors in pain clinics are so anxious to talk about OIH that they give away their true motivation. Those who believe that opioid prescriptions are uniformly too high and are the cause of an epidemic feel justified in using any evidence they can find to justify lowering the dose. If doctors have a reason to suspect hyperalgesia, which is a neuropathic pain, then they could test these using drugs, such as amitriptyline, that can reduce neuropathic pain in some patients. If the goal is meeting the pain needs of the patient, the first course of action should be to treat the symptom. If the symptom really is a neuropathic pain, then there could be better treatments than simply reducing the opioid dose, an option that may bring on more pain for a patient living with an incurable or serious disease. Patient Z would prefer if he could have a conversation in which the doctor would try to understand his pain and work with him to manage it. He has never asked for the dose to be increased. He has asked numerous times if there is an alternative to the opioids that would relieve his pain. Unfortunately, no pain clinic has presented him with a viable option. Yet they were determined to reduce his dose despite the fact that they could see that he was clearly in pain.

Patient Z has come to the conclusion that he will have residual pain no matter how high the dose. From long experience, he knows that inflammatory pain is poorly controlled by opioids alone, but his nociceptive pain from damaged joints, ligaments, skin and organs could only be controlled by opioids. Like many patients who suffer from inflammatory arthritic conditions, he has mechanical pain, sharp joint pain, and a general inflammatory discomfort. The latter is best treated using antibody drugs that intercept inflammatory cytokines in the blood. But when he has discussed this at the pain clinics, doctors repeatedly suggested that the residual pain is hyperalgesia. It would be best to have a forthright discussion about this, but the pain specialist today has an ulterior motive. The pain specialist should be an ally in trying to deal with the pain, but instead the issue today is the dose, not the pain. In a climate where any reason is seized upon as a justification to taper the patient, patients need to know that admitting that they have residual pain may result in a doctor pronouncing that the pain is caused by OIH, thus recommending a decrease in the prescribed dose. Of course, if a patient were to say that they had less pain, then the pain specialist could question their need for the opioids to begin with.

Although OIH has been observed in laboratory animals since the early 1970s, evidence of pain hypersensitivity in humans is still limited because there is no unified definition and the condition has been confused with opioid tolerance, allodynia, and withdrawal-associated hyperalgesia. Allodynia is the experience of pain from a benign stimulus, whereas hyperalgesia is an exacerbation of an existing pain. A recent meta-analysis of twenty-six relevant studies culled from a total of 6,167 hits in the database search state, "There was no evidence of OIH when assessing pain detection thresholds.

OIH was more evident in patients with opioid use disorder than in patients with pain, and in patient groups treated [calcium channel] receptor antagonists (primarily evidenced in methadone-maintained populations)."[779] It is reasonable that patients with drug use disorders may have a tendency to have OIH because they are likely to be taking higher opioid doses than persistent-pain patients. However, the reaction to methadone is curious since studies differ in their interpretation, some saying that methadone is a cure for OIH and others suggesting that methadone causes OIH.

The evidence suggests variation among patients, and OIH occurs in a small group of patients. A study of eighty-one patients treated with intravenous morphine observed that twelve of them showed symptoms of thermal hyperalgesia after treatment.[780] Another study of OIH during tapering using heat pain perception test to investigate the relationship between morphine equivalent dose and heat pain perception in chronic pain patients undergoing opioid tapering.[781] The mean dose was 192 MEDD at the outset. The study found that a greater baseline dose was correlated with hyperalgesia to heat. The heat response times were shorter, meaning that the patients felt the heat with greater sensitivity the higher the dose. Similar studies have been done with the cold pressor or thermode to test the effect of cold-temperature pain.[782] The two cold temperature tests are not perfectly correlated, and they both show significant variations from patient to patient. Cook and Nickerson noted that these acute pain studies are not representative for chronic pain and found that in other contexts morphine had antinociceptive and antihyperalgesic properties.[783] No correlation was found between the cold pressor test and electric shock test for chronic pain patients on opioid therapy or patients on methadone therapy.[784] Studies of both electrically and mechanically induced pain failed to find evidence of OIH in a range of subjects.[785–787] In summary, the effect is far from general for different types of pain or patient groups. Even heat block and cold pressor tests are inconclusive when all the studies are examined. We can distinguish the use of opioids for persistent pain from their administration for surgery. Stronger opioids such as remifentanil are often used in surgery, and there is stronger evidence for OIH in that case. In summary, studies of OIH in humans provide insufficient evidence that opioid-induced hyperalgesia is an important factor in common treatments with opioids for pain.

The data in the medical literature are not sufficiently strong to use OIH as a reason to shut down the conversation about the appropriate opioid dose for relief of a patient's pain. However, many physicians today will claim that they observe hyperalgesia in patients, and this is a justification to reduce their dose.[6672] There is a motive for bias in how doctors approach human hyperalgesia.[778] Pain management and primary care physicians who prescribe opioids frequently have at least one patient who seems to need medication without an obvious somatic cause and who complains of pain even once they have received opioids. One of the stereotypical examples is a fibromyalgia patient who complains of pain and yet does not show any obvious symptoms after testing. The fact that a patient continues to complain of pain after receiving treatment could be hyperalgesia. However, it is also possible that the patient has some other source of neuropathic pain that is poorly responsive to opioids. It is also possible that the patient has psychological problems.

Patient Z has observed how the hyperalgesia narrative is used as a subterfuge to avoid having to admit the underlying reasons for a doctor's decision to taper a patient. It is insidious because hyperalgesia is a real phenomenon, but patients have no way of knowing how little evidence there is to support that it happens in the course of routine treatment using opioids. Honest and careful patients will begin to question their own sensation of pain—where it comes from and how bad it really is. Patient Z's pain varies depending on what he is doing. On days when he has less pain, he starts to do more, and by the end of the day, he may end up with greater pain just because of the activity. The opioids permit him to do more, and that is essential for his health and psychological well-being. Instead of listening to Patient Z, the pain clinic staff continues to tell him on each visit that he is overmedicated and that any pain he has is caused by OIH. Behind these statements is a constant threat that refusal to cooperate will result in an opioid-use disorder diagnosis.

The Risk for Opioid Use Disorder

Many articles have been written to make the case that addiction is on the rise because of opioid prescribing. Some suggest that pain patients are particularly prone to opioid use disorder and dependence.[11,124,778] That completes the picture for those who want a simple solution. They propose to limit the dose to 90 MEDD and taper everyone down to that level as though that is known to solve the problem. Based on the evidence, the 90 MEDD dose is completely arbitrary.[269,471] In point of fact, the state legislature of the state of Washington set the threshold value at 50 MEDD. If 90 MEDD is in any way medically justified as a maximum dose for patients, then setting the statewide maximum at 50 MEDD is arbitrary and cruel for the tens of thousands of Washingtonians who have previously received higher doses to mitigate the pain of their disease. This report reveals the absurdity of arbitrary-dose maxima for people with serious diseases.

Looking at a wider range of recent studies on the tendency of pain patients to evolve toward opioid use disorder provides scant evidence that the tendency is relevant to the typical persistent-pain patient. Considering overdose death rates as evidence, in which 75% of prescription opioid overdoses involved diverted opioids, opioid use disorder tends to correlate with diverted opioids. Studies of the behavior of pain patients have attempted to find correlations, but this is a difficult subject to document because the behavior that constitutes use disorder is difficult to isolate. Researchers use the opioid-related behaviors in treatment (ORBIT) scale as an indicator of potential "extra-medical" opioid use. A study of opioid prescribed for chronic noncancer pain (CNCP) in Australia with 1,505 participants found 38% who reported at least one indicator of potential *extramedical opioid use*. The patients suffered from back and neck pain (76%) and arthritis and rheumatism (62%). The most common of these were asking for extra medication (21%) and early prescription renewal (12%). Indicators of potential extramedical opioid use were associated with younger age, male sex, lifetime pharmaceutical opioid use disorder, and lifetime illicit drug use disorder. Here lifetime means that it has occurred in the lifetime of the individual. According to the authors, longer time monitoring would be required to determine whether these behaviors are indicative of actual opioid use disorder.[789] In any study of this type, the assumption is that the reason for needing more medication is improper use—that is, it is not related to the pain. A patient in pain is always supposed to wait for the next appointment to discuss their pain. How can we know whether some of those requesting more medication actually had a legitimate reason? Since asking for more medication can be interpreted as aberrant behavior, a person in great pain runs the risk of appearing to have a disorder by mentioning an unmet pain need. Another study found that former addicts with pain relapsed from abstinence at a three to five times higher rate than addicts who lacked pain.[790] Here, too, one is left with the obvious question whether pain itself is the driver for their behavior rather addiction. In looking for a solution to the overprescribing, Volkow and coworkers note that even if overprescribing contributed to the population of patients with opioid use disorder, the solution is not to further restrict prescribing, as that may trigger depressed and suicidal patients to turn to heroin and fentanyl, which are the acknowledged drugs of addiction today. The finding is that increased use of methadone and buprenorphine could help to reduce drug overdoses.[791] Currently there is a push to recommend buprenorphine even for pain patients who have never been heroin or fentanyl users.[588] Prior to considering use of buprenorphine to treat chronic pain, a significant amount of work needs to be done to destigmatize that medication and to show that it is effective for long-term pain relief.

Dr. Lynn Webster developed an opioid risk tool (ORT) as a predictor of opioid use disorder based on the patient's history of substance abuse, preadolescent sexual abuse, and psychological diseases.[401] The tool was predictive in three categories (low, medium, and high) after observation of new patients for twelve months on opioid therapy. Of a total of 195 patients, the low-risk group consisted of 9%, with medium-risk group at 68% and high-risk group at 23%. The study found that 94% of the patients in the low-risk category had no incidence of use disorder, whereas 90% of the patients in the high-risk category did have at least one event indicative of a disorder. For the medium category, 72% of patients had no aberrant events. Webster clarified that the purpose of screening was not to deny treatment but to be prepared to offer additional specialized treatment for those patients who begin to show signs of opioid use disorder. Previous studies had estimated the percentage of patients who will misuse their prescription as 34% for one risk factor and 27% for three or more.[792] On the other hand, Weaver and coworkers concluded the risk of addiction in the patient population is approximately the same in the pain patient population as in the population in general.[793] Anxiety, anger, and depression were found to correlate with opioid misuse.[794] Fishman commented on potential use of such studies to deny treatment[795]:

> Solutions must factor in the full complexity of drug abuse, addiction and all the related social and medical disorders, to avoid penalizing those with legitimate needs. In particular, we must be careful with implications that these data inadvertently suggest that prescription drug abuse is mostly related to prescribers and their patients, implying that limiting medically appropriate use will have any effect on reversing this disturbing trend.

In trying to save pain patients from themselves, the discussion inevitably focuses on whether the pain patient is an addict. For those with severe pain, this literally becomes a question of life and death. Since addicts are stigmatized, and their services are poor. The fear of receiving an opioid use disorder diagnosis is a real concern for any pain patient since it could negatively affect their chances for treatment. Dr. Ballantyne's suggestion that patients should consider voluntarily seeking an opioid dependence diagnosis to qualify for insurance coverage of buprenorphine is unlikely to receive any kind of endorsement from pain patients or their advocates until addiction is treated as a medical condition.[10,124]

Differences in the Allostatic Effect in Addiction and in Pain

Addiction has been explained in the context of opponent process theory.[796] A *desirable* drug experience tends to cause a person to seek to repeat the experience, which leads to habituation. Habituation in turn leads to tolerance, which decreases the pleasure of the experience after repeated stimulus. After frequent repetition of the desirable experience, termination of that experience results in withdrawal each time the effect of the drug wears off. Opponent-process theory describes the effect of affective (mood enhancing) or hedonistic (pleasure enhancing) drug experiences in three phases: (1) contrast, (2) habituation, and (3) withdrawal (abstinence).[797] The cycle may generate new motives and behaviors because withdrawal is undesirable, and the subject will often look forward to returning to the contrast state. The opponent concept refers to the concept of the withdrawal being a reaction or *antireward* to the euphoria of the desirable state. More recent scientific descriptions use different language to describe the phases of a cycle of dependence: (1) anticipation, (2) intoxication, and (3) withdrawal.[798] The neurological and endocrinal changes caused by the drug remain after the drug has lost its effect. Withdrawal is a state of stress, depression, and anxiety that increases in intensity the longer the subject must wait for the next dose. The cycle of dysregulation gets progressively worse, arising from the factors of tolerance, need for the drug, social isolation, and depression.[799] These lead to dysregulation of opioid, dopamine, and adrenal receptors in the synapse of neurons in the brain, which results in hormone release in a stress response. Adrenocorticotropic hormone (ACTH) is released from the pituitary gland. Efferents from the thalamus to the amygdala are thought to be responsible for the harmful stress response to pain.[410] The altered neuronal structure because of plasticity and the secretion of stress hormones produces an *allostatic state*.[797] The drug user in this state of existence has no interest in anything other than the drug.

The pain-naive drug user enters the cycle of dysregulation, which tends to become more harmful as the person cycles into the *antireward* state.[798] The subject has a strong impetus to return to the pleasure state often with a level of desperation that leads to irrational and potentially self-destructive behavior. The speed of the onset of the stimulus is important to a subject who is seeking the euphoric state. This is associated with what drug users refer to as the "high." As the user pursues this state and cycles through the euphoric state and its opponent withdrawal, neural plasticity leads to changes in nerve cells that are adapting to these changes. The memory of the effect can be relatively long-term, which means that it will also take a long time to unlearn the changes, the physiological responses, and the associated behavior.

A large medical literature considers this cycle of addiction to be distinct from the pain-relief process. For a persistent-pain patient, the shift from normal homeostasis to an *allostatic state* occurs because of persistent pain, not the opioid drug. As described in chapter 3, the *allostatic state* caused by pain has some similarities to the effect of opioid drugs on pain-naive users. The desensitization of dopamine receptors and increase in stress hormone levels are observed in both.[800] The allostatic load consists of pain, which accumulates over a lifetime.[711] In some patients chronic pain refers to pain that has "taken on a life of its own," persisting after wounds or injuries have healed.[801] This type of pain does not have an obvious cause but is nonetheless very real to the patient. This pain is related to central pain, which is pain located in the brain following stroke or other injuries in the brain itself.[15,16] Central pain may serve as a model for chronic pain, but is not necessarily applicable to persistent pain that originates from ongoing inflammation or tissue, organ, or joint damage caused by disease. Regardless of origin, persistent pain never loses its effect, and the pain patient has no normal or balanced (homeostatic) reference state. When persistent pain is severe enough, a patient has no choice but to seek pain relief. Opioids provide the main medical route to shift the painful, *allostatic state* back toward a normal state. Because the nervous system of the persistent-pain patient is already in an advanced *allostatic state* that has certain similarity with the effects of non-natural opioid use, the effects of opioids do not create a cycle of dysregulation that mimics the drug user's experience. Rather the opponent process in pain relief is considered to be pain itself, and consequently tolerance is the main effect. Leknes writes the following[802]:

> The rewarding effect of relief from unpleasant states other than pain is well documented. For instance, food tastes better when it relieves hunger.[803,804] In general, the reward value (pleasantness) of a stimulus increases the more effective that stimulus is in restoring bodily equilibrium (homeostasis).[15,805]

The articles claiming that pain patients are dependent on their medication imply that the patients do not actually need the medication for pain relief.[10–12] Evidence shows that only a small minority feign their pain in the hopes of a higher dose. The patient population that appears to be the focus of PROP's concerns are those with minor pain who were overmedicated during a period of excessive prescribing, which ended a decade ago. When Drs. Ballantyne and Kolodny admit that patients do not conform to the definitions of aberrant behavior according to the DSM-5, they must at least pause to ask whether pain might be the explanation for the observed behavior of the patients who do not respond well to tapering. It is not ethical to disregard patient's pain.

Differentiating the Long-Term Treatment of Persistent Pain from Opioid Use Disorder

Since 2016 an arbitrary dose limit has been the criterion by which the clinicians judge all pain patients. Those who require more than the predefined maximum dose are overmedicated by definition. If they have difficulty complying with the arbitrary limit or a taper toward that limit, they are suspected of having opioid use disorder.[11,124] The 2019 article entitled "Rethinking Dose Tapering" suggests that buprenorphine, normally used for recovering addicts, should be prescribed to pain patients to help them to taper.[10] Although the articles speak in a tone suggesting clinicians will be compassionate, writing a publication to suggest that patients who appear to be pain patients are in reality suffering from opioid use disorder only strengthens the feeling among pain management specialists that the tapers should be mandatory and rapid. In many clinics, compassion is not part of the program. Meanwhile, Chou and coauthors admit that the criteria applied to opioid use disorder are not appropriate for pain patients when they write,[10]

> Some patients with difficulty tapering may have developed [opioid use disorder], but many do not neatly fit the [opioid use disorder] criteria in the Diagnostic and Statistical Manual of Mental Disorders, Fifth Edition (DSM-5). The DSM-5 eliminated opioid dependence as a separate diagnosis; excluded withdrawal and tolerance as [opioid use disorder] criteria when opioids are taken as prescribed; and requires that patients meet at least 1 criterion other than difficulty tapering, including craving, compulsive use, or harmful use.

Of course, it is difficult for someone in pain to avoid compulsive use. I find the inclusion of compulsive use in this quote to be inappropriate. The terms *craving* and *harmful use* seldom apply to pain patients. Nonetheless, Drs. Ballantyne and Kolodny have each used the DSM-5 criteria to "argue that some patients who have persistent difficulty in tapering and withdrawal but do not meet other DSM-5 criteria have a complex form of prescription opioid dependence." The new type of dependence, prescription opioid dependence, has the harms of "negative affect, reward deficiency, and social isolation." If these are the symptoms of prescription opioid dependence, then pain patients have no chance. Very ill people overwhelmingly have these symptoms. Patient Z is often depressed. He cannot work or even walk. He can barely get out of his chair to make a cup of tea. His physical disability is mainly exacerbated by the extreme pain of every move he makes. Thinking about Patient Z as an archetype for those patients who have incurable inflammatory diseases, it is rather insulting to suggest that research is needed to determine whether "a diagnosis of prescription opioid dependence results in fewer negative legal, work, and social consequences; is perceived as less stigmatizing than an opioid-use disorder diagnosis; or increases acceptance of buprenorphine use." Obviously, the authors have a different archetype in mind, but which one? Their writing does not inform us how to differentiate pain patients according to their diagnosis or any other criterion. Patient Z commented that the idea of research to substantiate a new type of "dependence" diagnosis is a way to depersonalize the issue and make it easier to put all patients into a single category. For whatever reason, buprenorphine has become the drug of choice for those who think all patients should taper down to a low level.

The description of the opponent process in pain management in a recent publication gives us insight into how the authors view tapers to low opioids levels or even down to abstinence. Dr. Ballantyne's article states,[124]

> It is not well recognized that allostatic opponent process involved in development of opioid dependence can cause worsening pain, functional status, sleep, and psychiatric symptoms over time, and significant fluctuation of pain and other affective symptoms because of their bidirectional dynamic interaction with opioid dependence ("affective dynamism"). These elements of complex persistent dependence (CPD), the gray area between simple dependence and addiction, can lead to escalating and labile opioid need, often generating aberrant behaviors. Opioid tapering, a seemingly logical intervention in this situation, may lead to worsening of pain, function, and psychiatric symptoms because of development of protracted abstinence syndrome.

Is this the fate that awaits Patient Z? To someone who is sick with various seriously painful conditions, destroyed joints, inflamed tendons, severely swollen legs, skin damage, and wounds from swelling and so on, it is frightening to hear that those debilitating comorbidities would be lumped into a "protracted abstinence syndrome" by the pain specialist.

There is yet another name for the new type of *dependence*. The experts have called it *complex persistent dependence*. The above description was written as though it applies to pain patients in general. Perhaps the authors had an overmedicated patient in mind, but they did not specify that. The clinical research and articles reviewed in this book made a clear case that pain patients are less likely than pain-naive people to succumb to addiction. In reality, the pain and personal proclivity toward addiction both comprise distributions. The generalizations provided by Drs. Kolodny and Ballantyne are not helpful[52] because they do not define the patient population or consider the role played by pain and disease in the behaviors they describe.[11,52]. Starting with Patient Z as an archetypal example, the idea of talking about patients worsening pain, functional status, and sleep as evidence of an *allostatic opponent process* do not apply.[796] In applying the tools used by psychiatrists to identify addiction, the doctor should answer the question, Why is the patient's disease not the primary concern? Many pain patients have cancer, inflammatory arthritis, or degenerative diseases. Their pain may, and probably will, worsen over a period of years, as a result of the disease. Alternatively, psychiatric symptoms may arise from feelings of depression at being unable to lead a normal life and witnessing one's own decline in health. In a person with a complex disease, these are almost impossible to distinguish. Yet the authors claim that "awareness of the science of the neuroplasticity effects of repeated use of opioids is necessary to better manage these patients with complex challenges" as though the major challenge is because of the opioids themselves. Are the authors aware of the science that addresses the neuroplasticity of pain itself? Pain alters the neurophysiology in an opioid-like manner because it involves the natural opioid system. In a person with persistent pain, opioids consequently lack an opponent process other than pain itself. For many, the effect of opioid treatment is the only hope they have that they could overcome their pain enough to work or have a family life. Of course, life is a struggle for someone who is very sick. However, labeling that person an addict and moving to a rehabilitation setting is likely to have an extremely negative psychological impact on the person. No one today has addressed a plan to remove the stigma of addiction. To talk as though there is a kinder, gentler version of the term *addict* is dangerous for the welfare of pain patients. Indeed, in this paper Ballantyne and coworkers admit that such attitudes have destabilized patients who had been managing their pain for years.[124]

Stable patients who have relatively high doses may experience certain chronic problems, but decreasing the dose often makes the situation worse. This is told in an "archetypal patient story" as follows[124]:

> A 61-year-old patient with posttraumatic stress disorder (PTSD) and chronic pain because of degenerative spine disease was able to maintain a business and provide for his family with fentanyl patches (>400 MEDD) to control his debilitating pain for over a decade. Over time, pain and function worsened; insomnia, anger, and depression slowly emerged, and PTSD worsened. He sought more opioids from physicians for better pain control and to maintain his functional life. He interpreted multiple failed attempts by himself to stop opioids as evidence that they were helping to manage the pain driven by advancing spine disease, which in turn was driving his psychiatric worsening. However, radiographic investigations revealed stable spine disease. He got no clear answers from physicians why his pain was increasing despite this and wondered if they missed something. On one of the visits with his primary care provider (PCP), he was told

about the new CDC guideline and the concerns about safety and inefficacy of high opioid doses and an opioid taper was offered. He was assured that the pain would be stable with dose reduction and he might actually do better. He reluctantly agreed, and the fentanyl dose was slowly tapered in half over next 3 months. However, his pain, function, mood, anger, insomnia, anxiety, and PTSD all worsened. His PCP advised him to stay the course, and he was offered additional support, including referral to substance abuse treatment. Neither the patient nor the substance abuse treatment program felt that he was addicted to opioids. He eventually decided to change the PCP, and during the transition he obtained overlapping opioid prescriptions from 2 doctors. Interpreting this as opioid contract violation, his old PCP tapered him off opioids completely over a month, providing medications for opioid withdrawal symptoms that lasted over a week after the last opioid dose. Hearing about this, his new PCP also refused to prescribe him any opioids. Over the next month, his pain and physical function continued to worsen, as did his emotional health. He became confined to a wheel chair, unable to work, severely limited by pain the whole day. He became despondent and suicidal. He could sleep only an hour and a half a night and was exhausted. He thought about getting heroin from the streets, but his moral upbringing and military training prevented him from doing so. He could not understand why the doctors would do this to him and leave him helpless. He wondered whether this was all because of pain that was not effectively treated. Patient progress: Recognizing severe protracted withdrawals, he was initially restarted on long-acting morphine tablets 90 mg 3 times a day. His pain and psychiatric symptoms came under some control, but not back to his baseline. Gabapentin and duloxetine were tried, but he could not tolerate them. He was still confined to a wheelchair after 2 months. Morphine was discontinued, and he was started on buprenorphine/naloxone 8/2 mg sublingually 3 times a day. Within several weeks, his overall function markedly improved, including abandoning his wheelchair. He was more engaged in multimodal chronic pain treatment with increased physical activation and willing to explore psychotherapy for pain and opioid dependence. His psychiatric distress abated considerably, and he started having up to 6 hours of uninterrupted sleep on most nights. From the patient's perspective, he describes "getting my life back."

The authors wrote that "the logical therapeutic intervention of opioid tapering and discontinuation [...] can cause persistent worsening of [pain, psychosocial status, function, misuse, etc.] (archetypal patient story [above]), leading to confusing clinical scenarios and sometimes disastrous consequences, including death." The frank admission that tapering a patient in this way could have such negative consequences as patient death was reported with clinical detachment. Instead of concern for patients who are victims of perverse system that can arbitrarily terminate them and send them into withdrawal despite their best intentions to comply, the authors focused only on the lesson that patients could successfully scale back their dose if sufficient pressure was applied. However, in this instance it apparently caused great misery and an unnecessary classification of the patient as having an opioid use disorder but fortunately did not result in death. Patient Z commented that from a pain patient's perspective, the archetypal patient appeared to have undergone a very painful and poorly executed opioid rotation from fentanyl patch to oral morphine to the buprenorphine-(1%)-naloxone mixture. First, the patient was stable, working and supporting a family for ten years on an opioid dose of 400 MEDD fentanyl patch. The patient's complaints of worsening pain were not explained by imaging, which is frequently the case when inflammation is involved. Aside from the mention of PTSD, the description has much in common with Patient Z's current situation. Rather than suggesting an opioid rotation, the doctor convinced the patient that tapering would improve the symptoms. "He was assured that the pain would be stable with dose reduction and he might actually do better." The archetypal patient was clearly given bad advice. But when a doctor recommends the reduction in dose for "safety" and compliance reasons, a patient may feel that there is no choice. Instead of addressing the patient's sense of anxiety and reassuring them, they are told they must taper at within a few weeks to 50 MEDD. After ten years on a fentanyl patch the patient may have built up a tolerance and perhaps could have benefitted from an opioid rotation. Instead of offering some alternative that might address the pain, the patient was told about the new recommendations to lower the dose in such a way that would only increase the patient's sense of shame about being on such a high dose. As a *reward* for following the physician's advice and reducing the dose, the patient was ultimately discharged without any pain medicine at all. Of course, there are terrible consequences for someone who has serious pain, and the shock to a person's system of being cut off in that way can be life threatening. At the end of all that, to find some relief on a combination of buprenorphine-(1%)-naloxone is touted as success because the patient says he is "getting [his] life back." After facing the prospect of living in pain for the rest of his life, the patient is probably happy to have any kind of pain medication. Does the life refer to the ten-year period of stability on a dose of 400 MME fentanyl patch or some other life?

At a minimum, this archetypal case study raises serious questions about why tapering is considered a good idea for patients with serious pain. In fact, the recommendation by CDC and HHS is not to taper if the patient is stable, has no side effects, and is compliant.

If this case is intended to illustrate a complex, but successful, voluntary taper, I shudder to think what the involuntary taper looks like. Patient Z has commented that playing on a patient's sense of shame is not voluntary but manipulation of the patient. One can infer that the patient was probably introduced to buprenorphine by Dr. Ballantyne, Dr. Manhapra, and their co-workers. In other words, her clinic is perhaps that one that brought back the patient who had been cast aside. If that is correct, then kudos to Dr. Ballantyne for ethical treatment of patients. If only that level of care could be extended to the masses of patients who have been terminated in the past four years. Under the circumstances, it was that humane action that probably rescued this patient. However, the treatment that preceded the buprenorphine prescription was irresponsible. The archetypal cases and generalizations made in this and other articles would lead one to believe that the majority of pain patients are overmedicated and many are addicted to their medications. It is remarkable to me that these archetypes are so different from the ones that I know of from conversations with doctors, pain support groups, and Patient Z. The literature is the best arbiter of the typical patient, and there is no publication I am aware of that presents evidence that a significant percentage of pain patients is addicted to their medication. Based on extensive evidence, conservative estimates suggest that <3% of pain patients[133,137,138,141,142] and <8% of the general pain-naive population go on to become addicted or have a use disorder.[4,9,139,141,300]

There appears to be an implication that pain itself is not debilitating for the archetypal patient. On the contrary, pain is often a crucial issue, a life-determining issue. The issue that is not stated openly is whether or not the *overmedicated* patient has a severe and debilitating disease or disability. A patient who has severe pain may be practically incapacitated by a significant taper or abstinence. To discuss these measures as necessary to reduce risk of overdose or other side effects is to assume that the patient does not have such severe pain that the health of the patient will be compromised by being in pain.

The application of opponent process theory to pain patients is purely speculative. The drug addict also experiences tolerance, and the drug addict must dose escalate. Yet a pain patient may be stable for decades on a fixed dose, as shown by the archetypal study above. Evidence suggests that tolerance is significantly less of an effect when treating pain compared to seeking euphoria.[62,148,154] Data comparing dose escalation and withdrawal between persistent-pain patients and heroin users was obtained by Cowan and coworkers. Their results are summarized as follows[154]:

> [Persistent pain] patients started therapy in the low dose range for oral morphine (approx. 60 mg/day) and most (83%) did not move into a higher dose range once adequate levels of analgesia were attained. Street users started smoking heroin intermittently, before daily use. Most escalated their dose by increasing the amount used and by switching from smoking to injecting. Unlike CNCP patients, street users demonstrated patterns of compulsive drug use, social problems and intoxication. Only 3/31 (9.5%) pain patients that discontinued opioid therapy reported withdrawal symptoms on abstaining from the drug compared to 35 (89.5%) of street users.

These data show the large difference between street users of heroin and pain patients. It is common sense that persistent-pain patients fear returning to a state of pain, and if their pain is severe enough, they fear the health consequences and ultimately a premature death. The physiological changes that street drug users undergo are different from the persistent-pain patient in large measure because of the stress response that is inherent to pain but is absent in the street users until they may have a stress that arises caused by withdrawal from a high heroin dose.

Dr. Ballantyne's proposal that persistent-pain patients could be considered *opioid-use dependents* is developed further in an administrative dimension. With regard to the fact that insurance companies may refuse to pay for buprenorphine for pain patients, they write that[124]

> misinformed local insurance and pharmacy formulary restrictions may often disallow such use of buprenorphine for pain. In that case, we recommend making a clinical diagnosis of opioid dependence collaboratively with the patient and then starting the buprenorphine substitution when indicated.

Cowan and coworkers were adamant about the harms of calling pain patients addicts. They cite the following example[154]:

> The following case history demonstrates that fears of addiction still exist and stigmatization is still experienced by some pain patients. A 35-year-old man with inoperable spondylolisthesis was prescribed controlled-release morphine sulphate 60 mg twice daily at a pain clinic. He was subsequently able to return to his work as a car mechanic. On attempting to renew his prescription at his General Practitioner surgery, he was told by the doctor on duty that he was the same as a "junkie" and that morphine was available for only those dying of cancer. On another occasion, he was also described as a junkie by a clinic nurse. This misidentification has previously been discussed. This man then saw a neurologist who believed that morphine was the main cause of the patient's problem and that the patient should stop the treatment by gradually reducing the dose to minimize withdrawal symptoms. The patient claimed that he had not suffered such symptoms when his painkillers had been unavailable previ-

ously and to prove this decided to abruptly stop taking all morphine.

Although the patient had no withdrawal effects, the pain returned. The pain specialists encouraged him to resume taking morphine. Regarding the criticisms of their study, Cowan and coworkers responded with a commentary of their own[154]:

> The typical chronic pain patient is simply different from the typical street user. They differ in many ways including age, sex, opiate drug used, route, dose escalation, experience of withdrawal symptoms, and other signs of problematic drug use including drug seeking behaviours. We agree that there are some problems with this simplistic approach to comparison, for example it would be preferable to compare groups who had taken opiates for similar lengths of time. However the argument we seek to counter is equally simplistic but hugely damaging. Chronic pain patients taking prescribed opiate drugs are accused by their health care providers of being similar to street users by virtue of the fact that they take opiates. This has led to stigmatization and, in some cases, the withholding of effective pain control. Our paper simply shows that the assumption upon which these judgments are made is false.

We see the different points of view in the medical community are in stark contrast with one another. At least Cowan and coworkers conducted a study as the basis for their statements.[154] The policy and prescribing recommendations made in numerous publications by Ballantyne and coworkers were opinion without underlying data.[11,132]

CHAPTER 15

꧁꧂

Are We Learning from History or Repeating the Mistakes of the Past?

Opioids have a long history starting with their cultivation by the Sumerians in Mesopotamia more than five thousand years ago.[151] The medicinal value of opioids was recognized in ancient India and is part of Ayurvedic medicine. Despite this long history of use, there has been considerable misinformation about the subject in recent years, even among trained doctors.[119] The solution to a high heroin overdose rate proposed by the CDC has been to limit prescribing and taper pain patients to a fixed dose. That solution has made the problem worse by leading to such poor treatment of pain patients that some of them have fallen victim to suicide or overdose. This is not happening because of human weakness, but because of the unspeakable tragedy of medical abandonment on a massive scale. The idea of arbitrarily limiting all pain patients' doses smacks of abolition. The punitive approach to opioids has failed for over one hundred years. Addiction has been a national obsession periodically over that time, until people become inured to an increasing drug-overdose rate. We have wasted enormous resources, using failed ideas, and ignored the scientific reality that addiction is a disease. Addiction should be treated by a doctor with the same confidentiality we afford all patients. Abstinence has failed as a form of rehabilitation, and the punitive policies of the DEA and state law enforcement have made every aspect of the drug problem worse—greater addiction, more overdoses, and more people in prison for possession. Morphine is one of the oldest drugs known, and yet it is one of the least well understood in terms of its effect on humans. We know a great deal about its mechanism of action and increasingly about the neurophysiology. Yet we seem to be incapable of confronting the variability in human response to opioids.

Today, many doctors receive poor training in pain management.[806] As a result, there is a common misconception that opioids have no beneficial use in medicine. Recent graduates from medical schools have only negative associations with words *opioid* or *morphine*. We have taken a step backward on the path toward learning how to use this powerful medicine that has both beneficial uses and formidable risks. The undertreatment of pain patients began to receive recognition in the 1970s, and attitudes began to change as the collective experience with opioids was publicized.[807] Now that we have enough experience to say that opioid therapies work for some patients, we need to find a comprehensive solution to opioids as both medications and drugs. While many patients in severe pain benefit from opioid therapy, other patients have been harmed. The only way to solve the issue humanely is to treat pain according to its severity while treating addiction as a disease.[297] The is no *shortcut* to personalized medicine. It is sensible to end the DEA's jurisdiction over doctors. Instead, medical boards should have a leading role in ensuring standards of care. Many countries in western Europe have shown that this idea is feasible. The statistics are much better in those countries, lower addiction and overdose rates than in the US, and good access to pain medication for patients with serious diseases.

The Lessons of History

One of the important insights that the history of opioids provides us is that criminalization of opioids (as well as cocaine and marijuana) occurred in the context of racism and populist nationalism. It is disturbing to read an echo of that shameful history in the *Annual Review* article written by Dr. Kolodny and coworkers.[12] When authors write about Chinese opium dens in the United States in the late 1800s as a source of the problem in the US, they should put the matter in the perspective of the illegal policy by the Western powers to force the sale of British opium, grown in India, throughout China. In the Opium Wars of the 1840s, the British and Americans forced the sale of British opium on the Qing Dynasty of China in order to settle the balance of payments. It is very unfair to the Chinese to bring up the opium dens run by some Chinese immigrants in North America without acknowledging the role of the Western powers in imposing opium on China. That history has made it extremely difficult for the Chinese to use opioids for the treatment of pain. If addiction is stigmatized in the United States, one can only begin to imagine the stigma felt by the Chinese since addiction was a scourge that was forced on them by American and British cannons in devastating naval attacks. China finally has begun to move past that history and to use opioids for medical purposes. A recent Chinese study evaluated untreated cancer pain and concluded that China needs to increase opioid medications to come up to international norms for treatment of cancer pain in the WHO standards.[808] A 2014 study of cancer patients in Fujian Province described treatment of pain in 257 cancer patients using doses of up to 105 MEDD. Good efficacy was found, and the study suggested methods for other hospitals to emulate.[25] China is overcoming the barriers to opioid use for pain at a time when the United States is pulling back strongly from the commitments made to pain patients. Given the burden of a very negative history with opioids imposed from colonial times, this is a big step forward for China and a step backward for the United States.

The opium used in the United States during the latter part of the nineteenth century was mostly homegrown. Chinese immigrants purchased opium the same way everyone else did. This was a time when a person could order Bayer Corporation's new heroin formulation from the Sears and Roebuck catalog. Morphine was used for amputations and other surgeries during the Civil War. The medicinal value became clear to millions following that wartime experience. Toward the end of the nineteenth century, injectable morphine became widely used in American medicine and became one of the most popular medicines in a doctor's satchel. Since morphine was legal, that use continued, and eventually addiction followed. Historians debated the extent to which addiction was a social problem during the Civil War. Perhaps, the narrative that addiction started in the Civil War was used to explain why White men in the United States were so much more prone to take opium compared to Europeans.[809] Certainly, by the end of the nineteenth century, there was an addiction problem in the United States. The debate at that time was between those who thought it should be treated as a medical problem and those who wanted to criminalize morphine and heroin.

The Criminalization of Opioids in the Early Twentieth Century Caused Social Turmoil

The fear of addiction permeated the American response to opioids. Addiction was a concept that grew out of the perceived moral failing of those who drank too much or took opium on a regular basis. The modern debate about the historical record occurred around the end of the Vietnam War when there was a great fear of the effect of thousands of veterans who had become addicted to heroin returning to the United States. Those who wanted a new law and tougher measures argued that there were large numbers of addicts during the Civil War who had caused the initial wave of addiction.[810] Irrespective of the cause, the rate of opioid addiction around 1900 was 0.25–0.3%, which was similar to the rates of addiction from 1960 to 2010. Ironically, the heroin addiction rate began to increase again in 2011 for the first time in many years after the crackdown on prescription opioids was implemented.[507,617]

Unlike the typical addict in more recent times, prior to the change in law that made it a crime, many people addicted to morphine were active in society. In the early years, women addicts outnumbered men by three to one.[811] Women are afflicted disproportionately by many of the rheumatic and autoimmune diseases, which was as true one hundred years ago as it is today. Some of the reported addiction probably was medical use. Of course, the growth of addiction was not a healthy development. However, it was not the health issue that was foremost in people's minds. It was seen by many as a moral failing.[809] The moral arguments combined with racist fears about the "opium dens of the Chinaman" and "cocaine-snorting negro" led to the change in law and effectively ended any hope of medical treatment for addiction. These absurdly racist justifications were used to conjure a fear of addiction in the American public and the legislators who would have to support the new laws. The racist tropes were completely false. The majority of drug users in the United States had always been White and middle class or wealthy. But in 1914, these racist ideas were sufficient justification for a new act of Congress to criminalize opioids and cocaine.[811]

The Harrison Narcotics Act of 1914 was actually a tax act, and as such was not popular. The members of Congress in southern states were convinced to vote for it because of the use of racist tropes about Blacks. In the western states, it was the anti-Chinese sentiment that garnered support. Following passage of the act, morphine became increasingly expensive and difficult to obtain.[799] The Harrison Act was ruled unconstitutional in 1919 in the Supreme Court decision the *United States v. Doremus [249 US 86]*, but de facto the process of criminalizing morphine was well underway. Shortly thereafter, the ruling in *Webb et al. v. the United States [249 US 96]* outlawed maintenance therapy for addicts and began to close the door for addicts to receive medical treatment. Many of the prescribing doctors who continued to support wealthier patients were prosecuted. The prosecution of doctors continued until 1925 when the Supreme Court decision in *Linder v. the United States* ruled in favor of the doctors.[812] By that time some thirty-five thousand physicians had been prosecuted and many sentenced to prison.[485] Many former addicts were incarcerated or forced to live in a criminal underworld created by the combination of abolition and the antinarcotics legislation. Many women who had used morphine ended up in brothels.[811]

In an admonition to learn the lesson of history, the *Annual Review*[12] discusses the prosecution of physicians and tragedy of the patients as follows:

> The development of alternative analgesics such as aspirin; stricter prescription laws; and admonitions about morphine in the lay and professional literature stemmed the addiction tide. One important lesson of the first narcotic epidemic is that physicians were educable. Indeed, by 1919, narcotic overprescribing was the hallmark of older, less-competent physicians. The younger, better-trained practitioners who replaced them were more circumspect about administering and prescribing opioids.

By 1919, the doctors were indeed circumspect if they did not want to go to prison. If we want to learn the lessons of history, we would do well to consider that abolition was a failure and criminalization of addiction had long-lasting negative social consequences.[485] Racism had been an integral part of the concept of addiction from the beginning, and it continued to the present. The proof was in the statistics of incarceration in the United States. Although the vast majority of addicts were White, the vast majority of people prosecuted and incarcerated under the Controlled Substances Act were people of color.

The law-and-order view of history misses the plain fact that it is *because* of the criminalization that addiction continued untreated for the next one hundred years. The crackdown of 1919 did not solve the problem. From a public health standpoint, the crackdown created the problem. From the beginning, the US government had been quick to punish and slow to provide rehabilitation. The prohibition of alcohol and drugs had been shown repeatedly to be a failed policy that brought misery and exacerbated the original problem. An aggressive campaign to stamp out addiction lowered the rate of addiction significantly by World War II. But heroin addiction surged again after World War II. By the 1960s the rate was as high as it had been prior to the Harrison Act. PROP's proposal of hard limits is a prohibition that is in line with the DEA's *war on prescription drugs.* Yet the reasoning behind this prohibition is flawed. To eliminate prescription drugs when 80% of the deaths are caused by heroin and fentanyl will do nothing to change the status of current drug users. Of the small portion of overdoses that involve prescription drugs, the majority comes from diversion not from pain patients using their prescriptions. The argument that new drug users are starting because of prescription drugs fails to explain the origin of the major drug abuse problem for the past fifty years or why ten years of decrease in the prescription rate has only exacerbated the overdose rate. We are punishing pain patients for the actions of others, and "responsible prescribing," as defined by PROP, is only making the problem worse.

The failure of the *war on drugs* stems from the fact that we cannot eliminate addiction by cutting off the supply of drugs. In fact, the lesson is that we will only make the addiction problem worse by trying to cut off the supply.[421–423,813] What is true for illicit drugs is also true for prescription drugs. If we eliminated prescribing altogether, there would still be sources of illicit drugs and addiction from those routes. A more prudent idea is to regard both pain treatment and addiction as diseases that require medical treatment.[360,813] Criminalizing addiction in 1914 merely changed the addicts and their doctors into criminals. Today we know that addiction is part of the human condition with genetic and sociological aspects affecting a small minority of patients. Society plays a major role in how addiction manifests itself, but if we want to cure addiction, we must treat it as a disease, which means with the same compassion, privacy, and advice that a patient would receive for any other disease. Rather than learn the lesson that punitive approaches fail,[557] the US has continued on the same path with an even greater waste of financial resources and human life.

Sickle Cell Disease—Pain Crisis in a Microcosm

Sickle cell disease (SCD) is an important case for understanding opioid-prescribing trends and the issues that prevent pain patients from receiving treatment. Sickle cell disease arises because of an inherited genetic mutation in hemoglobin in African or African American populations at a rate of approximately 1 in 365 live births.[814] There are approximately 90,000 SCD patients in the United States. Yet far fewer resources are devoted to the study and treatment of SCD compared to cystic fibrosis, which afflicts 30,000 primarily Caucasian patients. SCD causes proteins to aggregate in red blood cells. SCD impedes the ability of hemoglobin to bind and release oxygen normally and can also affect the blood flow in capillaries. The blockage or friction in the capillaries is very painful. The pain of SCD has been underestimated and undertreated. SCD patients have been stigmatized by race, which has limited their access to medical care. Most SCD patients receive opioids to manage pain by going to the emergency room (ER).[815] This corresponds to a widely held idea that SCD has acute crises when the symptoms become much worse. The medical community has only recently acknowledged the fact that SCD is accompanied significant untreated chronic pain. One way to understand the severity of the disease is to realize that SCD patients' life expectancy is in the midfifties.

It is not easy to see an organic reason for sickle cell pain without looking inside the patient's red blood cell or seeing tiny blockages in capillaries. A patient who presents himself or herself to the ER will not have an outward manifestation of pain that a doctor can recognize. The doctor must know the diagnosis and believe the patient report. The pain caused by aggregation of hemoglobin molecules inside red blood cells and the corresponding change in cell dynamics in capillaries cannot be directly detected by any simple test. Patients who come to the emergency room (ER) typically receive injections of hydromorphone or other opioids to relieve the pain.[68] Patients report frequently to being subject to discrimination in the ER because of their race, but also because they do not have obvious lesions. Studies show that SCD patients wait 60% longer to receive medications than other patients.[308]

Over time, clinicians became aware that SCD patients were feeling pain a great deal of the time and that their pain was undertreated. An article describing treatment with opioid therapy and several commenting letters in 1992 began the discussion of opioid treatment of SCD in the literature.[28,67] At that time patients typically waited until they had a crisis and were admitted to the hospital. They often received parenteral opioids for several days until the crisis subsided. Apparently, many doctors assumed that the rest of the time SCD did not have severe pain. However, records indicate that patients were in severe pain 56% of the time.[69] This realization began to change treatment protocols. Change has been hampered by the restrictive policies mandated by the CDC guidelines. Following the implementation of the CDC guidelines, it became more difficult for patients to receive treatment in the emergency room or to receive prescriptions that they had been able to fill prior to 2016. Interviews with patients revealed a perception of discrimination [816] As with other diseases, the revisions to the CDC guidelines have done little to help patients whose care was diminished by the original CDC guidelines.[817]

There are psychological consequences of the stigma of SCD that can be generalized to the stigma felt by all pain patients. Studies have found that African American patients generally tend to under-report the unpleasantness of pain to physicians. They were also more likely to attribute their pain to a personal inadequacy.[818] This self-effacing attitude has not been met with understanding, but rather with a reticence to prescribe opioids because of the stereotype that African Americans are more likely to be drug users. This prejudice is completely inaccurate. In fact, numerous studies show that the vast majority of opioid drug users per capita are White. Studies have shown that African Americans on average fear addiction much more than Whites do. Despite the pain of SCD and, of course, other diseases that affect all races, on average Whites receive significantly better pain care compared to African Americans.[818] The particular plight of SCD patients is described in medical detail addressing the injustice of the current legal and ethical climate[26]:

> Despite the trust required of patients by physicians prescribing opioids in SCD, or the risks associated with prescribing opioids, physicians must adhere to ethical prescribing practices in

SCD or any disease. The Hippocratic Oath and other creeds dictate that underprescription is not ethical. Though unsafe prescribing or overprescribing is potentially harmful and therefore not ethical as well, in general, the legal and regulatory climate now appears to favor underprescribing.

Doses that previously were considered normal are now above the limit in many places. Whether pain patients have SCD or Patient Z's disease, current practice favors underprescribing. Rather than learning from past experience, the trend in the U.S. has been to turn the clock back to a time when most of the pain of serious diseases remained untreated.

Opioid Policies Around the Globe

The best evidence that the punitive approach is not necessary and creates problems is found in the example provided by other countries. The point of discussing what works elsewhere is not to say that we should do exactly what others do. But the mere fact that there are industrialized countries where the addiction and overdose rate are vastly lower compared to the US should give us hope that this problem can be solved in a rational way.

Canada is the closest country to the United States in terms of attitudes and culture. However, one major difference concerns health care because Canada has a national health-care system. The study by Furlan and coworkers formed the basis for the Canadian Guidelines for CNCP of 2010.[819] The study by Furlan et al. found good efficacy for high-strength opioids for long-term use. This study was questioned by Busse et al., whose later recommendation became the basis for the 2017 revised guidelines.[820] The 2013 study was based on the initiative on methods, measurement, and pain assessment in clinical trials (IMMPACT) and used the grading of recommendations, assessment, development, and evaluation (GRADE) system to evaluate confidence in the evidence. The final recommendation in the

Canadian guidelines are similar to those put in place in the CDC guidelines.[281] Because Canada lacks a DEA, the recommendations are less rigidly implemented compared to many places in the United States.[821,822] The Canadian guidelines acknowledge that the EU has taken a more liberal stance toward pain management.

The EU community-wide guideline is a remarkably lucid and comprehensive document.[311] It discusses the social responsibility and the need in such a way that there can be no doubt that patients will be treated with dignity. It also discusses many side effects and treatment issues with alacrity. A publication of prescribing guidelines for nine EU countries has many commonsense statements concerning the need for prescribing to be a conversation between patient and doctor.[823] The importance of careful listening by doctors is emphasized. These guidelines make it clear that opioid therapy is considered on an individual basis. Some patients do not tolerate opioids as is well known. But for those who do, the issues discussed in the guidelines are mainly concerned with making sure that there is a plan to treat the disease and not just the pain (no opioid monotherapy) and that patients understand that the lowest possible dose is always desired.[824]

The Canadian guideline for treatment of cancer pain published in 2019 expresses the relationship of the above Canadian and EU guidelines and the ethical considerations that apply to treatment of cancer patients in Canada[825]:

> Two guidelines about opioid use in chronic pain management were published in 2017: the Canadian Guideline for Opioids for Chronic Non-Cancer Pain and the European Pain Federation position paper on appropriate opioid use in chronic pain management. Though the target populations for the guidelines are the same, their recommendations differ depending on their purpose. The intent of the Canadian guideline is to reduce the incidence of serious adverse effects. Its goal was therefore to set limits

on the use of opioids. In contrast, the European Pain Federation position paper is meant to promote safe and appropriate opioid use for chronic pain. The content of the two guidelines could have unintentional consequences on other populations that receive opioid therapy for symptom management, such as patients with cancer. In this article, we present expert opinion about those chronic pain management guidelines and their impact on patients with cancer diagnoses, especially those with histories of substance use disorder and psychiatric conditions. Though some principles of chronic pain management can be extrapolated, we recommend that guidelines for cancer pain management should be developed using empirical data primarily from patients with cancer who are receiving opioid therapy.

This abstract from the Canadian guidelines is worth providing in its entirety because it so accurately distinguishes the intent of the various guidelines in official language and because it clarifies what I have been calling "clinical ethics," which is the ethical requirement to treat patients on an individual basis in the absence of complete information on efficacy. This is the opposite of the approach taken by CDC guideline as actually implemented, which is to apply a single limit to every patient. The reasoning used by PROP is that there is insufficient information on efficacy and some information on harms, and therefore we should not treat pain with opioids or strictly limit that treatment. They ignore the harm of pain itself, which outweighs the harms of responsible opioid use for patients whose pain results from extensive tissue damage and the inflammation of a severe disease. If the disease is incurable, there is no hope of resolution through curing the symptoms.

The overdose death rate in the United Kingdom is less than half that in the United States per capita, but it has grown in parallel. The documentation provided by Gallagher and Galvin shows that the vast majority of overdose deaths are from illegal drugs or from methadone, which is provided to recovering addicts.[824] Nonetheless, a significant degree of caution pervades the recommendations. Unlike the proposal of PROP in North America, there is no suggestion of a mandatory maximum or that patients should be tapered rapidly down to a particular level. Nonetheless, measures are discussed throughout to prevent diversion, prevent prescribing from leading to addiction, and above all to ensure that patient needs are met.

The German guidelines have recently followed the lead of the American guidelines in the sense that they have instituted a limit, which could become a hard limit of 120 MEDD.[826] However, 0.8% of prescriptions were at higher levels. Rather than discussing diseases or outcomes for pain patients, the focus is on abuse, which is discussed with explicit reference to the North American situation.

The French guidelines are similar to the Korean and Canadian in level of specificity. There are a number of quite specific recommendations regarding useful opioids, their appropriate dose, their morphine equivalency, and even the price.[827] The guidelines are specific about how to screen for and monitor addictive behavior and when to recommend an alternative treatment. One difference with respect to the more conservative dose in other countries is that the maximum recommended cutoff dose before special justification is required is set at 150 MEDD. Many examples of successes with various persistent noncancer pain conditions have been described.[828] A few disease-specific recommendations are made for the use of strong-opioid treatment. Inflammatory arthritis of the lower joints (sacroiliac, hips, knees), lower back pain, and neuropathic pain are recommended for high-dose therapy, while fibromyalgia and headaches are not. France has also recently made buprenorphine available by prescription of any primary care doctor. Under the new law, addicts can see the doctor privately like any patient. This change alone cut the overdose rate by a factor of five in four years' time.[829]

We should study Portugal's policy toward opioid drugs carefully.[830] Portugal has decriminalized opioid drugs, which is now the recommendation of an increasing number of think tanks.[270] In Portugal, addicts are encouraged to seek treatment, which is provided free of charge. Even those who refuse treatment are given clean needles to prevent the spread of disease. The rates of addiction plummeted. The rate of opioid overdose deaths is 2% of the per capita overdose death rate in the US.[831] This kind of success at least warrants study when death rates in the US are soaring and the draconian reductions in the prescriptions deny relief to hundreds of thousands of patients in pain. Solutions that work in one society are not necessarily transferrable to another. But we should consider the fact that Portugal was able to turn around a serious opioid crisis in a short time. While there are piecemeal attempts to implement needle-sharing programs and to expand methadone clinics in the US, these are so few and far between that it is clearly not going to make a dent in the problem.

The Japanese guidelines have a great deal of precision in terms of the questions and deliberations for various treatment options.[832] While the Japanese see themselves as traditionally very conservative in their administration of pain medication, their limit has been 120 MEDD since 2012.[833] The Korean guidelines[834] have followed the lead of the American, Canadian, and Japanese recommendations of 2016, 2017, and 2018, respectively (90 MEDD, 90 MEDD, and 120 MEDD).[281,820] The Korean approach is precise in saying that these are initial maximum doses. The Korean literature also draws on the historical perspective that doses up to 200 MEDD are considered moderate, but that higher levels have a greater risk of accidental overdose or addiction.[10] The target diseases are not specified in these guidelines, but by implication they are using a case-by-case approach. In a thoughtful commentary that follows the guidelines, Baik writes that Korean medicine has little experience with opioids and that it is time to overcome *opioidophobia*. Ironically, today there are many in the US who mock the term *opioidophobia*, which was first coined in the US to describe the fear of addiction as a reason to avoid prescribing opioids for pain. The Korean approach is rational and recognizes that fear of addiction has impeded the use of medications that can treat people in pain. Even China is waking up to the reality that their history with the ill effects of opium forced on them by the colonial powers does not need to prevent humane treatment of pain patients.

Many countries are cautiously moving forward with more permissive prescribing guidelines. They are cognizant of addiction, which they treat as a medical condition and not as a reason to deny care to a person with persistent pain. The American guidelines are now among the most restrictive in the industrialized world. Those who think that this is a good development had better hope that they do not contract a painful inflammatory degenerative disease. Any of us could be Patient Z.

EPILOGUE

⤔

How Patient Z Survived

There were many days when Patient Z wanted to give up. He had such pain that he could not move and he felt that there was no point in remaining alive. However, his hope was combined with his determination to overcome the problems that he had encountered in receiving appropriate medical care. Patient Z was sufficiently strong that he did not seriously contemplate suicide. Many patients do, but Patient Z managed to overcome the depression and desperation. His will to live was seriously challenged for a long period, during which he attempted to reason with the pain clinic or find another pain clinic that would treat him as a patient, rather than as a client who needed to adopt to the limits set by an opioid dispensary. For more than one year, he convinced the doctors to wait or proceed very slowly with his taper. He was quite sick, had operations, spent time in the hospital because of his lymphedema. During that year, he also learned of the need for neck surgery to prevent paralysis. Some of the staff at the pain clinic were sympathetic, while others told him he was "making excuses." However, he was persuasive enough, and perhaps evidently suffering enough, that he was able to avoid a rapid taper down to the clinic limit. Nonetheless, his dose had been cut significantly, and his pain had increased. He was often scared of what life would be like on the dose they intended him to reach. He was also intensely worried that the clinic would abandon him since he had already received one threat. He knew that patient abandonment laws do not protect pain patients. Even the state medical board personnel had warned him of that fact. Patient Z understood that he would need to find another way to survive with his terrible disease. But what could he do? The pain clinic and university hospital offered no services or help. Every pain clinic he contacted was limited in the same way as the university pain clinic.

Patient Z contacted his congressman. He wrote a detailed letter describing the situation, the poor care, and the threats. Congressman A was nervous about the conversation. It is clear that popular opinion against opioids weighs heavily in the mind of any politician. No congressman wants to be seen as being weak on drugs. In the eyes of many, Patient Z was nothing more than a drug user. But Congressman A was a compassionate person, and he agreed to help Patient Z contact the state medical board. Patient Z formulated his message as a petition to the Board. He asked what a patient can do when doctors recognize the pain but refuse to treat it. Everyone agrees that this should not happen, but it is precisely what is happening in the United States. Once Patient Z had formulated his petition, the congressman's staff worked to quickly contact the medical board. Then there was a wait of approximately one month for the response. At the end of the wait, the congressman's staff member called Patient Z with good news and bad news. The bad news was that they had could not change clinic policies or intervene in any way to help a patient. The good news was that they suggested that Patient Z was a candidate for palliative care.

When Patient Z heard this proposal, he was skeptical at first. He had thought of palliative care as end-of-life care. He was not well and he was miserable, but there was no imminent threat to his life. In fact, he felt the irony that he could be kept alive for many years, but without pain medication, he would be wishing for an early death. Fortunately, palliative care has evolved to include patients who do not have cancer and patients who are not in a terminal stage of their disease. If a disease is sufficiently serious and has no cure, then patients can qualify. However, many current providers still do not recognize the expanded mission of palliative care identified in the CARA law of 2016. Although the federal laws have called for an expansion of palliative care and Medicare and Medicaid will cover some of the costs, many providers still follow the model that palliative care is for patients with a terminal diagnosis. Unfortunately, the state medical board provided no guidance. One might think that one function of a medical board would be to organize the information on providers so that patients would be able to find an appropriate provider. That is not how the medical board is designed. Instead, Patient Z spent several months contacting various providers until, finally, he spoke with a sympathetic nurse practitioner who explained that she treats patients with conditions like ankylosing spondylitis. She understood rheumatologic diseases. She was authorized to write opioid prescriptions, and her mandate was to treat pain, as well as symptoms of advanced disease.

Palliative care is not a solution for all the problems that have developed for millions of patients, but it could be, and should be, an option for patients like Patient Z whose disease has no cure and only expect a life in severe pain. Once Patient Z had received a dose of opioids that managed his pain, he could come to terms with his pain. He knew his limitations, but the pain became tolerable, and he regained a sense of hope that life could be more than the prison of being trapped in a chair in his apartment. He needed to use a walker and a wheelchair. It was still painful to move and even more painful to go out to doctor visits or to do the shopping, but with assistance, he could manage. If he had not received the higher dose of opioids, he would not have even tried to move. The pain had been too severe. After receiving medication at the higher level, the same level he had used historically for a period of years, he regained a sense of confidence and a relative sense of well-being. Sometimes, when he sat in his special chair, he could say to himself that he actually felt comfortable. He could accept the discomfort and deterioration of his terrible disease because of the relief valve provided by the opioid medications. Life is never easy for a patient with ankylosing spondylitis, but it does not have to be total misery. Patient Z became obsessed with the disturbing reality that people are being denied this humane option of treatment for their disease.

There are many patients whose pain is not easily diagnosed. In some cases, pain is not an obvious consequence of a disease. Such patients are most likely not eligible for palliative care. Perhaps they should be. Clearly, the medical community needs to revisit how it regards pain. The current system often fails to treat those patients who do not have easily recognizable symptoms with dignity. For those who have symptoms that are diagnosed as an incurable disease, palliative care should be an option, although many patients either do not know or do not have the means to find appropriate care. Patient Z's struggle to find care convinced him that there is a great shortage of training and information. The irony is that none of the doctors Z ever saw suggested a path for him. He had to petition the state medical board. While the board was sympathetic, they offered no specific advice or help. Patient Z was on his own. The guidelines and medical practice need to be revised for the benefit of all patients so that pain is no longer undertreated or ignored. The goal is not to encourage opioid therapy, but neither is it discourage use of opioids where they are needed. The treatment decision should be between doctor and patient without the involvement of the DEA, law enforcement, pharmaceutical companies or zealots. We should rely on medical boards and medical societies for education and enforcement where necessary.

Patient Z has always been a private person, and he never sought attention. However, the experience he had suffered caused him to become a public person and to advocate for patients' rights. This book is a tribute to Patient Z's inner strength and to his tenacity. The spirit of the book follows conversations with Patient Z and formulates the message that Patient Z has wanted to spread to as many pain patients, doctors, regulators, lawmakers, and citizens as possible. Thanks to Patient Z, I feel I have come to understand pain in a way that few healthy people can. As I began to understand the reality of persistent pain and how it feels to be alone and to have no one believe that the pain is real, I came to understand that a crime against humanity is being committed by our legal and political framework that prevents doctors from treating pain in a responsible but compassionate way. I have focused on the situation in the United States since that is where all of this took place, but the problem is global.

It is my hope that the United States realizes the need for reform, and that this reform should be spread throughout the world. We can treat pain responsibly. We do not need to rely on a policy of deprivation and cruel indifference to suffering.

APPENDIX

❧

Literature Review of Meta-Analyses

There are more than 100 studies on the efficacy and safety of opioids for long-term treatment of chronic pain, including both RCT and observational studies. Over one hundred independent studies have been conducted over the past thirty-five years. The major criticism has been that they are not of sufficient duration to obtain meaningful results. However, it was in 2014 in an *NIH Evidence Review*[9] that the requirement for a long-term study to be valid was set to one year. None of the prior studies had been conducted longer than approximately four months, except observational studies. The one-year requirement was a paper tiger since no pain drug has ever have been studied in a one-year RCT for the simple reason that the FDA only requires twelve weeks. In this appendix, I document how repeated meta-analyses were conducted with changing criteria for validity and changing conclusions. Moreover, I will compare the most recent meta-analyses done in Germany, Canada, and the US to show how different authors in different countries explain the conclusions of nearly identical quantitative results, specifically, the reduction in pain scores for common conditions, such as low back pain and osteoarthritis, which were treated with standard opioid treatments of approximately 30–60 MEDD, giving an average of 0.8 points improvement on the eleven-point scale, correcting for placebo. This is a robust result from the average of dozens of studies in each meta-analysis. In Germany, the recommendation is to

treat pain using opioids (cautiously with consultation of each individual patient); whereas, in the US, the conclusion is that opioids
have no efficacy. It is hard to avoid the conclusion that there is bias
in these reviews, since the review authors lobby government agencies
and make strong public statements to attempt to justify a rule that
would tell pain clinics what they are permitted to prescribe.

Comparing the Methods, Criteria, and Conclusions of Meta-Analyses Over Time

The comparison made in the text of chapter 6 follows meta-analyses
authored by Dr. Roger Chou with various coauthors starting with
the study by Chou et al. published in 2003.[6] Dr. Chou was the lead
author on a series of meta-analyses, evidence reviews, recommendations, and the CDC guidelines over the years. This provides an
opportunity to see the changes in perceptions and attitudes—that
is, potential bias in the presentation of the evidence in the literature.
The data on pain in all studies are derived from patient reporting. To
clarify how this is usually done, as distinct from a clinical evaluation,
the precise language from the study is quoted below[6]:

> Most studies measure pain intensity using either
> visual analogue or categorical pain scales. Visual
> analogue scales (VAS) consist of a line on a piece
> of paper labeled 0 at one end, indicating no pain,
> and a maximum number (commonly 100) at the
> other, indicating excruciating or most severe pain.
> Patients designate their current pain level on the
> line. An advantage of VAS is that they provide
> a continuous range of values for relative sever-
> ity. A disadvantage is that the meaning of a pain
> score for any individual patient remains arbitrary.
> Categorical pain scales, on the other hand, con-
> sist of several pain category options from which
> a patient must choose (e.g., no pain, mild, mod-

erate, or severe). A disadvantage of categorical scales is that patients must chose [*sic*] between categories that may not accurately describe their pain. The best approach may be to utilize both methods.

In addition, the studies used a questionnaire to obtain quality of life (QOL) information. A common one, which was used in this study, is the SF-36 (Medical Outcomes Study Short Form-36). This type of form is designed to "measure how well an individual functions physically, socially, cognitively, and psychologically." It asks general questions about health, function, and abilities with a ranking from 1 to 10, or similar scale. If a patient is feeling worse at the end of the study for any reason, such as their disease's progression, this will, of course, register as a lower QOL score. Does this really inform us on whether a pain medication made a difference in any of these categories? But one cannot ask the patient directly whether the opioid medication was beneficial since the answer could be biased. Other measures are how well a person sleeps or performs on the job.

The study also looked on the harm side of the balance and determined "abuse, addiction, respiratory depression, nausea, vomiting, constipation, dizziness, somnolence, and confusion." The authors recorded events and serious events, noting that many studies did not make this distinction. They also recorded how many patients dropped out of the study because of one or more of the adverse side effects. This meta-analysis study included sixteen RCT studies of efficacy with 1,427 patients and eight RCT studies of adverse effects studies with 1,109 patients. The authors noted that the most accurate way to determine an adverse effect was a withdrawal from the study. They mentioned that those subjects who received placebo often withdrew because of inadequate pain relief. The criterion for all studies required pain that had lasted for longer than six months and that all subjects were over eighteen years old. The trials ranged in size from 12 to 295 evaluable enrollees, with an average of 79 enrollees. The trials ranged from five days to sixteen weeks. Five of the trials focused on osteoarthritis, five on back pain, two on neuropathic pain, one on phantom limb pain, and three on heterogeneous chronic noncancer pain. None of these are debilitating types of pain associated with degenerative or severe autoimmune diseases. This is not to belittle anyone's pain, but both at that time and certainly today, these types of pain would be treated with low-dose opioids. Today, many of them might not be treated at all.

The studies that were included were rated as poor, fair, or good. Poor-quality studies were considered invalid because they had at least one fatal flaw. Fair-quality studies may be valid. A first study question was concerned on whether time-release morphine was better than a transdermal fentanyl patch. The authors noted one study was poor and flawed because 76% of the patients had been on morphine at the beginning of the study and it was not blinded. There were fourteen studies that compared long-acting and short-acting formulations to placebo, and all were rated as fair. The studies were not consistent in their findings. The withdrawal rates varied substantially, but a rough average was that one-third of participants dropped out because of side effects.

Part 2 of the Chou et al. study focused on adverse effects.[6] There is less to say here since many of the studies were considered of poor quality. One interesting statement made was, "Constipation was significantly lower for transdermal fentanyl compared to long-acting morphine (29% vs. 48%) only as assessed by a bowel function questionnaire, and not by patient-reported or investigator-observed symptoms." The dropout rates for opioid-naive patients were the most informative data on side effects. These varied from study to study but were in the range of one-third of participants.

The two studies comparing extended-release morphine and transdermal fentanyl were of interest despite their poor and fair ratings by Chou et al.[6] The morphine dose used in the Allan et al. 2001 study of 256 patients from the United Kingdom, Belgium, Finland, and several other countries was 120–130 MEDD.[835] The type of chronic pain was not specified. The Allan study was rated as poor, which means that there was no conclusion regarding the comparison of two extended-release forms (ER morphine or transdermal patch fentanyl), but either one was considered since the majority of the patients on the study had been receiving the medication for an average of nine years. The Allan study cited five previous studies that supported the efficacy of opioid treatments for long-term or persistent pain, including neuropathic pain.[332,333,824,837] As one delves into the supporting literature cited in this 2003 Oregon study, one finds that following one path back in the literature there is ample evidence of efficacy of opioids for the treatment of pain. But we have actually only scratched the surface.

The Caldwell et al. 2002 study[331] had doses in a range from 20 to 200 MEDD for treatment of osteoarthritis pain. By today's standards, the high end of this dose range for osteoarthritis pain would probably not be recommended because most osteoarthritis is reasonably well controlled at lower doses and there are numerous interventions possible to relieve arthritis pain. Osteoarthritis has an inflammatory component, but the severity tends to be less than in diseases such as rheumatoid arthritis and psoriatic arthritis. Each of these has a wide variation from mild discomfort to extreme pain.

The Chou et al. study[6] also cited fourteen RCT studies that compared morphine or fentanyl to placebo. The types of pain range from lower back pain, to severe osteoarthritis, and even some more severe neuropathic pain.[334,335,396l Arkinstall, 332,838] Doses were in the range from 90 to 130 MEDD, which would be acceptable for these types of pain, by today's standard. Good efficacy was reported. A particularly interesting study by Harke et al. reported on severe neuropathic pain. The patients had electrical stimulators to relieve the pain. These could be switched off, and the study could be carried out using either morphine (90 MEDD) or carbamazepine (600 milligrams daily) compared to a nonactive placebo. Carbamazepine is an anticonvulsant and is not an opioid. If the patients on placebo found the pain to be intolerable, they could switch on their electrical stimulators.[839] This method permitted ethical study of severe pain. They found that carbamazepine was an effective drug. Morphine was not effective, but that was attributed to the "low" dose used. Of course, today 90 MEDD is the CDC limit. Neuropathic pain is a particularly difficult type of pain, and for many years it was thought that opioids were ineffective. In fact, opioids can be used, but for some types of neuropathic pain, the required dose is high. If nonopioid alternatives are effective, then these would probably be preferable to very high-dose opioids. Nonetheless, these studies and others cited in the Chou et al. study from 2003 support the basic premise that opioids are effective for pain relief of a broad spectrum of pain.[6] It appears that patients may have had different preferences for extended-release morphine or a fentanyl patch, but the basic premise that opioids are effective for treating pain was confirmed in the eighteen studies cited in this review. At the time, the efficacy of opioids was not studied since everyone in the field accepted that efficacy was established. In 2003, the major issue was finding the best methods to deliver opioids.

Treating Neuropathic Pain Using Opioids— Prospects for Long-Term Opioid Therapy

The 2008 review by Ballantyne and Shin summarizing the results of twenty-five RCT studies[321–342] was one of the first to summarize the use of opioid treatment for neuropathic pain containing six RCT studies. The other studies in the review covered lower back pain (five) and osteoarthritis (eight). There were two studies covering musculo-skeletal pain, one for fibromyalgia, one for rheumatoid arthritis, and one for phantom limb pain. Most of the studies used oxycodone, which was found to be effective in all cases. One study used codeine and acetaminophen combination as the trial and acetaminophen as the control.[321] This study was discontinued because of side effects. One study used Oxytrex, which is an oxycodone formation with ultralow dose of naltrexone (one microgram). The addition of a tiny amount of MOR antagonist actually increased the potency of the oxycodone and reduced the tolerance and dependence.

For many years, it was believed that opioids had no efficacy for neuropathic pain. However, McQuay conducted some preliminary trials showing that neuropathic pain responded to opioids in 2001.[355] The Ballantyne and Shin review includes six RCT studies[337–342] that showed efficacy for various kinds of neuropathic pain, diabetic, pos-therpetic, and mixed neuropathy.

A note of concern was sounded regarding a Danish population-wide epidemiological study.[840] Denmark had the most liberal opioid prescription policies in the world at the time. The cohort of 1,906 individuals with chronic pain who used opioid therapy was compared to a control group. By their own self-assessment, the opioid group did worse on pain level, function, and quality of life scores. However, there was no information provided on the diseases treated or reasons for the prescriptions, which complicates the interpretation.

Revisionist History

Following the 2011 systematic review and position paper announcing the formation of PROP,[8] a new review was conducted in 2015 by Chou et al. to reevaluate previous findings.[4] The title of the study was "The Effectiveness and Risks of Long-Term Opioid Therapy for Chronic Pain." The review included thirty-nine studies considered the highest level available. A meta-analysis was not attempted because the disparity in studies was considered too large. However, the efficacy did not require any analysis since no study was found that satisfied the criteria that the trial must have duration of at least one year. The authors did find multiple studies that compared harms, such as fractures, cardiovascular events, erectile dysfunction, and motor vehicle accidents. The increase in harms was modest in all cases, barely above the level of statistical significance. The conclusion read as follows[4]:

> Evidence is insufficient to determine the effectiveness of long-term opioid therapy for improving persistent pain and function. Evidence supports a dose-dependent risk for serious harms.

This statement has a ring of authority, but it is incumbent on the authors to explain why their conclusion contradicts their own earlier studies that did find efficacy. We can examine the methods of this study compared to the 2003 Oregon Health System study by

Chou et al. to understand the shifts in thinking and the extent to which they are based on hard data.[6] A number of the individual studies were also part of the 2003 review on the efficacy of short- vs. long-term formulations, yet the 2015 study could not find a single study that showed any efficacy of long-term opioid therapy. We see the evolution from evidence of efficacy from (1) efficacy is assumed to be good and only delivery is studied (2003),[6] to (2) lack of strong evidence (2011),[8] to now (3) "insufficient evidence of efficacy" (2015).[4] The authors summarized these findings as follows[4]:

> We identified no studies of long-term opioid therapy for persistent pain versus no opioid therapy or nonopioid therapies that evaluated effects on pain, function, or quality of life at 1 year or longer. Most placebo-controlled, randomized trials were shorter than 6 weeks, and almost all were shorter than 16 weeks. We did not include uncontrolled studies for these outcomes; reliable conclusions cannot be drawn from such studies because of the lack of a nonopioid comparison group and heterogeneity of the results.[4]

This statement is remarkable since the same author(s) had located eighteen acceptable RCTs (including ones with a nonopioid comparison) in the 2003 study. The difference is a result of the new requirement that the studies be conducted for one year or longer. Using that criterion, none of the drugs for pain relief on the market would have been accepted into the study. Applying these same criteria, there is no evidence for efficacy of aspirin, acetaminophen, ibuprofen, drugs, which result in over 15,000 deaths annually in the U.S.[404] The authors of a critique of the Chou et al. studies wrote the following[404]:

> No common non-opioid treatment for persistent pain has been studied in aggregate over longer intervals of active treatment than opioids. To

dismiss trials as "inadequate" if their observation period is a year or less is inconsistent with current regulatory standards. The literature on major drug and nondrug treatments for persistent pain reveals similarly shaped distributions across modalities. Considering only duration of active treatment in efficacy or effectiveness trials, published evidence is no stronger for any major drug category or behavioral therapy than for opioids.

The list of harms in the 2015 study was significantly longer and included new harms, such as falls and heart attacks, which had not been included in the previous study. In coming to their conclusion, the authors examined studies in categories of (1) initiation of therapy (two studies), (2) comparative effectiveness and harms (three studies), and (3) dose escalation (one study).

In category 1, the initiation of therapy, two studies showed excellent efficacy and low side effects, with a very low incidence of abuse (< 1% in each study). Salzmann et al. wrote that for 105 patients studied "among cancer patients, 85% achieved stable analgesia, 92% with the controlled-release (CR) formulation and 79% with the immediate-release (IR) formulation. Among noncancer patients, 91% achieved stable pain control, 87% with the CR formulation and 96% with the IR formulation."[396]

The study be Jamison and coworkers[334] on thirty-six patients found that "weekly reports during the experimental phase [twelve weeks] showed the titrated-dose group to have less pain and less emotional distress than the other two groups. Both opioid groups were significantly different from the naproxen-only group. During the titration phase, patients also reported significantly less pain and improved mood."[334] Note that this study had been included in all the reviews and meta-analyses in this chapter. The interpretation changed significantly as time progressed. The Jamison et al. study reported that there was no long-term benefit after the patients were tapered off the therapy. This simply means that the patient must keep taking the drug to get any benefit, like any drug. Yet Chou and coworkers wrote that "results were inconsistent and difficult to interpret because of differences between treatment groups in dosing protocols (titrated vs. fixed dosing) and opioid doses." What is difficult to interpret about the above results? The Jamison et al. study showed clear evidence for efficacy as Ballantyne and Shin clearly stated in 2008. Both the Salzmann and Jamison studies were part of the Chou 2003 study where they were accepted as part the conclusion. But the overall conclusions grew weaker, and in 2015, Chou declared that these studies were "inconsistent and difficult to interpret." Essentially, the studies were being reinterpreted, not based on their individual merits but on their perceived compatibility with the definitions set forth in the review protocol.

In category 2, comparative effectiveness and harms, the first study by Allan and coworkers stated the following[371]:

> **Results.** Data from 680 patients showed that (transdermal fentanyl) TDF and (sustained release morphine) SRM provided similar levels of pain relief [dose = 60 MEDD], but TDF was associated with significantly less constipation than SRM, indicating a greater likelihood of satisfactory pain relief without unmanageable constipation for patients receiving TDF. Other ratings were similar for TDF and SRM, but TDF provided greater relief of pain at rest and at night.
>
> **Conclusions.** TDF and SRM provided equivalent levels of pain relief, but TDF was associated with less constipation. This study indicates that sustained-release strong opioids can safely be used in strong-opioid naive patients.[371]

These studies and others indicate that intrathecal opioid delivery systems can provide long-term relief for many of those patients who do not have side effects. In this category, as well, the individual studies provide good evidence that the opioids are effective in reducing pain, but they are not able to discern the difference between extended-release morphine and a transdermal patch.

In the second study by Wild et al. under this subsection of the meta-analysis, 1,117 patients with lower back, osteoarthritic hip, or knee pain were treated with tapentadol or oxycodone (40–100 MEDD) for up to one year.[403] The pain intensity scores in both groups were 7.6 initially and 4.4 to 4.5 at the end of the study period. Some adverse events arising from gastrointestinal intolerance and other events led to discontinuation of 22.5% and 36.1% of patients, respectively.[403] A third study of transdermal fentanyl and buprenorphine patches found that nearly 40% of patients with severe pain from back and joints withdrew from the long-term study, but 50% experienced long-term relief up to six months. Beyond six months, the number dropped to 11% experiencing good relief, but rotation of the patches appeared to help.[390] Here was an example of the roughly one-third of patients who had unacceptable side effects, but for the others, the study reported "long-term relief." A third study compared opioid deaths from methadone and morphine and found that overdose deaths were higher for morphine. This study had little in common with the other studies, and it was not clear why it was even included in the category.

The authors dismissed all positive findings in these studies because of *heterogeneity*. Yet with regard to harms, these authors were able to draw conclusions using the same studies. Apparently, heterogeneity is a concern for the consideration of the relief of pain reported in the studies, but not for consideration of the adverse side effects. The authors concluded that opioids led to increased risk of fracture and heart attack based on the limited data. Although the authors mentioned the risk of addiction numerous times, only one study was identified as having "fair quality" of evidence to determine that the rate of opioid use disorder was 0.7% and 6.1% for dosing over 90 days at 36 MEDD and >120 MEDD, respectively.[4,300]

Meta-Analyses on the Efficacy of Opioids for Long-Term Treatment of Cancer Pain

A Cochrane database study by Wiffen and coworkers[841] from University of Oslo, Norway, is worth a brief description to illustrate the points made regarding inherent limitations of these studies. The study selected four independent studies with 1,029 patients for meta-analysis in the treatment of cancer pain. These studies all compared tapentadol to morphine/oxycodone as the control for treatment of cancer pain. The control group was taking the standard pain medicine. It would have been unthinkable to ask the control group to be without pain medication. Ultimately, according to Wiffen, the study concluded that pain control was similar and the side effects of nausea and constipation were slightly improved with Tapentadol. The words of the authors of the largest study with 374 patients (of whom 236 completed the study) were as follows[842]:

> Tapentadol ER (25–200 mg bid) provides analgesic efficacy that is non-inferior to that provided by oxycodone HCl CR (5–40 mg bid) for the management of moderate to severe, chronic malignant tumor-related pain, and is well tolerated overall, with a better gastrointestinal tolerability profile than oxycodone CR.

Chou and coworkers were outliers in terms of redefining criteria for inclusion and emphasizing harms in their selection process.[9]

The Gold Standard—a Twelve-Month RCT Study with Two Fatal Flaws

The requirement for a one-year minimum observation for an RCT study made by Chou and coworkers in the 2014 *NIH Evidence Assessment*[9] effectively excluded all studies on pain medication of any type from consideration as valid studies.[404] In this manner, a single study of sufficient duration to meet the criteria becomes extremely important. Krebs and coworkers attempted to meet this challenge with the SPACE study comparing opioid to nonopioid therapy for back pain as well as hip and knee pain from osteoarthritis.[351] Their conclusion was that there was little difference between the opioid and nonopioid therapy. The ailments in this study were relatively low on the scale of pain—that is, compared to inflammatory arthritis diseases, degenerative diseases, sickle cell disease, and cancer. There were numerous potential flaws in the study pointed out in a comment written by Wang and Macaulay.[350] Among these were the fact that radiographic imaging is not always indicative of pain in osteo-arthritis, and there are numerous other common interventions that may work better than either of the indicated therapies. The nonopi-oid medications had acetaminophen and NSAIDs (e.g. ibuprofen, naproxen) as the first line of treatment. The study listed tramadol as the third-line medication under the nonopioid category. This was an apparent contradiction since tramadol is an opioid, yet it was placed in the nonopioid control. The opioid doses were titrated to a maximum dose of 100 MMED. *Titrated* means that "the dose was increased until the patient indicated that pain was controlled, which determined the stopping point." If the same approach was employed using the control arm, then any patient who had severe enough pain to require an opioid could have received tramadol. This study was cited as a high-quality study by those who were supportive of limiting opioid doses for all patients. However, since the opioid tramadol was present in the nonopioid arm, the study has a fatal flaw.

Meta-Analyses from the United States and Canada

The opioid crisis in the United States has taken on a dimension that is unlike that in any other country. Perhaps the closest is Canada, which has many cultural similarities. Still Canada has a National Health Service and does not have a Drug Enforcement Agency. Nonetheless, one can see a pattern in which the methods and attitudes that are prevalent in the United States tend to spill over. One amusing example is the meta-analysis of Els et al. from Edmonton, Alberta, in Canada that found zero studies that met the search criteria for studies of high-dose opioids in long-term therapy. In many fields of research, it is impossible to publish a study that does not have any data. However, the meta-analysis in the Cochrane database by Els and coworkers begins with 735 articles identified as potential candidates, and after evaluation using the selection criteria, there were *zero* articles accepted for study.[405] The same authors who found zero studies that satisfy their efficacy criteria simultaneously published a second study on side effects and found fourteen studies that met the selection criteria in the side-effect category.[407] Indeed, these studies parallel very closely the methods and findings of the Chou and coworkers study done in 2015.[4]

A recent meta-analysis of 96 RCT studies was carried out by a team led by Dr. Jason Busse of McMaster University.[38] This study has one of clearest tables showing which studies found opioid versus placebo to be superior.

> In this meta-analysis of RCTs of patients with chronic noncancer pain, evidence from high-quality studies showed that opioid use was associated with statistically significant but small improvements in pain and physical functioning, and increased risk of vomiting compared with placebo. Comparisons of opioids with nonopioid alternatives suggested that the benefit for pain and functioning may be similar, although the evidence was from studies of only low to moderate quality.

When writing about the conclusion of the study in the *Daily Globe and Mail*, "Health Report" Carly Weeks's title was "Opioids No More Effective for Treating Chronic Pain than Over-The-Counter Options, Study Finds."[39] To be precise, the study took the average of the pain improvement scores for 42 studies with 16,617 subjects. All except two of the studies found that the opioid was superior to placebo. After correcting for the placebo effect, the average reduction in pain score was -0.79 (out of 10) with a 95% confidence interval between -0.68 and -0.90. This was a high-quality finding on a large data set. The reason that the meta-analysis stated that there were "small improvements" is because the arbitrary definition of *what was significant moderate improvement* is when the pain score changes by -1.0. However, this result was not reported in the *Globe and Mail*, but instead, the finding of nine RCTs where an NSAID was compared to an opioid was the headline. In those studies on 1,431 subjects, the net improvement because of opioids was -0.6 with a large 95% confidence limit from 0.34 to -1.51. Because the spread in the statistics was relatively large, this was called low- to moderate-quality data. Nonetheless, the low-quality data on a small data set that did not give meaningful improvement was reported in the mainstream news, while the solid finding with high-quality data that showed a "small improvement" was not. Perhaps the on-line commentary by a reader named Chris summed up the lesson from this article the best:

> I can only speak for myself and my chronic non cancer degenerative facet joint pain: Opioid therapy (oxycontin) is the hands down winner for a pain free better life. I know this isn't politically correct to say this. Naproxen makes me nauseous and ibuprofen raises blood pressure and is not advised for hypertensives such as myself. In any case, neither is strong enough to counteract my pain. [...] You just have to be judicious in what you use and not succumb to the hysteria and misinformation you read in the media. I will review the cited journal article but patients have to deal with their own pain, not someone else's.

Patients are increasingly aware of the fact that opioid prescription has become politicized. It is remarkable that the Busse and coworker's study has been interpreted to make a statement about recommended treatment, when it is not sufficient for that purpose.

The Busse and coworker study is the most thorough meta-analysis that I am aware of, and it does not appear to have a great deal of bias. It finds that opioid therapy has efficacy for the types of pain studied (which are mostly the usual low back pain, osteoarthritis, and neuropathic pain). Yet despite the lack of bias in the study itself, the presentation of the study in the media suffers from an incorrect interpretation.

The studies by a collaborative group in Switzerland, Canada, and United States on the Cochrane database compared oral oxycodone and transdermal opioids for osteoarthritis pain.[47,318] Ten trials with a total of 2,043 subjects were included in the analysis.[47] The opioids used in the oral study were morphine (30 MEDD), oxycodone (15–60 MEDD), and oxymorphone (80 MEDD). The conclusion was that the net reduction in pain scores was approximately –0.9 point after controlling for placebo. Actually, placebo resulted in a –1.8 point decrease and the opioid in a –2.7 point decrease. The standard deviation was large, and there was no correlation between increasing MEDD and pain scores. Side effects of nausea and constipation were observed. The conclusion of both studies was that non-tramadol opioids are not recommended for osteoarthritis pain despite the small-to-moderate reduction in pain and increase in function. A Cochrane database study on tramadol (dose of 200 mg or 20 MEDD) for osteoarthritis concluded that side effects were minor and pain control was acceptable (–0.85 relative to placebo).[319]

Rauck and coworkers from Wake Forest University in Winston-Salem, North Carolina, conducted a meta-analysis of twelve studies and more than 2,000 patients. Dr. Rauck's goal was to study the difference between short-acting and long-acting (time-release) formulations on quality of life.[320] The studies uniformly supported a strong patient preference for extended-release formulations. These helped both with sleep and had reduced side effects of nausea and constipation. The study was unusually detailed in discussing different types of pain, which is a feature often missing despite its central importance. For example, in an illuminating section on lower back pain, Rauck points out that there were many studies showing the efficacy of opioids for treatment of pain, but one dissenting study was that of

Martell et al.[301] The interesting insight here was that the reason for dissent is not lack of efficacy, but the relatively high diversion and opioid use disorder rate (circa 24%) that was found. Of course, lower back pain was the most common pain complaint, and this type of pain that is the easiest to fake. In this context, it is relevant to remind the reader that the Martell et al. outlier was the only study[301] cited by Dr. Lembke in her book *Drug Dealer MD* to support her contention that the rate of addiction among pain patients was 56%.[18]

Meta-Analyses from the European Union

The meta-analysis by Kalso and coworkers[315] published in 2004 included eleven studies with 1,025 patients up to eight weeks of oral administration, and four of the studies used intravenous administration. This international collaboration involved the United Kingdom, Finland, Spain, Germany, Belgium, the Netherlands, Austria, Denmark, and France. Six studies had a follow-up phase from 6 to 24 months. Fifteen randomized double-blind placebo-controlled trials were included. Four investigations with 120 patients studied intravenous opioid testing. Only 44% of the patients opted to continue to do the follow-up. The average reduction in pain was 30%. The side effects reported were nausea (32%), constipation (41%), and somnolence (29%). The short-term efficacy of opioids was good in both neuropathic and musculoskeletal pain conditions. However, only a minority of patients in these studies went on to long-term management with opioids. The small number of selected patients and the short follow-ups did not allow conclusions concerning problems such as tolerance and addiction.

Eisenberg et al. conducted a meta-analysis in Haifa, Israel.[316] They found efficacy in the use opioids to treat neuropathic pain in eight RCT studies of up to 28 days.[316] Devulder et al. focused on quality of life and found that function and quality of life improved overall for opioid therapy of chronic pain.[843] Furlan and coworkers reviewed 41 RCTs including 6,019 patients for up to 16 weeks.[819] They found that pain control was improved for high-dose opioids, but not for low-dose opioids, while function improved for low-dose opioids, but not for high dose.

The group of Noble and coworkers from Oxford University in the United Kingdom conducted a meta-analysis that had a final tally of 17 studies with 3,079 patients and found the following[317]:

> We conclude that many patients discontinue long-term opioid therapy because of adverse events (32% and 18%) or insufficient pain relief (12% and 11%); however, weak evidence suggests that oral and intrathecal opioids reduce pain long-term (by 38%) in the relatively small proportion (56% and 71%) of individuals with CNCP who continue treatment.

The addiction rate they found in this particular study of persistent-pain patients was approximately <0.3%. Even when discussing individual studies, similar patterns of caution were observed. In the study by Milligan et al. on transdermal fentanyl patches, 57% completed the one-year study at 48–90 micrograms/hour and more 66% reported better results than with other methods and improved quality of life.[844] Concerning this particular study, Noble writes, "[the] study showed minimal change on both the mental and physical subscales," but the change was a comparison of transdermal patches to other methods. One of studies included in Noble's meta-analysis was that of Mystakidou and coworkers, who found both efficacy and improved quality of life for patients using transdermal fentanyl patches.[314]

A French meta-analysis published in 2007 included 18 RCTs with a total of 3,244 patients with a trial duration of 13±8 weeks. The average pain reduction was –0.79 for the opioid arm and –0.31 for the placebo. Side effects were non-life-threatening and were not considered serious. The conclusion of the authors was that "opioids significantly decrease pain intensity and have small benefits on function compared with placebo."[313] This was interesting because the value of the pain reduction for osteoarthritis (and low back pain as well in studies below) is consistently in the vicinity of –0.8.

One of the early German clinical groups was Dr. Strumpf, who passed away unexpectedly at the age of fifty-two. Dr. Strumpf's view of treatment with opioids was that chronic and extreme pain should be considered *malignant* on the basis of its quality and intensity even if its origin was not cancer.[845] When other therapy fails, clinical studies demonstrate that patients with pain of noncancer origin may benefit from opioid therapy. Opioid therapy can fail to be effective if the choice of opioid is inappropriate or if dosages are inadequate. Of course, prescribing restrictions in many countries prevent application of opioid therapy. The lack of success of opioid therapy is largely because of factors other than the responsiveness of pain. Strumpf's research addressed side effects and function.[846] He found that patients who received strong opioids tested more poorly for concentration but better for coordination than healthy controls. The results in tests for reaction time, vigilance, and perception did not significantly differ between the two groups.

Dr. Strumpf's studies of low back pain are relevant for American medicine. He used a multidisciplinary approach and believed that drugs should never be the mainstay of a back pain treatment program. NSAIDs prescribed at regular intervals can be effective to reduce simple back pain. However, they have serious adverse effects, particularly at high doses and for long-term care. The new cyclooxygenase 2 (COX-2) inhibitors have fewer gastrointestinal complications. Writing in 2001, Dr. Strumpf pointed out that long-term experiences with opioids had been limited in Germany up to that time and that considerable controversy existed about their use in chronic noncancer pain.[847] Dr. Strumpf's clinical research addressed use of opioids to treat chronic low back pain. He observed a low incidence of organ toxicity and that addiction was likewise relatively low risk. The potential for increased function and improved quality of life seems to outweigh the risks. However, there was a lack of RCTs on opioid therapy in a multimodal pain treatment approach. Clinical experience and some studies suggest administration of sustained release opioids because of better comfort for the patient and less risk for addiction.

There has been a series of meta-analyses from German clinical groups in the past five years that indicate a climate for use of opioid therapy that is much like the beginning of the compassionate care movement.[40–46,312,352] Ueberall and coworkers found that oxycodone was noninferior to tapentadol for treatment of low back pain.[46]

Lauche and coworkers included thirteen RCTs with 6,748 participants. Median study duration was fifteen weeks (range four to fifty-six weeks). Hydromorphone, morphine, oxymorphone, and tapentadol were compared to oxycodone; fentanyl to morphine; and buprenorphine to tramadol. In pooled analysis, there were no significant differences between the two groups of opioids in terms of mean pain reduction (low-quality evidence), the patient global impression to be much or very much improved outcome (low-quality evidence), physical function (very low-quality evidence), serious adverse events (moderate-quality evidence), or mortality (moderate-quality evidence). There was no significant difference between transdermal and oral application of opioids in terms of mean pain reduction, physical function, serious adverse events, mortality (all low-quality evidence), or dropout because of adverse events (very low-quality).[41]

Hauser and coworkers included eleven open-label extension studies with 2,445 participants with nociceptive (low back, osteoarthritis) and neuropathic (radicular, polyneuropathy) pain. Median study duration was twenty-six (range 26 to 108) weeks. Four studies tested oxycodone, two studies tramadol and buprenorphine; hydromorphone, morphine, oxymorphone, and tapentadol were each tested in one study. A total of 4.9% of patients dropped out due lack of efficacy, 16.8% dropped out to due adverse events (AE) in the open-label period, and 0.08% (95% CI 0.001–0.05%) of patients died during the open-label period. Only one study systematically assessed aberrant drug behavior of the patients: 5.7% showed aberrant drug behavior in the opinion of the investigators, and 2.6% were judged to show aberrant drug behavior by independent expert assessment. There was no significant change in pain intensity between the end of the randomized period and the end of open-label phase. Only a minority of patients selected for opioid therapy at randomization finished the long-term open-label study. However, sustained effects of pain reduction could be demonstrated in these patients.[40]

Sommer and coworkers included twelve RCTs with 1,192 participants. The included conditions were painful diabetic neuropathy (four studies), postherpetic neuralgia (three studies), mixed polyneuropathic pain (two studies), and lumbar root, spinal cord injury, and postamputation pain (one study each). The mean study duration was six weeks. Four studies tested morphine, three studies tramadol, two studies oxycodone, and one study tapentadol. These were the pooled results of the studies with a parallel or crossover design: opioids were superior to placebo in reducing pain intensity and in improving physical functioning. Opioids were not superior to placebo in 50% pain reduction or very much improved pain. The authors concluded that short-term opioid therapy may be considered in selected neuropathic pain patients.[45]

A second meta-analysis by Sommer and coworkers in 2019 included sixteen primary studies and 2,199 patients analyzed for pain reduction and side effects for four to twelve weeks. It concluded that there was significant evidence of opioid efficacy for pain reduction.[848] There was no analysis of addiction rates or other side effects. The average dosages reported were 148 MEDD, 78 MEDD, and 60 MEDD for hydromorphone, morphine, and oxycodone, respectively. This study included diabetic neuropathy, postherpetic neuralgia, lumbar root lesion, and spinal cord injury.

A study of 42 out of 1,389 pain patients in Singapore who received strong opioids for a period of more than three months a year for two years with doses mostly <60 MEDD daily reported that fifteen (36%) had improvement, twenty-one (50%) stayed the same, and six (14%) had worse symptoms on the opioids.[849] Most of the patients had some form of back pain, although there was one patient with an autoimmune disease. Ten of the patients reported improved ability to work (24%), fourteen reported no improvement (33%), fourteen others (33%) reported a decrease in their ability to work, and three stopped working (7%).

Welsch and coworkers included ten RCTs with 3,046 participants with a median study duration of six weeks (range four to twelve weeks). Five studies compared tramadol with NSAIDs in osteoarthritis pain, and one trial compared tramadol to flupirtine in low back pain. Morphine was compared to antidepressants (two studies), an anticonvulsant (one study), and an antiarrhythmic (one study) in different neuropathic pain syndromes. There was no significant difference between opioids and nonopioid analgesics in pain reduction. Nonopioid analgesics were superior to opioids in improving physical function.[352]

A second study by Welsch and coworkers in 2020, which analyzed data from nearly four hundred patients with osteoarthritis was not able to make conclusions about either the efficacy of treatment or side effects.[850] A study of morphine as an analgesic for rheumatoid arthritis found no evidence for efficacy.[851] On the other hand, a study of the application of the fentanyl transdermal patch showed good efficacy in controlling pain in rheumatoid arthritis and osteoarthritis patients.[663,852] Noble et al. conducted a meta-analysis that had a final tally of seventeen studies comparing oral vs. intrathecal delivery for 3,079 patients and found the following: [317]

> We conclude that many patients discontinue long-term opioid therapy because of adverse events (32% and 18%) or insufficient pain relief (12% and 11%); however, weak evidence suggests that oral and intrathecal opioids reduce pain long-term (by 38%) in the relatively small proportion (56% and 71%) of individuals with CNCP who continue treatment.

Schaefert and coworkers conducted a meta-analysis on opioid therapy in chronic osteoarthritis pain that included twenty RCTs with 8,545 participants and a median study duration of twelve weeks. Oxycodone and tramadol were each tested in six studies; buprenorphine, hydromorphone, morphine, and tapentadol each in two studies; and codeine, fentanyl, and oxymorphone in one study each. Opioids were superior to placebo in reducing pain intensity but not physical function. The conclusion on the safety of opioids compared to placebo was limited by the low number of adverse events and deaths. No current evidence-based guideline recommends opioids as the first-line treatment option for chronic osteoarthritis pain. While the authors cautiously endorsed opioid therapy, they added that RCTs must directly compare existing pharmacological and non-pharmacological therapies and administer these in various combinations and sequences to provide superior evidence for future treatment guidelines.[44]

Petzke and coworkers included twelve RCTs with 4,375 participants with a median study duration of twelve weeks. Seven (41.2%) used oxycodone; four (23.6%) tramadol; buprenorphine and oxymorphone were each used in two (11.8%), and hydromorphone and tapentadol each in one (5.8%). Opioids were superior to placebo in reducing pain intensity, in 50% pain reduction, and in improving physical functioning. Opioids were superior to placebo in terms of efficacy and inferior in terms of tolerability.[43]

Bialas and coworkers conducted extension trials including a total of fifteen studies with 3,590 participants and a study duration of >= 26 weeks of RCTs with >= 2 weeks' duration. Study duration ranged between 26 and 156 weeks. Studies included patients with low back, osteoarthritis, and neuropathic pain. They found 2.7% aberrant drug behavior was noted and 0.5% of patients died. Opioids maintained the reduction of pain and disability and were rather well tolerated and safe. There was very low-quality evidence of the long-term efficacy, tolerability, and safety of opioids for chronic low back, osteoarthritis, and diabetic polyneuropathic pain.[312]

In summary, these EU studies covered the same range of painful conditions studied in US clinical RCTs. The great majority of the studies found efficacy relative to placebo, which was also found by Busse and coworkers. When comparing opioids to NSAIDs for certain conditions, there was no clear conclusion. There was low-quality evidence in some studies that favored opioids. However, the side effects of NSAIDs were a serious problem for some patients. The German and Scandinavian studies cited here recommended opioid use on low back pain, osteoarthritis, and neuropathic pain, which is precisely the point that US studies have begun to question.

In making the case that the harms outweigh the benefits, the US studies conducted since 2014 found "no efficacy" but found harms. One of the most common is nausea. A recent German study had suggested that there may be a way to manage opioid-induced nausea, which consisted of avoiding vigorous head movements.[42] This study and a similar type of approach taken by the Italian group of Coluzzi and coworkers toward the risk of falls was indicative of a difference in attitude. The EU groups tended look at side effects as disadvantages to be overcome, while the US researchers appeared to be searching for disadvantages that will recommend against use. Finally, the problem of opioid use disorder in pain patients was studied by one recent French study. The study proposed buprenorphine/naloxone as a replacement for oxycodone in patients who have abused their medications.[853] This was, at least, a reasonable application of buprenorphine compared to studies in the US that propose to diagnose compliant patients with an opioid dependence in order to switch them to buprenorphine.

REFERENCES

[1] Kertesz, S.G., Satel, S.L., DeMicco, J., Dart, R.C. & Alford, D.P. Opioid discontinuation as an institutional mandate: Questions and answers on why we wrote to the Centers for Disease Control and Prevention. *Substance Abuse* 40, 4–6 (2019).

[2] Kroenke, K., *et al.* Challenges with implementing the Centers for Disease Control and Prevention Opioid Guideline: A consensus panel report. *Pain Medicine* 20, 724–735 (2019).

[3] Darnall, B.D., *et al.* International stakeholder community of pain experts and leaders call for an urgent action on forced opioid tapering. *Pain Medicine* 20, 429–433 (2019).

[4] Chou, R., *et al.* The effectiveness and risks of long-term opioid therapy for chronic pain: A systematic review for a National Institutes of Health pathways to prevention workshop. *Annals of Internal Medicine* 162, 276–286 (2015).

[5] Cohen, M.J. & Jangro, W.C. A clinical ethics approach to opioid treatment of chronic noncancer pain *American Medical Association Journal of Ethics* 17, 521–529 (2015).

[6] Chou, R., Clark, E. & Helfand, M. Comparative efficacy and safety of long-acting oral Opioids for chronic non-cancer pain: A systematic review. *Journal of Pain and Symptom Management* 26, 1026–1048 (2003).

[7] Chou, R., Ballantyne, J.C., Fanciullo, G.J., Fine, P.G. & Miaskowski, C. Research gaps on use of opioids for chronic noncancer pain: Findings from a review of the evidence for an American Pain Society and American Academy of Pain Medicine clinical practice guideline. *Journal of Pain* 10, 147–159 (2009).

[8] Von Korff, M., Kolodny, A., Deyo, R.A. & Chou, R. Long-term opioid therapy reconsidered. *Annals of Internal Medicine* 155, 325–328 (2011).

[9] Chou, R., *et al.* The effectiveness and risks of long-term opioid treatment of chronic pain. *Evidence report/technology assessment No. 218. AHRQ publication No. 14-E005-EF. Rockville, MD: Agency for Healthcare Research and Quality;* September 2014. www.effectivehealthcare.ahrq.gov/ reports/final.cfm (2014).

[10] Chou, R., Ballantyne, J. & Lembke, A. Rethinking opioid dose tapering, prescription opioid dependence, and indications for buprenorphine. *Annals of Internal Medicine* 171, 427–429 (2019).

11 Ballantyne, J.C., Sullivan, M.D. & Kolodny, A. Opioid dependence vs addiction: A distinction without a difference? *Archives of Internal Medicine* 172, 1342–1343 (2012).

12 Kolodny, A., *et al.* The prescription opioid and heroin crisis: A public health approach to an epidemic of addiction. in *Annual Review of Public Health,* Vol. 36 (ed. Fielding, J.E.), 559–574 (2015).

13 American Psychiatric Association, T. *Diagnostic and Statistical Manual of Mental Disorders* (*DSM-5*). Fifth Edition, Sheridan Books, Inc. (2013).

14 Kertesz, S.G. & Gordon, A.I. A crisis of opioids and the limits of prescription control: United States. *Addiction* 114, 169–180 (2019).

15 Craig, A.D.B. A new version of the thalamic disinhibition hypothesis of central pain. *Pain Forum* 7, 1–14 (1998).

16 Head, H. & Holmes, G. Sensory disturbances from cerebral lesions. *Brain* 34, 102–254 (1911).

17 Meldrum, M.L. A capsule history of pain management. *JAMA—Journal of the American Medical Association* 290, 2470–2475 (2003).

18 Lembke, A. *Drug Dealer, MD.* Johns Hopkins Press (2016).

19 Apkarian, A.V., Baliki, M.N. & Farmer, M.A. Predicting transition to chronic pain. *Current Opinion in Neurology* 26, 360–367 (2013).

20 Stein, C. Opioids, sensory systems and chronic pain. *European Journal of Pharmacology* 716, 179–187 (2013).

21 Anonymous. The use of opioids for the treatment of chronic pain. A consensus statement from the American Academy of Pain Medicine and the American Pain Society. *Clinical Pain Journal* 13, 6–8 (1997).

22 Anonymous. The management of chronic pain in older persons. AGS Panel on Chronic Pain in Older Persons. American Geriatrics Society. *Geriatrics* 53 (Suppl 3), S8–24 (1998).

23 Cherny, N.I. & Portenoy, R.K. Cancer pain management: Current strategy. *Cancer* 72, 3393–3415 (1993).

24 WHO. Cancer Pain Relief with a Guide to Opioid Availability. Second Edition (1996).

25 Zhao, S., Xu, C.W. & Lin, R.B. Controlled release of oxycodone as an opioid titration for cancer pain relief: A retrospective study. *Medical Science Monitor* 26 (2020).

26 Smith, W.R. Treating pain in sickle cell disease with opioids: Clinical advances, ethical pitfalls. *Journal of Law Medicine & Ethics* 42, 139–146 (2014).

27 Zempsky, W.T. Treatment of sickle cell pain: Fostering trust and justice. *J. Am. Med. Assoc.* 302, 2479–2480 (2009).

28 Portenoy, R.K. Treating sickle cell pain like cancer pain. *Annals of Internal Medicine* 117, 264–265 (1992).

29 IASP. IASP Statement on Opioids. *IASP Website.* February (2018).

30 Anson, P. Prominent pain doctor faces hundreds of lawsuits. *Pain News Network.* April 3, 2018.

[31] Hall, R. Attorney General announces lawsuit against three opioid distributors. *Arkansas Times.* April 25, 2019.

[32] Joseph, A. Purdue Pharma filed for bankruptcy. What does it mean for lawsuits against the opioid manufacturer? *STAT.* September 16, 2019.

[33] Mann, B. Lawsuits highlight government failures in opioid crisis. *National Public Radio.* September 16, 2019.

[34] Fischer, D. At opioid trial, Johnson & Johnson moves to strike Oklahoma witness as 'de facto member of State's legal team.' *Legal Newsline.* June 18, 2019.

[35] Mann, B. Doctors and dentists still flooding US with opioid prescriptions. *National Public Radio.* July 17, 2020.

[36] Lopez, G. The thousands of lawsuits against opioid companies, explained. *Vox.* October. 17, 2019.

[37] Hyde, J. & Chen, D. The untold story of how Utah doctors and Big Pharma helped drive the national opioid epidemic. *Deseret News.* October 26, 2017.

[38] Busse, J.W., *et al.* Opioids for chronic noncancer pain: A systematic review and meta-analysis. *JAMA—Journal of the American Medical Association* 320, 2448–2460 (2018).

[39] Weeks, C. Opioids no more effective for treating chronic pain than over-the-counter options, study finds. *Daily Globe and Mail.* December 18, 2018.

[40] Hauser, W., Bernardy, K. & Maier, C. Long-term opioid therapy in chronic noncancer pain. A systematic review and meta-analysis of efficacy, tolerability and safety in open-label extension trials with study duration of at least 26 weeks. *Schmerz* 29, 96–108 (2015).

[41] Lauche, R., Klose, P., Radbruch, L., Welsch, P. & Hauser, W. Opioids in chronic noncancer pain—are opioids different? A systematic review and meta-analysis of efficacy, tolerability and safety in randomized head-to-head comparisons of opioids of at least four weeks' duration. *Schmerz* 29, 73–84 (2015).

[42] Lehnen, N., *et al.* Opioid-induced nausea involves a vestibular problem preventable by head-rest. *PLOS One* 10, Art. No. e0135263 (2015).

[43] Petzke, F., *et al.* Opioids in chronic low back pain. A systematic review and meta-analysis of efficacy, tolerability and safety in randomized placebo-controlled studies of at least 4 weeks' duration. *Schmerz* 29, 60–72 (2015).

[44] Schaefert, R., *et al.* Opioids in chronic osteoarthritis pain. A systematic review and meta-analysis of efficacy, tolerability and safety in randomized placebo-controlled studies of at least 4 weeks' duration. *Schmerz* 29, 47–59 (2015).

[45] Sommer, C., *et al.* Opioids in chronic neuropathic pain. A systematic review and meta-analysis of efficacy, tolerability and safety in randomized placebo-controlled studies of at least 4 weeks' duration. *Schmerz* 29, 35–46 (2015).

[46] Ueberall, M.A. & Mueller-Schwefe, G.H.H. Efficacy and tolerability balance of oxycodone/naloxone and tapentadol in chronic low back pain with a neuropathic component: A blinded end point analysis of randomly selected routine data from 12-week prospective open-label observations. *Journal of Pain Research* 9, 1001–1020 (2016).

47 Nuesch, E., *et al.* Oral or transdermal opioids for osteoarthritis of the knee or hip. *Cochrane Database of Systematic Reviews* (2014).

48 NCQA, National Committee for Quality Assurance. Updates Quality Measures for HEDIS. Washington, D.C.: National Committee for Quality Assurance available at https://www.ncqa.org/hedis/measures/use-of-opioids-at-high-dosage/. July 11, 2017.

49 Beall, P. Florida cuts off oxy: Death, devastation follow. *West Palm Beach Post.* July 13, 2018.

50 Dowell, D., Noonan, R.K. & Houry, D. Underlying factors in drug overdose deaths. *JAMA-Journal of the American Medical Association* 318, 2295–2296 (2017).

51 Ballantyne, J.C., Murinova, N. & Krashin, D.L. Opioid guidelines are a necessary response to the opioid crisis. *Clinical Pharmacology & Therapeutics* 103, 946–949 (2018).

52 Ballantyne, J.C. & Kolodny, A. Preventing prescription opioid abuse. *JAMA-Journal of the American Medical Association* 313, 1059 (2015).

53 Mark, T.L. & Parish, W. Opioid medication discontinuation and risk of adverse opioid-related health care events. *Journal of Substance Abuse Treatment* 103, 58–63 (2019).

54 O'Rourke, M. Doctors tell all—and it's bad. *The Atlantic.* November (2014).

55 Choi, Y., Mayer, T.G., Williams, M. & Gatchel, R.J. The clinical utility of the Multidimensional Pain Inventory (MPI) in characterizing chronic disabling occupational musculoskeletal disorders. *Journal of Occupational Rehabilitation* 23, 239–247 (2013).

56 Gatchel, R.J., *et al.* A preliminary study of multidimensional pain inventory profile differences in predicting treatment outcome in a heterogeneous cohort of patients with chronic pain. *Clinical Journal of Pain* 18, 139–143 (2002).

57 Harlacher, U., Persson, A.L., Rivano-Fischer, M. & Sjolund, B.H. Using data from Multidimensional Pain Inventory subscales to assess functioning in pain rehabilitation. *International Journal of Rehabilitation Research* 34, 14–21 (2011).

58 Kerns, R.D., Turk, D.C. & Rudy, T.E. The West Haven Yale multidimensional pain inventory (WHYMPI). *Pain* 23, 345–356 (1985).

59 Bernstein, I.H., Jaremko, M.E. & Hinkley, B.S. On the utility of the West Haven Yale Multidimensional pain inventory. *Spine* 20, 956–963 (1995).

60 Melzack, R. McGill pain questionnaire—major properties and scoring methods. *Pain* 1, 277–299 (1975).

61 Greco, C.M., Rudy, T.E. & Manzi, S. Adaptation to chronic pain in systemic lupus erythematosus: Applicability of the multidimensional pain inventory. *Pain Medicine* 4, 39–50 (2003).

62 Collett, B.J. Opioid tolerance: The clinical perspective. *British Journal of Anaesthesia* 81, 58–68 (1998).

63 Ventafridda, V., Tamburini, M., Caraceni, A., Deconno, F. & Naldi, F. A validation study of the WHO method for cancer pain relief. *Cancer* 59, 850–856 (1987).

64 Twycross, R.G. Clinical experience with diamorphine in advanced malignant disease. *International Journal of Clinical Pharmacology and Therapeutics* 9, 184–198 (1974).

65 Hill, H.F., *et al.* Self-administration of morphine in bone-marrow transplant patients reduces drug requirement. *Pain* 40, 121–129 (1990).

66 Portenoy, R.K. & Lesage, P. Management of cancer pain. *Lancet* 353, 1695–1700 (1999).

67 Brookoff, D. & Polomano, R. Treating sickle-cell pain like cancer pain. *Annals of Internal Medicine* 116, 364–368 (1992).

68 Whitehead, S. Effort To control opioids in an ER leaves some sickle cell patients in pain. *National Public Radio.* January 6, 2020.

69 Mitchell, B.L. Navigating the pain, psychosocial and racial dynamics of hospitalized patients with sickle cell disease. *Archives of Medicine* 10, 1–6 (2018).

70 Tan, G., Jensen, M.P., Thornby, J.I. & Shanti, B.F. Validation of the brief pain inventory for chronic nonmalignant pain. *Journal of Pain* 5, 133–137 (2004).

71 Keller, S., *et al.* Validity of the brief pain inventory for use in documenting the outcomes of patients with noncancer pain. *Clinical Journal of Pain* 20, 309–318 (2004).

72 Cleeland, C.S. Measurement of pain by subjective report. In *Advances in Pain Research Therapy Vol. 12 Boca Raton Press*, 391–403 (1989).

73 Melzack, R. From the gate to the neuromatrix. *Pain*, S121–S126 (1999).

74 Mandell, B.F. The fifth vital sign: A complex story of politics and patient care. *Cleveland Clinic Journal of Medicine* 83, 400–401 (2016).

75 Niculescu, A.B., *et al.* Towards precision medicine for pain: Diagnostic biomarkers and repurposed drugs. *Molecular Psychiatry* 24, 501–522 (2019).

76 Denes, K., *et al.* Serum biomarkers in acute low back pain and sciatica. *Orvosi Hetilap* 161, 483–490 (2020).

77 Melzack, R. *Pain and stress: Clues toward understanding chronic pain* (1998).

78 Baliki, M.N., Geha, P.Y., Fields, H.L. & Apkarian, A.V. Predicting value of pain and analgesia: Nucleus accumbens response to noxious stimuli changes in the presence of chronic pain. *Neuron* 66, 149–160 (2010).

79 Apkarian, A.V. The brain in chronic pain: Clinical implications. *Pain Management* 1, 577–586 (2011).

80 Bruehl, S., *et al.* Personalized medicine and opioid analgesic prescribing for chronic pain: Opportunities and challenges. *Journal of Pain* 14, 103–113 (2013).

81 Reckziegel, D., *et al.* Deconstructing biomarkers for chronic pain: Context- and hypothesis-dependent biomarker types in relation to chronic pain. *Pain* 160, S37–S48 (2019).

82 Apkarian, A.V., Hashmi, J.A. & Baliki, M.N. Pain and the brain: Specificity and plasticity of the brain in clinical chronic pain. *Pain* 152, S49–S64 (2011).

83 Farmer, M.A., *et al.* Brain functional and anatomical changes in chronic prostatitis/chronic pelvic pain syndrome. *Journal of Urology* 186, 117–124 (2011).

84 Mutso, A.A., *et al.* Abnormalities in hippocampal functioning with persistent pain. *Journal of Neuroscience* 32, 5747–5756 (2012).

85 Grace, A.A., Floresco, S.B., Goto, Y. & Lodge, D.J. Regulation of firing of dopaminergic neurons and control of goal-directed behaviors. *Trends in Neurosciences* 30, 220–227 (2007).

86 Zweifel, L.S., *et al.* Disruption of NMDAR-dependent burst firing by dopamine neurons provides selective assessment of phasic dopamine-dependent behavior. *Proceedings of the National Academy of Sciences of the United States of America* 106, 7281–7288 (2009).

87 Tsai, H.C., *et al.* Phasic firing in dopaminergic neurons is sufficient for behavioral conditioning. *Science* 324, 1080–1084 (2009).

88 Navratilova, E., Atcherley, C.W. & Porreca, F. Brain circuits encoding reward from pain relief. *Trends in Neurosciences* 38, 741–750 (2015).

89 Tennant, F. Treat the pain…save a heart. *Practical Pain Management* 10, March 7, 2011 (2011).

90 Tennant, F. The physiologic effects of pain on the endocrine system. *Pain and Therapy* 2, 75–86 (2013).

91 Tennant, F. Adrenocorticotropin (ACTH) as a biomarker of uncontrolled pain. *Journal of Pain* 14, S88–S88 (2013).

92 Tennant, F. Hormone abnormalities in patients with severe and chronic pain who fail standard treatments. *Postgraduate Medicine* 127, 1–4 (2015).

93 Tennant, F. Adrenocorticotropin (ACTH) in chronic pain. *Journal of Applied Biobehavioral Research* 22(2017).

94 FDA. The voice of the patient. https://www.fda.gov/media/124390/download (2019).

95 Marks, L.J., Sallade, R.L. & Chute, R. Rapid functional suppression of the adrenal cortex due to prednisone therapy. *New England Journal of Medicine* 264, 10–13 (1961).

96 Dhital, S.M., Shenker, Y., Meredith, M. & Davis, D.B. A retrospective study comparing neutral protamine hagedorn insulin with glargine as basal therapy in prednisone-associated diabetes mellitus in hospitalized patients. *Endocrine Practice* 18, 712–719 (2012).

97 Scott, K.D., Bishop, M.A. & Cook, A.K. Development of diabetes mellitus in dogs administered a combination of cyclosporine and prednisone for immune-mediated disease. *Journal of Veterinary Internal Medicine* 27, 749–749 (2013).

98 Pate, D. & Huslig, E.L. Atypical presentation of ankylosing spondylitis—a case study. *Journal of Manipulative and Physiological Therapeutics* 8, 105–108 (1985).

99 Mader, R. Atypical clinical presentation of ankylosing spondylitis. *Seminars in Arthritis and Rheumatism* 29, 191–196 (1999).

100 Danve, A. & Deodhar, A. Axial spondyloarthritis in the USA: Diagnostic challenges and missed opportunities. *Clinical Rheumatology* 38, 625–634 (2019).

101 Simon, T.A., *et al.* Prevalence of co-existing autoimmune disease in rheumatoid arthritis: A cross-sectional study. *Advances in Therapy* 34, 2481–2490 (2017).

102 Nash, P. Psoriatic arthritis: Novel targets add to a therapeutic renaissance. *Lancet* 391, 2187–2189 (2018).

103 Cauli, A. & Mathieu, A. Th17 and interleukin 23 in the pathogenesis of psoriatic arthritis and spondyloarthritis. *Journal of Rheumatology* 39, 15–18 (2012).

104 Frleta, M., Siebert, S. & McInnes, I.B. The interleukin-17 pathway in psoriasis and psoriatic arthritis: Disease pathogenesis and possibilities of treatment. *Current Rheumatology Reports* 16, Art. No. 414 (2014).

105 Blauvelt, A. & Chiricozzi, A. The immunologic role of IL-17 in psoriasis and psoriatic arthritis pathogenesis. *Clinical Reviews in Allergy & Immunology* 55, 379–390 (2018).

106 Walsh, J.A., Song, X., Kim, G. & Park, Y. Healthcare utilization and direct costs in patients with ankylosing spondylitis using a large US administrative claims database. *Rheumatology and Therapy* 5, 463–474 (2018).

107 Schemoul, J., Poulain, C. & Claudepierre, P. Treatment strategies for psoriatic arthritis. *Joint Bone Spine* 85, 537–544 (2018).

108 Libby, R. The criminalization of medicine: America's war on doctors. Greenwood Publishing Group (2007).

109 Helmick, C.G., *et al.* Estimates of the prevalence of arthritis and other rheumatic conditions in the United States. *Arthritis and Rheumatism* 58, 15–25 (2008).

110 Lawrence, R.C., *et al.* Estimates of the prevalence of arthritis and other rheumatic conditions in the United States. *Arthritis and Rheumatism* 58, 26–35 (2008).

111 Knaack, L. & Janicki, J. Rheumatological diseases and sleep: Somnological aspects of diagnostics and therapy. *Aktuelle Rheumatologie* 43, 277–288 (2018).

112 Thiels, C.A., Habermann, E.B., Hooten, W.M. & Jeffery, M.M. Chronic use of tramadol after acute pain episode: Cohort study. *BMJ-British Medical Journal* 365, Art. No. l1849 (2019).

113 Ballantyne, J.C. & Mao, J.R. Opioid therapy for chronic pain. *New England Journal of Medicine* 349, 1943–1953 (2003).

114 Joranson, D.E., Ryan, K.M., Gilson, A.M. & Dahl, J.L. Trends in medical use and abuse of opioid analgesics. *JAMA-Journal of the American Medical Association* 283, 1710–1714 (2000).

115 Wu, J.J., *et al.* The risk of depression, suicidal ideation and suicide attempt in patients with psoriasis, psoriatic arthritis or ankylosing spondylitis. *Journal of the European Academy of Dermatology and Venereology* 31, 1168–1175 (2017).

116 Dellemijn, P.L.I. Opioids in non-cancer pain: A life-time sentence? *European Journal of Pain-London* 5, 333–339 (2001).

117 Sloan, V.S., Sheahan, A., Stark, J.L. & Suruki, R.Y. Opioid use in patients with ankylosing spondylitis is common in the United States: Outcomes of a retrospective cohort study. *Journal of Rheumatology* 46, 1450–1457 (2019).

118 Dau, J.D., *et al.* Opioid analgesic use in patients with ankylosing spondylitis: An analysis of the prospective study of outcomes in an ankylosing spondylitis cohort. *Journal of Rheumatology* 45, 188–194 (2018).

119 Marks, R.M. & Sachar, E.J. Undertreatment of medical inpatients with narcotic analgesics. *Annals of Internal Medicine* 78, 173–181 (1973).

120 Cohen, S.P. & Hooten, W.M. Balancing the risks and benefits of opioid therapy: The pill and the pendulum. *Mayo Clinic Proceedings* 94, 2385–2389 (2019).

121 Melzack, R. Pain and stress: Clues toward understanding chronic pain in Advances in Psychological Science, Vol 2: Biological and Cognitive Aspects from the 26th International Congress of Psychology, NRC Canada; Sabourin, M., Craik, F., and Robert, M. Eds. (1998).

122 Cole, B.E. Just how responsible is PROP? *MD Magazine.* December 11 (2012).

123 Chisholm-Burns, M.A., Spivey, C.A., Sherwin, E., Wheeler, J. & Hohmeier, K. The opioid crisis: Origins, trends, policies, and the roles of pharmacists. *American Journal of Health-System Pharmacy* 76, 424–435 (2019).

124 Manhapra, A., Arias, A.J. & Ballantyne, J.C. The conundrum of opioid tapering in long-term opioid therapy for chronic pain: A commentary. *Substance Abuse* 39, 152–161 (2018).

125 Tick MD, H. The opioid band-aid: The state of pain pills, Congressional bills, and healthcare in the US. *Practical Pain Management* 18, 6–8 (2018).

126 Fudin, J., Cleary, J.P. & Schatman, M.E. The MEDD myth: The impact of pseudoscience on pain research and prescribing-guideline development. *Journal of Pain Research* 9, 153–156 (2016).

127 Rennick, A., *et al.* Variability in opioid equivalence calculations. *Pain Medicine* 17, 892–898 (2016).

128 Christensen, A.W., *et al.* Temporal summation of pain and ultrasound Doppler activity as predictors of treatment response in patients with rheumatoid arthritis: Protocol for the Frederiksberg hospitals: Rheumatoid arthritis, pain assessment and medical evaluation (FRAME-cohort) study. *BMJ Open* 4, Art. No. e004313 (2014).

129 Adlan, A.M., *et al.* Cardiovascular autonomic regulation, inflammation and pain in rheumatoid arthritis. *Autonomic Neuroscience-Basic & Clinical* 208, 137–145 (2017).

130 Ballantyne, J.C. & Fleisher, L.A. Ethical issues in opioid prescribing for chronic pain. *Pain* 148, 365–367 (2010).

131 McQuay, H. Opioids in pain management. *Lancet* 353, 2229–2232 (1999).

132 Ballantyne, J.C. "Safe and effective when used as directed": The case of chronic use of opioid analgesics. *Journal of Medical Toxicology* 8, 417–423 (2012).

[133] Portenoy, R.K. & Foley, K.M. Chronic use of opioid analgesics in nonmalignant pain—report of 38 cases. *Pain* 25, 171–186 (1986).

[134] Melzack, R. The tragedy of needless pain. *Scientific American* 262, 27–33 (1990).

[135] Urban, B.J., France, R.D., Steinberger, E.K., Scott, D.L. & Maltbie, A.A. Long-term use of narcotic antidepressant medication in the management of phantom limb pain. *Pain* 24, 191–196 (1986).

[136] Taub, A. Opioid analgesics in the treatment of chronic intractable pain of non-neoplastic origin. In Kitahata LM, Collins JG, eds. *Narcotic Analgesics in Anaesthesiology.* Baltimore/London: Williams & Wilkins 199–208 (1982).

[137] Porter, J. & Jick, H. Addiction rare in patients treated with narcotics. *New Eng. J. Med.* 302, 123 (1980).

[138] Brat, G.A., *et al.* Postsurgical prescriptions for opioid naive patients and association with overdose and misuse: Retrospective cohort study. *BMJ-British Medical Journal* 360, Art. No. j5790(2018).

[139] Edlund, M.J., *et al.* The role of opioid prescription in incident opioid abuse and dependence among individuals with chronic noncancer pain: The role of opioid prescription. *Clinical Journal of Pain* 30, 557–564 (2014).

[140] Fishbain, D.A., Cole, B., Lewis, J., Rosomoff, H.L. & Rosomoff, R.S. What percentage of chronic nonmalignant pain patients exposed to chronic opioid analgesic therapy develop abuse/addiction and/or aberrant drug-related behaviors? A structured evidence-based review. *Pain Medicine* 9, 444–459 (2008).

[141] Noble, M., *et al.* Long-term opioid management for chronic noncancer pain. *Cochrane Database of Systematic Reviews* (2010).

[142] Passik, S.D., Messina, J., Golsorkhi, A. & Xie, F. Aberrant drug-related behavior observed during clinical studies involving patients taking chronic opioid therapy for persistent pain and fentanyl buccal tablet for breakthrough pain. *Journal of Pain and Symptom Management* 41, 116–125 (2011).

[143] Boscarino, J.A., *et al.* Prevalence of prescription opioid-use disorder among chronic pain patients: Comparison of the DSM-5 vs. DSM-4 diagnostic criteria. *Journal of Addictive Diseases* 30, 185–194 (2011).

[144] Cheatle, M.D., Gallagher, R.M. & O'Brien, C.P. Low risk of producing an opioid use disorder in primary care by prescribing opioids to prescreened patients with chronic noncancer pain. *Pain Medicine* 19, 764–773 (2018).

[145] Jacobs, M.M., *et al.* Dopamine receptor D1 and postsynaptic density gene variants associate with opiate abuse and striatal expression levels. *Molecular Psychiatry* 18, 1205–1210 (2013).

[146] Baldacchino, A., Gilchrist, G., Fleming, R. & Bannister, J. Guilty until proven innocent: A qualitative study of the management of chronic non-cancer pain among patients with a history of substance abuse. *Addictive Behaviors* 35, 270–272 (2010).

[147] Cheatle, M., Comer, D., Wunsch, M., Skoufalos, A. & Reddy, Y. Treating pain in addicted patients: Recommendations from an expert panel. *Population Health Management* 17, 79–89 (2014).

[148] Colpaert, F.C. System theory of pain and of opiate analgesia: No tolerance to opiates. *Pharmacological Reviews* 48, 355–402 (1996).

[149] Franklin, K.B.J. Analgesia and abuse potential: An accidental association or a common substrate? *Pharmacology Biochemistry and Behavior* 59, 993–1002 (1998).

[150] Breitbart, W., et al. Patient-related barriers to pain management in ambulatory AIDS patients. *Pain* 76, 9–16 (1998).

[151] Rosenblum, A., Marsch, L.A., Joseph, H. & Portenoy, R.K. Opioids and the treatment of chronic pain: Controversies, current status, and future directions. *Experimental and Clinical Psychopharmacology* 16, 405–416 (2008).

[152] Portenoy, R.K., et al. Long-term use of controlled-release oxycodone for noncancer pain: Results of a 3-year registry study. *Clinical Journal of Pain* 23, 287–299 (2007).

[153] Savage, S.R. Opioid medications in the management of pain. In Graham, A.W., Shultz, T.K., Mayo-Smith, M.F., eds. *Principles of Addiction Medicine*. 3rd ed. Chevy Chase, MD: American Society of Addiction Medicine, 1451–1463 (2003).

[154] Cowan, D.T., Allan, L.G., Libretto, S.E. & Griffiths, P. Opioid drugs: A comparative survey of therapeutic and "street" use. *Pain Medicine* 2, 193–203 (2001).

[155] Griffiths, P., Cowan, D.T., Allan, L.G. & Libretto, S.E. Therapeutic and "street" opioid users: Compare the comparables. Response. *Pain Medicine* 3, 78–79 (2002).

[156] Huang, C.J. On being the "right" kind of chronic pain patient. *Narrat Inq Bioeth.* 8, 239–245 (2018).

[157] Sullivan, M.D., et al. Trends in use of opioids for non-cancer pain conditions 2000–2005 in Commercial and Medicaid insurance plans: The TROUP study. *Pain* 138, 440–449 (2008).

[158] Alltucker, K. & O'Donnell, J. "Fighting the wrong war": Chronic pain patients push feds to change opioid policies. *USA Today.* July 12, 2019.

[159] O'Donnell, J. & Alltucker, K. Pain patients left in anguish by doctors "terrified" of opioid addiction, despite CDC change. *USA Today.* June 30, 2019.

[160] Mahmoud, S., et al. Pharmacological consequence of the A118G mu opioid receptor polymorphism on morphine- and fentanyl-mediated modulation of Ca2+ channels in humanized mouse sensory neurons. *Anesthesiology* 115, 1054–1062 (2011).

[161] Koijam, A.S., Chakraborty, B., Mukhopadhyay, K., Rajamma, U. & Haobam, R. A single nucleotide polymorphism in OPRM1 (rs483481) and risk for heroin use disorder. *Journal of Addictive Diseases* 38, 214–222 (2020).

[162] Colloca, L., *et al.* OPRM1 rs1799971, COMT rs4680, and FAAH rs324420 genes interact with placebo procedures to induce hypoalgesia. *Pain* 160, 1824–1834 (2019).

[163] Cheuk, D.K.L. & Wong, V. Meta-analysis of association between a catechol-O-methyltransferase gene polymorphism and attention deficit hyperactivity disorder. *Behavior Genetics* 36, 651–659 (2006).

[164] Zhang, X.Y., *et al.* The relevance of the OPRM1 118A>G genetic variant for opioid requirement in pain treatment: A meta-analysis. *Pain Physician* 22, 331–340 (2019).

[165] Xu, F., *et al.* COMT gene variants and beta-endorphin levels contribute to ethnic differences in experimental pain sensitivity. *Molecular Pain* 16, PMC7036500 (2020).

[166] Persson, E., *et al.* Variation in the mu-opioid receptor gene (OPRM1) does not moderate social-rejection sensitivity in humans. *Psychological Science* 30, 1050–1062 (2019).

[167] Glauser, W. Against the tide in an ocean of opioids. *New Scientist* 237, 35–37 (2018).

[168] The author acknowledges the use of Wikipedia for the image in Figure 1B, which has been used in accord with instructions at https://commons.wikimedia.org/wiki/File:1206_The_Neuron.jpg by OpenStax / CC BY (https://creativecommons.org/licenses/by/4.0).

[169] Wenzel, J.M., Rauscher, N.A., Cheer, J.F. & Oleson, E.B. A role for phasic dopamine release within the nucleus accumbens in encoding aversion: A review of the neurochemical literature. *Acs Chemical Neuroscience* 6, 16–26 (2015).

[170] Cheng, M.H. & Bahar, I. Monoamine transporters: Structure, intrinsic dynamics and allosteric regulation. *Nature Structural & Molecular Biology* 26, 545–556 (2019).

[171] Henry, M.S., Gendron, L., Tremblay, M.E. & Drolet, G. Enkephalins: Endogenous analgesics with an emerging role in stress resilience. *Neural Plasticity* Art. No. 1546125 (2017).

[172] Meldrum, B.S. Glutamate as a neurotransmitter in the brain: Review of physiology and pathology. *Journal of Nutrition* 130, 1007S-1015S (2000).

[173] Bannister, K. & Dickenson, A.H. What do monoamines do in pain modulation? *Current Opinion in Supportive and Palliative Care* 10, 143–148 (2016).

[174] Berridge, K.C., Robinson, T.E. & Aldridge, J.W. Dissecting components of reward: "liking", "wanting", and learning. *Current Opinion in Pharmacology* 9, 65–73 (2009).

[175] Rice, M.E., Patel, J.C. & Cragg, S.J. Dopamine release in the basal ganglia. *Neuroscience* 198, 112–137 (2011).

[176] Schultz, W. Multiple dopamine functions at different time courses. *Annual Review of Neuroscience* 30, 259–288 (2007).

[177] Bjorklund, A. & Dunnett, S.B. Dopamine neuron systems in the brain: An update. *Trends in Neurosciences* 30, 194–202 (2007).

[178] Melzack, R. & Wall, P.D. Pain mechanisms—a new theory. *Science* 150, 971–979 (1965).

[179] Keefe, F.J., Lefebvre, J.C. & Starr, K.R. From the gate Control Theory to the neuromatrix: Revolution or evolution? *Pain Forum* 5, 143–146 (1996).

[180] Allouche, S., Noble, F. & Marie, N. Opioid receptor desensitization: Mechanisms and its link to tolerance. *Frontiers in Pharmacology* 5 (2014)

[181] Ni, Q., *et al.* Opioid peptide receptor studies. 9. Identification of a novel non-mu- non-delta-like opioid peptide binding site in rat brain. *Peptides* 19, 1079–1090 (1998).

[182] Martin, W.R. Multiple opioid receptors. *Life Sciences* 28, 1547–1554 (1981).

[183] Martin, W.J. & Wallace, T.L. The nociceptive opioid peptide receptor system and posttraumatic stress disorder: An enigma wrapped around a conundrum. *Biological Psychiatry* 85, 986–988 (2019).

[184] Footnote. For the interested reader, the two transcription factors that are most important are the cyclic adenosine monophosphate response element binding (CREB) protein and Delta-FosB. CREB is upregulated both in pain patients and drug users. It is also activated by cAMP (cyclic adenosine monophosphate), a signaling molecule triggered by stimulatory binding of dopamine to D1, but inhibited by binding to D2. CREB upregulation is associated with pain and depression. Therefore, I call it a transcription factor for pain and depression in the text. Its presence decreases the dopamine receptor density as seen in both pain patients and drug users. Thus, it is part of the long-term effects of high cross-tolerance for the euphoric effect by pain patients. Stated simply, CREB in pain patients inhibits euphoria, which is also what happens to drug users over time as they develop tolerance. Delta-FosB is upregulated in drug users. It is a more complicated transcription factor, but very important in the study of addiction. Therefore, I call Delta-FosB the transcription factor for addiction in the text.

[185] Iasevoli, F., Tomasetti, C. & de Bartolomeis, A. Scaffolding proteins of the post-synaptic density contribute to synaptic plasticity by regulating receptor localization and distribution: Relevance for neuropsychiatric diseases. *Neurochemical Research* 38, 1–22 (2013).

[186] Cochin, J. & Kornetsky, C. Development and loss of tolerance to morphine in rat after single and multiple injections. *Journal of Pharmacology and Experimental Therapeutics* 145, 1–10 (1964).

[187] Matthes, H.W.D., *et al.* Loss of morphine-induced analgesia, reward effect and withdrawal symptoms in mice lacking the mu-opioid-receptor gene. *Nature* 383, 819–823 (1996).

[188] Footnote. Each gene comes in a pair of alleles. Alleles can code for different proteins (which lead to different appearance or phenotype). There are heterozygous (single allele of mutant) knockouts that produce approximately 50% of the MOR and then homozygous (both alleles of mutant) knockouts that have no MOR at all. MOR is 100% eliminated.

[189] Bodnar, R.J. Endogenous opiates and behavior: 2017. *Peptides* 124, Art. No. 170223.

[190] Sora, I., *et al.* Opiate receptor knockout mice define mu receptor roles in endogenous nociceptive responses and morphine-induced analgesia. *Proceedings of the National Academy of Sciences of the United States of America* 94, 1544–1549 (1997).

[191] Footnote. The fact that there is still some effect of morphine tells us that the MOR is not the only mechanism of action to inhibit pain. However, it is still the main mechanism.

[192] Grim, T.W., *et al.* A G protein signaling-biased agonist at the mu-opioid receptor reverses morphine tolerance while preventing morphine withdrawal. *Neuropsychopharmacology* 45, 416–425 (2020).

[193] Bohn, L.M., Gainetdinov, R.R., Lin, F.T., Lefkowitz, R.J. & Caron, M.G. mu-Opioid receptor desensitization by beta-arrestin-2 determines morphine tolerance but not dependence. *Nature* 408, 720–723 (2000).

[194] Paterson, C., *et al.* Resisting prescribed opioids: A qualitative study of decision making in patients taking opioids for chronic noncancer pain. *Pain Medicine* 17, 717–727 (2016).

[195] Walentiny, D.M., Moisa, L.T. & Beardsley, P.M. Oxycodone-like discriminative stimulus effects of fentanyl-related emerging drugs of abuse in mice. *Neuropharmacology* 150, 210–216 (2019).

[196] Olson, K.M., Duron, D.I., Womer, D., Fell, R. & Streicher, J.M. Comprehensive molecular pharmacology screening reveals potential new receptor interactions for clinically relevant opioids. *PLOS One* 14, Art. No. e217371 (2019).

[197] Kitchen, I., Slowe, S.J., Matthes, H.W.D. & Kieffer, B. Quantitative autoradiographic mapping of mu-, delta- and kappa-opioid receptors in knockout mice lacking the mu-opioid receptor gene. *Brain Research* 778, 73–88 (1997).

[198] Loh, H.H., *et al.* mu opioid receptor knockout in mice: Effects on ligand-induced analgesia and morphine lethality. *Molecular Brain Research* 54, 321–326 (1998).

[199] Sora, I., Funada, M. & Uhl, G.R. The mu-opioid receptor is necessary for D-Pen(2),D-Pen(5) enkephalin-induced analgesia. *European Journal of Pharmacology* 324, R1–R2 (1997).

[200] Baliki, M.N. & Apkarian, A.V. Nociception, pain, negative moods, and behavior selection. *Neuron* 87, 474–491 (2015).

[201] Selley, D.E., *et al.* Attenuated dopamine receptor signaling in nucleus accumbens core in a rat model of chemically-induced neuropathy. *Neuropharmacology* 166, Art. No. 107935 (2020).

[202] Sternini, C., *et al.* Agonist-selective endocytosis of mu-opioid receptor by neurons in vivo. *Proceedings of the National Academy of Sciences of the United States of America* 93, 9241–9246 (1996).

203 J. L. Whistler, H. Chuang, P. Chu, L. Y. Jan & von Zastrow, M. Functional dissociation of mu opioid receptor signaling and endocytosis: Implications for the biology of opiate tolerance and addiction. *Neuron* 23, 737–746 (1999).

204 Perrotti, L.I., *et al.* Distinct patterns of Delta FosB induction in brain by drugs of abuse. *Synapse* 62, 358–369 (2008).

205 Pollema-Mays, S.L., Centeno, M.V., Chang, Z., Apkarian, A.V. & Martina, M. Reduced Delta FosB expression in the rat nucleus accumbens has causal role in the neuropathic pain phenotype. *Neuroscience Letters* 702, 77–83 (2019).

206 Akil, H., *et al.* Endogenous opioids—biology and function. *Annual Review of Neuroscience* 7, 223–255 (1984).

207 Harris, H.N. & Peng, Y.B. Evidence and explanation for the involvement of the nucleus accumbens in pain processing. *Neural Regeneration Research* 15, 597–605 (2020).

208 Graziane, N.M., *et al.* Opposing mechanisms mediate morphine- and cocaine-induced generation of silent synapses. *Nature Neuroscience* 19, 915–925 (2016).

209 Nestler, E.J. Reflections on: "A general role for adaptations in G-Proteins and the cyclic AMP system in mediating the chronic actions of morphine and cocaine on neuronal function". *Brain Research* 1645, 71–74 (2016).

210 Hagelberg, N., *et al.* Striatal dopamine D2 receptors in modulation of pain in humans: A review. *European Journal of Pharmacology* 500, 187–192 (2004).

211 Pertovaara, A., *et al.* Striatal dopamine D2/D3 receptor availability correlates with individual response characteristics to pain. *European Journal of Neuroscience* 20, 1587–1592 (2004).

212 Chang, P.C., *et al.* Role of nucleus accumbens in neuropathic pain: Linked multi-scale evidence in the rat transitioning to neuropathic pain. *Pain* 155, 1128–1139 (2014).

213 Ren, W.J., *et al.* The indirect pathway of the nucleus accumbens shell amplifies neuropathic pain. *Nature Neuroscience* 19, 220–222 (2016).

214 Franklin, K.B.J. Analgesia and the neural substrate of reward. *Neuroscience and Biobehavioral Reviews* 13, 149–154 (1989).

215 Jones, A.K.P., *et al.* Changes in central opioid receptor-binding in relation to inflammation and pain in patients with rheumatoid arthritis. *British Journal of Rheumatology* 33, 909–916 (1994).

216 Lemagnen, J., Marfaingjallat, P., Miceli, D. & Devos, M. Pain modulating and reward systems—a single brain mechanism. *Pharmacology Biochemistry and Behavior* 12, 729–733 (1980).

217 Akil, H., Mayer, D.J. & Liebeskind, J.C. Antagonism of stimulation produced analgesia by naloxone, a narcotic antagonist. *Science* 191, 961–962 (1976).

218 Jacob, J.J.C. & Ramabadran, K. Enhancement of a nociceptive reaction by opioid antagonists in mice. *British Journal of Pharmacology* 64, 91–98 (1978).

219 Bodnar, R.J., Kelly, D.D., Steiner, S.S. & Glusman, M. Stress-produced analgesia and morphine-produced analgesia—lack of cross-tolerance. *Pharmacology Biochemistry and Behavior* 8, 661–666 (1978).

[220] Reynolds, D.V. Surgery in rat during electrical analgesia by focal brain stimulations. *Science* 164, 444–445 (1969).

[221] Eippert, F., *et al.* Activation of the opioidergic descending pain control system underlies placebo analgesia. *Neuron* 63, 533–543 (2009).

[222] Cahill, C.M., Holdridge, S.V. & Morinville, A. Trafficking of delta-opioid receptors and other G-protein-coupled receptors: Implications for pain and analgesia. *Trends in Pharmacological Sciences* 28, 23–31 (2007).

[223] Basbaum, A.I. & Fields, H.L. Endogenous pain control mechanisms: Review and hypotheses. *Annals of Neurology* 4, 451–462 (1978).

[224] Bai, Y., *et al.* Enkephalinergic circuit involved in nociceptive modulation in the spinal dorsal horn. *Neuroscience* 429, 78–91 (2020).

[225] Braz, J., Solorzano, C., Wang, X.D. & Basbaum, A.I. Transmitting pain and itch messages: A contemporary view of the spinal cord circuits that generate gate control. *Neuron* 82, 522–536 (2014).

[226] Garland, E.L. Pain processing in the human nervous system: A selective review of nociceptive and biobehavioral pathways. *Primary Care* 39, 561–571 (2012).

[227] Baliki, M.N., Geha, P.Y. & Apkarian, A.V. Parsing pain perception between nociceptive representation and magnitude estimation. *Journal of Neurophysiology* 101, 875–887 (2009).

[228] Kato, T., Ide, S. & Minami, M. Pain relief induces dopamine release in the rat nucleus accumbens during the early but not late phase of neuropathic pain. *Neuroscience Letters* 629, 73–78 (2016).

[229] DiNieri, J.A., *et al.* Altered sensitivity to rewarding and aversive drugs in mice with inducible disruption of cAMP response element-binding protein function within the nucleus accumbens. *Journal of Neuroscience* 29, 1855–1859 (2009).

[230] Grenier, P., Mailhiot, M.C., Cahill, C.M. & Olmstead, M.C. Blockade of dopamine D1 receptors in male rats disrupts morphine reward in pain naive but not in chronic pain states. *Journal of Neuroscience Research* 00: 1–13 (2019).

[231] Footnote. There is distinction between antinociception and analgesia, which can be detected by separate tests in the mouse spine and brain, respectively. The tail flick test shows that morphine is antinociceptive in the spinal cord where there is a high density of MOR on the inhibitory cells. In the dorsal horn (back corner) there are many such cells that are located in the region where the incoming fibers from the periphery with a pain message will relay that message to projecting cells to carry it up to the thalamus in the brain. On the other hand, the formalin test reveals that morphine can also produce analgesia by a mechanism that is analogous to the euphoria induced by release of a particular neurotransmitter in the reward center of the brain.

[232] Chen, J.T., Fagan, M.J., Diaz, J.A. & Reinert, S.E. Is treating chronic pain torture? Internal medicine residents' experience with patients with chronic nonmalignant pain. *Teaching and Learning in Medicine* 19, 101–105 (2007).

[233] Not allowed to be compassionate. Human Rights Watch. December 18, 2018.

234 Berg, K.M., Arnsten, J.H., Sacajiu, G. & Karasz, A. Providers' experiences treating chronic pain among opioid-dependent drug users. *Journal of General Internal Medicine* 24, 482–488 (2009).

235 Rastegar, D.A. Providers' experiences treating chronic pain among opioid-dependent drug users. *Journal of General Internal Medicine* 24, 1081 (2009).

236 Berg, K.M., Arnsten, J.H., Sacajiu, G. & Karasz, A. Providers' experiences treating chronic pain among opioid-dependent drug users—reply. *Journal of General Internal Medicine* 24, 1082 (2009).

237 Barry, C.L., *et al.* Understanding Americans' views on opioid pain reliever abuse. *Addiction* 111, 85–93 (2016).

238 Kessler, A., Cohen, E., Griese, K. & Bonifeld, J. The more opioids doctors prescribe, the more money they make. *CNN.* March 12, 2018.

239 Stewart, K. Prominent Utah pain doc no longer under scrutiny for patient deaths. *The Salt Lake Tribune.* June 30, 2014.

240 Wight, P. Doctors in Maine say halt in OxyContin marketing comes "20 years too late." *National Public Radio.* February 11, 2018.

241 Booker, B. Doctor gets 40 years for illegally prescribing more than half a million opioid doses. *National Public Radio.* October 2, 2019.

242 Dwyer, C. & Fortier, J. Oklahoma judge shaves $107 million off opioid decision against Johnson & Johnson. *National Public Radio.* November 21, 2019.

243 Smith, S.E. War on prescription drugs: what if you depend on opioids to live a decent life? *The Guardian.* July 12, 2016.

244 Walters, J. Sackler family members face mass litigation and criminal investigations over opioids crisis. *The Guardian.* November 19, 2018.

245 McGreal, C. Doctor who was paid by Purdue to push opioids to testify against drugmaker. *The Guardian.* April 10, 2019.

246 Reuters. Purdue is unnamed company in investigation of illegal kickbacks, insiders say. *The Guardian.* January 28, 2020.

247 Markon, J. Va. pain doctor's prison term is cut to 57 months. *The Washington Post.* July 14, 2007.

248 Zapotsky, M. DEA mismanaged, overpaid confidential informants, Justice Department finds. *The Washington Post.* September 30, 2016.

249 Editorial Board, T. The government's shameful role in the opioid crisis. *The Washington Post.* October 16, 2017.

250 Higham, S. & Bernstein, L. The drug industry's triumph over the DEA. *The Washington Post.* October 15, 2017.

251 Achenbach, J. & Bernstein, L. Opioid crackdown forces pain patients to taper off drugs they say they need. *The Washington Post.* September 10, 2019.

252 Bernstein, L. DEA allowed huge growth in painkiller supply as overdose deaths rose, IG says. *The Washington Post.* October 1, 2019.

253 Higham, S., Horwitz, S. & Rich, S. 76 billion opioid pills: Newly released federal data unmasks the epidemic. *The Washington Post.* July 16, 2019.

[254] Merle, R. Judge in Purdue Pharma bankruptcy case extends lawsuit protection to Sacklers. *The Washington Post.* November 6, 2019.

[255] Editorial Board, T. Drilling into the DEA's pain pill database. *The Washington Post.* January 17, 2020.

[256] Hamblin, J. The opioid reckoning will not be just. *The Atlantic.* August 29, 2019.

[257] Satel, S. The truth about painkiller addiction. *The Atlantic.* August 4, 2019.

[258] Bromwich, J.E. Vermont governor proposes limits on painkiller prescriptions. *New York Times.* October 19, 2016.

[259] Karmasek, J. Plaintiffs firm consultant helped develop CDC's controversial opioid guidelines *Legal Newsline.* December 6, 2015.

[260] Anson, P. PROP president discloses conflicts of interest. *Pain News Network.* November 12, 2019.

[261] Anson, P. How opioid critics and law firms profit from litigation. *Pain News Network.* June 21, 2019.

[262] Kolodny, A. Clarification of reporting of potential conflicts of interest in JAMA articles. *JAMA-Journal of the American Medical Association* 322, 1214–1215 (2019).

[263] Drash, W. Expert witness: Johnson & Johnson's role in opioid crisis may be "worse" than Purdue's. *CNN.* June 11, 2019.

[264] American Medical Association. https://www.ama-assn.org/press-center/press-releases/ama-urges-cdc-revise-opioid-prescribing-guideline. *American Medical Association* Docket No. CDC-2020-0029 (2020).

[265] Joseph, A. Purdue cemented ties with universities and hospitals to expand opioid sales, documents contend. *STAT.* January 16, 2019.

[266] IOM. Relieving pain in America: A blueprint for transforming prevention, care, education, and research. Institute of Medicine: Committee on Advancing Pain Research, Care, and Education. National Academies Press (2011).

[267] Nicholson, K.M., Hoffman, D.E. & Kollas, C.D. Overzealous use of the CDC's opioid prescribing guideline is harming pain patients. *STAT.* December 6, 2018.

[268] Kertesz, S.G. Outcomes after opioid dose reductions and stoppage: It's time to start counting. *Journal of Substance Abuse Treatment* 103, 64–65 (2019).

[269] Fudin, J. & Atkinson, T.J. Opioid prescribing levels off, but is less really more? *Pain Medicine* 15, 184–187 (2014).

[270] Miron, J., Sollenberger, G. & Nicolae, L. Overdosing on regulation: How government caused the opioid epidemic. *Policy Analysis CATO Institute.* February 14, 2019.

[271] Ballantyne, J.C. Opioid controls: Regulate to educate. *Pain Medicine* 11, 480–481 (2010).

[272] Sullivan, M.D. & Ballantyne, J.C. What are we treating with long-term opioid therapy? *Archives of Internal Medicine* 172, 433–434 (2012).

[273] Ballantyne, J.C. & Sullivan, M.D. Why doctors prescribe opioids to known opioid abusers. *New England Journal of Medicine* 368, 484–485 (2013).

[274] Ballantyne, J.C. Opioid therapy in chronic pain. *Physical Medicine and Rehabilitation Clinics of North America* 26, 201–218 (2015).

[275] Ballantyne, J.C. Avoiding opioid analgesics for treatment of chronic low back pain. *JAMA-Journal of the American Medical Association* 315, 2459–2460 (2016).

[276] Kolodny, A. Chronic pain patients are not immune to opioid harms. *Journal of Pain & Palliative Care Pharmacotherapy* 30, 330–331 (2016).

[277] Joseph, A. Clinicians were told their patient had died of an overdose. Then opioid prescribing dropped. *STAT.* August 9, 2018.

[278] Lembke, A. Why doctors prescribe opioids to known opioid abusers. *New England Journal of Medicine* 367, 1580–1581 (2013).

[279] Anson, P. "You ruined my life": Patients blame CDC for poor pain care. *Pain News Network.* June 17, 2020.

[280] Anson, P. North Carolina investigating pain patient advocate. *Pain News Network.* February 19, 2020.

[281] Dowell, D., Haegerich, T.M. & Chou, R. CDC guideline for prescribing opioids for chronic pain—United States, 2016. *MMWR Recomm Rep* 65, 1–49 (2016).

[282] Darnall, B.D. The national imperative to align practice and policy with the actual CDC Opioid Guideline. *Pain Medicine* 21, 229–231 (2020).

[283] Anson, P. Opioid hysteria leading to patient abandonment. *Pain News Network.* March 28, 2018.

[284] Sullum, J. Punishing pain patients won't reduce opioid deaths. *Reason.* December 19, 2018.

[285] Hoffman, J. & Goodnough, A. Good news: Opioid prescribing fell. The bad? Pain patients suffer, doctors say. *New York Times* A16. March 6, 2019.

[286] Kertesz, S.G. An opioid quality metric based on dose alone—80 professionals respond to NCQA. Available at https://medium.com/@StefanKertesz/an-opioid-qualitymetric-based-on-dose-alone-80 (2017).

[287] Ballantyne, J.C. & Shin, N.S. Efficacy of opioids for chronic pain: A review of the evidence. *Clinical Journal of Pain* 24, 469–478 (2008).

[288] Hadland, S.E., Rivera-Aguirre, A., Marshall, B.D.L. & Cerda, M. Association of pharmaceutical industry marketing of opioid products with mortality from ppioid-related overdoses. *JAMA Network Open* 2, Art. No. e186007 (2019).

[289] Jones, C.M., Lurie, P. & Woodcock, J. Addressing prescription opioid overdose data support a comprehensive policy approach. *JAMA-Journal of the American Medical Association* 312, 1733–1734 (2014).

[290] Raji, M.A., Kuo, Y.F., Adhikari, D., Baillargeon, J. & Goodwin, J.S. Decline in opioid prescribing after federal rescheduling of hydrocodone products. *Pharmacoepidemiology and Drug Safety* 27, 513–519 (2018).

[291] Fleming, M.L., *et al.* Drug Enforcement Administration rescheduling of hydrocodone combination products is associated with changes in physician pain management prescribing preferences. *Journal of Pain & Palliative Care Pharmacotherapy* 33, 22–31 (2019).

292 Harrison, M.L. & Walsh, T.L. The effect of a more strict 2014 DEA schedule designation for hydrocodone products on opioid prescription rates in the United States. *Clinical Toxicology* 57, 1064–1072 (2019).

293 Dhalla, I.A., Persaud, N. & Juurlink, D.N. Facing up to the prescription opioid crisis. *BMJ-British Medical Journal* 343, Art. No. d5142 (2011).

294 Tedeschi, B. A "civil war" over painkillers rips apart the medical community—and leaves patients in fear. *STAT.* January 17, 2017.

295 Andrilla, C.H.A., Moore, T.E. & Patterson, D.G. Overcoming barriers to prescribing buprenorphine for the treatment of opioid use disorder: Recommendations from rural physicians. *Journal of Rural Health* 35, 113–121 (2019).

296 Andrilla, C.H.A., Jones, K.C. & Patterson, D.G. Prescribing practices of nurse practitioners and physician assistants waivered to prescribe buprenorphine and the barriers they experience prescribing buprenorphine. *Journal of Rural Health* 36, 187–195 (2020).

297 Bonnie, R.J., Ford, M.A. & Phillips, J.K. *Pain Management and the Opioid Epidemic: Balancing Societal and Individual Benefits and Risks of Prescription Opioid Use Summary* (National Academy of Sciences, Engineering and Medicine, Washington, DC, National Academies Press, 2017).

298 Reid, M.C., *et al.* Use of opioid medications for chronic noncancer pain syndromes in primary care. *Journal of General Internal Medicine* 17, 173–179 (2002).

299 Zee, A.V. The promotion and marketing of OxyContin: Commercial triumph, public health tragedy. *American Journal of Public Health* 99, 221–227 (2009).

300 Edlund, M.J., Steffick, D., Hudson, T., Harris, K.M. & Sullivan, M. Risk factors for clinically recognized opioid abuse and dependence among veterans using opioids for chronic non-cancer pain. *Pain* 129, 355–362 (2007).

301 Martell, B.A., *et al.* Systematic review: Opioid treatment for chronic back pain: Prevalence, efficacy, and association with addiction. *Annals of Internal Medicine* 146, 116–127 (2007).

302 Roosevelt, M. Why is the DEA hounding this doctor? *Time.* July 18, 2005.

303 Libby, R.T. Treating doctors as drug dealers: The DEA's war on prescription painkillers. *Cato Institute Policy Report.* June 16, 2005.

304 Goldenbaum, D.M., *et al.* Physicians charged with opioid analgesic-prescribing offenses. *Pain Medicine* 9, 737–747 (2008).

305 Anson, P. Death of pain patient blamed on DEA raid. *Pain News Network.* April 30, 2018.

306 Lord, R. & Silber, M. DEA is cracking down on physicians who overprescribe pills. *Pittsburgh Post-Gazette.* August 12, 2016.

307 Stanton, S. Murder case dissolved, but so did doctor's life. *Sacramento Bee.* May 23, 2004.

308 Begley, S. "Every time it's a battle": In excruciating pain, sickle cell patients are shunted aside. *STAT.* September 8, 2017.

[309] Marill, M.C. The unseen victims of the opioid crisis are starting to rebel. *Wired.* May 21, 2019.

[310] Bloom, J. Pain in the time of opioid denial: An interview with Aric Hausknecht, M.D. *American Council on Science and Health.* July 19 (2017).

[311] O'Brien, T., *et al.* European Pain Federation position paper on appropriate opioid use in chronic pain management. *European Journal of Pain* 21, 3–19 (2017).

[312] Bialas, P., Maier, C., Klose, P. & Häuser, W. Efficacy and harms of long-term opioid therapy in chronic non-cancer pain: Systematic review and meta-analysis of open-label extension trials with a study duration >= 26 weeks. *European Journal of Pain* 24, 265–278 (2020).

[313] Avouac, J., Gossec, L. & Dougados, M. Efficacy and safety of opioids for osteoarthritis: A meta-analysis of randomized controlled trials. *Osteoarthritis and Cartilage* 15, 957–965 (2007).

[314] Mystakidou, K., *et al.* Long-term management of noncancer pain with transdermal therapeutic system-fentanyl. *Journal of Pain* 4, 298–306 (2003).

[315] Kalso, E., Edwards, J.E., Moore, R.A. & McQuay, H.J. Opioids in chronic non-cancer pain: Systematic review of efficacy and safety. *Pain* 112, 372–380 (2004).

[316] Eisenberg, E., McNicol, E.D. & Carr, D.B. Efficacy and safety of opioid agonists in the treatment of neuropathic pain of nonmalignant origin: Systematic review and meta-analysis of randomized controlled trials. *JAMA-Journal of the American Medical Association* 293, 3043–3052 (2005).

[317] Noble, M., Tregear, S.J., Treadwell, J.R. & Schoelles, K. Long-term opioid therapy for chronic noncancer pain: A systematic review and meta-analysis of efficacy and safety. *Journal of Pain and Symptom Management* 35, 214–228 (2008).

[318] da Costa, B.R., *et al.* Oral or transdermal opioids for osteoarthritis of the knee or hip. *Cochrane Database of Systematic Reviews* (2014).

[319] Cepeda, M.S., Camargo, F., Zea, C. & Valencia, L. Tramadol for osteoarthritis. *Cochrane Database of Systematic Reviews* (2006).

[320] Rauck, R.L. What is the case for prescribing long-acting opioids over short-acting opioids for patients with chronic pain? A critical review. *Pain Practice* 9, 468–479 (2009).

[321] Kjaersgaardandersen, P., *et al.* Codeine plus paracetamol versus paracetamol in longer-term treatment of chronic pain due to osteoarthritis of the hip: A randomized, double-blind multicenter study. *Pain* 43, 309–318 (1990).

[322] Caldwell, J.R., *et al.* Treatment of osteoarthritis pain with controlled release oxycodone or fixed combination oxycodone plus acetaminophen added to nonsteroidal anti-inflammatory drugs: A double blind, randomized, multicenter, placebo controlled trial. *Journal of Rheumatology* 26, 862–869 (1999).

[323] Peloso, P.M., et al. Double blind randomized placebo control trial of controlled release codeine in the treatment of osteoarthritis of the hip or knee. *Journal of Rheumatology* 27, 764–771 (2000).

[324] Huse, E., Larbig, W., Flor, H. & Birbaumer, N. The effect of opioids on phantom limb pain and cortical reorganization. *Pain* 90, 47–55 (2001).

[325] Maier, C., et al. Morphine responsiveness, efficacy and tolerability in patients with chronic non-tumor associated pain: Results of a double-blind placebo-controlled trial (MONTAS). *Pain* 97, 223–233 (2002).

[326] Kivitz, A., Ma, C., Ahdieh, H. & Galer, B.S. A 2-week, multicenter, randomized, double-blind, placebo-controlled, dose-ranging, phase III trial comparing the efficacy of oxymorphone extended release and placebo in adults with pain associated with osteoarthritis of the hip or knee. *Clinical Therapeutics* 28, 352–364 (2006).

[327] Matsumoto, A.K., Babul, N. & Ahdieh, H. Oxymorphone extended-release tablets relieve moderate to severe pain and improve physical function in osteoarthritis: Results of a randomized, double-blind, placebo- and active-controlled phase III trial. *Pain Medicine* 6, 357–366 (2005).

[328] Markenson, J.A., Croft, J., Zhang, P.G. & Richards, P. Treatment of persistent pain associated with osteoarthritis with controlled-release oxycodone tablets in a randomized controlled clinical trial. *Clinical Journal of Pain* 21, 524–535 (2005).

[329] Webster, L.R., et al. Oxytrex minimizes physical dependence while providing effective analgesia: A randomized controlled trial in low back pain. *Journal of Pain* 7, 937–946 (2006).

[330] Hale, M.E., Ahdieh, H., Ma, T., Rauck, R. & Oxymorphone, E.R.S.G. Efficacy and safety of OPANA ER (oxymorphone extended release) for relief of moderate to severe chronic low back pain in opioid-experienced patients: A 12-week, randomized, double-blind, placebo-controlled study. *Journal of Pain* 8, 175–184 (2007).

[331] Caldwell, J.R., et al. Efficacy and safety of a once-daily morphine formulation in chronic, moderate-to-severe osteoarthritis pain: Results from a randomized, placebo-controlled, double-blind trial and an open-label extension trial. *Journal of Pain and Symptom Management* 23, 278–291 (2002).

[332] Arkinstall, W., et al. Efficacy of controlled-release codeine in chronic nonmalignant pain: A randomized placebo controlled clinical trial. *Pain* 62, 169–178 (1995).

[333] Moulin, D.E., et al. Randomized trial of oral morphine for chronic non-cancer pain. *Lancet* 347, 143–147 (1996).

[334] Jamison, R.N., Raymond, S.A., Slawsby, E.A., Nedeljkovic, S.S. & Katz, N.P. Opioid therapy for chronic noncancer back pain: A randomized prospective study. *Spine* 23, 2591–2600 (1998).

[335] Hale, M.E., Dvergsten, C. & Gimbel, J. Efficacy and safety of oxymorphone extended release in chronic low back pain: Results of a randomized, double-

blind, placebo- and active-controlled phase III study. *Journal of Pain* 6, 21–28 (2005).

[336] Roth, S.H., *et al.* Around-the-clock, controlled-release oxycodone therapy for osteoarthritis-related pain: Placebo-controlled trial and long-term evaluation. *Archives of Internal Medicine* 160, 853–860 (2000).

[337] Watson, C.P.N. & Babul, N. Efficacy of oxycodone in neuropathic pain: A randomized trial in postherpetic neuralgia. *Neurology* 50, 1837–1841 (1998).

[338] Raja, S.N., *et al.* Opioids versus antidepressants in postherpetic neuralgia: A randomized, placebo-controlled trial. *Neurology* 59, 1015–1021 (2002).

[339] Gimbel, J.S., Richards, P. & Portenoy, R.K. Controlled-release oxycodone for pain in diabetic neuropathy: A randomized controlled trial. *Neurology* 60, 927–934 (2003).

[340] Morley, J.S., *et al.* Low-dose methadone has an analgesic effect in neuropathic pain: A double-blind randomized controlled crossover trial. *Palliative Medicine* 17, 576–587 (2003).

[341] Rowbotham, M.C., *et al.* Oral opioid therapy for chronic peripheral and central neuropathic pain. *New England Journal of Medicine* 348, 1223–1232 (2003).

[342] Watson, C.P.N., Moulin, D., Watt-Watson, J., Gordon, A. & Eisenhoffer, J. Controlled-release oxycodone relieves neuropathic pain: A randomized controlled trial in painful diabetic neuropathy. *Pain* 105, 71–78 (2003).

[343] Meier, B. In guilty plea, OxyContin maker to pay $600 million. *New York Times*. May 10, 2007.

[344] Bonnie, R.J., Ford, M.A., Phillips, J.K. & editors. Pain management and the opioid epidemic: Balancing societal and individual benefits and risks of prescription opioid use. *National Academies of Sciences, Engineering, and Medicine; Health and Medicine Division; Board on Health Sciences Policy; Committee on Pain Management and Regulatory Strategies to Address Prescription Opioid Abuse.* Washington (DC): National Academies Press (US). July 13, 2017.

[345] Anson, P. PROP linked to new federal opioid study. *Pain News Network*. April 20, 2020.

[346] Levine, A. The real "Death Panels": Oregon Medicaid planned to cut off opioids to chronic pain patients. *Tarbell*. March 15, 2019.

[347] Chou, R., *et al.* Opioid treatments for chronic pain: Comparative effectiveness review no. 229. (Prepared by the Pacific Northwest Evidence-based Practice Center under Contract No. 290-2015-00009-I.) *AHRQ Publication No. 20-EHC011.* Rockville, MD: Agency for Healthcare Research and Quality. April (2020).

[348] Wakeland, W., Nielsen, A. & Geissert, P. Dynamic model of nonmedical opioid use trajectories and potential policy interventions. *American Journal of Drug and Alcohol Abuse* 41, 508–518 (2015).

[349] Lembke, A. Why doctors prescribe opioids to known opioid abusers reply. *New England Journal of Medicine* 368, 485–485 (2013).

[350] Krebs, E.E., Gravely, A. & Noorbaloochi, S. Opioids vs nonopioids for chronic back, hip, or knee pain: Reply. *JAMA-Journal of the American Medical Association* 320, 508–509 (2018).

[351] Krebs, E.E., *et al.* Effect of opioid vs nonopioid medications on pain-related function in patients with chronic back pain or hip or knee osteoarthritis pain: The SPACE randomized clinical trial. *JAMA-Journal of the American Medical Association* 319, 872–882 (2018).

[352] Welsch, P., Sommer, C., Schiltenwolf, M. & Hauser, W. Opioids in chronic noncancer pain—are opioids superior to nonopioid analgesics? A systematic review and meta-analysis of efficacy, tolerability and safety in randomized head-to-head comparisons of opioids versus nonopioid analgesics of at least four weeks' duration. *Schmerz* 29, 85–95 (2015).

[353] Hutton, B., *et al.* The PRISMA extension statement for reporting of systematic reviews incorporating network meta-analyses of health care Interventions: Checklist and explanations. *Annals of Internal Medicine* 162, 777–784 (2015).

[354] Diasso, P.D.K., *et al.* Patient reported outcomes and neuropsychological testing in patients with chronic non-cancer pain in long-term opioid therapy: A pilot study. *Scandinavian Journal of Pain* 19, 533–543 (2019).

[355] McQuay, H.J. Opioid use in chronic pain. *Acta Anaesthesiologica Scandinavica* 41, 175–183 (1997).

[356] Mercadante, S. & Bruera, E. Opioid switching: A systematic and critical review. *Cancer Treatment Reviews* 32, 304–315 (2006).

[357] McQuay, H. Dose optimisation in pain control. in *Optimal Dose Identification: Excerta Medica*, Vol. 1220 (ed. Brekenridge, A.) 99–115 (2001).

[358] Bartlett, G. & Gagnon, J. Physicians and knowledge translation of statistics: Mind the gap. *Canadian Medical Association Journal* 188, 11–12 (2016).

[359] Katz, N.P., *et al.* Prescription opioid abuse: Challenges and opportunities for payers. *American Journal of Managed Care* 19, 295–302 (2013).

[360] Saloner, B., *et al.* A public health strategy for the opioid crisis. *Public Health Reports* 133, 24S-34S (2018).

[361] Climent, M.d.C. Why doctors are bad at stats—and how that could affect your health. *Medium—The Winton Centre for Risk and Evidence Communication.* September 19, 2019.

[362] Geller, A.S. Clinician identification of appropriate long-term opioid therapy candidacy. *Archives of Internal Medicine* 172, 1113–1114 (2012).

[363] Shalhoup, D. Local pain management doctor fined. *The Nashua Telegraph.* October 18, 2018.

[364] Farrar, J.T., Portenoy, R.K., Berlin, J.A., Kinman, J.L. & Strom, B.L. Defining the clinically important difference in pain outcome measures. *Pain* 88, 287–294 (2000).

[365] Agarwal, D., Udoji, M.A. & Trescot, A. Genetic resting for opioid pain management: A primer. *Pain and Therapy* 6, 93–105 (2017).

[366] Chou, R. 2009 Clinical Guidelines from the American Pain Society and the American Academy of Pain Medicine on the use of chronic opioid therapy in chronic noncancer pain What are the key messages for clinical practice? *Polskie Archiwum Medycyny Wewnetrznej-Polish Archives of Internal Medicine* 119, 469–476 (2009).

[367] Schneberk, T., Raffetto, B., Kim, D. & Schriger, D.L. The supply of prescription opioids: Contributions of episodic-care prescribers and high-quantity prescribers. *Annals of Emergency Medicine* 71, 668–673 (2018).

[368] Barbor, M. Opioids for cancer pain: A review of the evidence and current challenges. *The ASCO Post.* August 25, 2019.

[369] Eccleston, C., *et al.* Interventions for the reduction of prescribed opioid use in chronic non-cancer pain. *Cochrane Database of Systematic Reviews* (2017).

[370] Akbik, H., *et al.* Validation and clinical application of the Screener and Opioid Assessment for Patients with Pain (SOAPP). *Journal of Pain and Symptom Management* 32, 287–293 (2006).

[371] Allan, L., Richarz, U., Simpson, K. & Slappendel, R. Transdermal fentanyl versus sustained release oral morphine in strong-opioid naive patients with chronic low back pain. *Spine* 30, 2484–2490 (2005).

[372] Ashburn, M.A., Slevin, K.A., Messina, J. & Xie, F. The efficacy and safety of fentanyl buccal tablet compared with immediate-release oxycodone for the management of breakthrough pain in opioid-tolerant patients with chronic pain. *Anesthesia and Analgesia* 112, 693–702 (2011).

[373] Banta-Green, C.J., Merrill, J.O., Doyle, S.R., Boudreau, D.M. & Calsyn, D.A. Opioid use behaviors, mental health and pain-Development of a typology of chronic pain patients. *Drug and Alcohol Dependence* 104, 34–42 (2009).

[374] Boscarino, J.A., *et al.* Risk factors for drug dependence among out-patients on opioid therapy in a large US health-care system. *Addiction* 105, 1776–1782 (2010).

[375] Carman, W.J., Su, S.H., Cook, S.F., Wurzelmann, J.I. & McAfee, A. Coronary heart disease outcomes among chronic opioid and cyclooxygenase-2 users compared with a general population cohort. *Pharmacoepidemiology and Drug Safety* 20, 754–762 (2011).

[376] Compton, P.A., Wu, S.M., Schieffer, B., Pham, Q. & Naliboff, B.D. Introduction of a self-report version of the prescription drug use questionnaire and relationship to medication agreement noncompliance. *Journal of Pain and Symptom Management* 36, 383–395 (2008).

[377] Cowan, D.T., Wilson-Barnett, J., Griffiths, P. & Allan, L.G. A survey of chronic noncancer pain patients prescribed opioid analgesics. *Pain Medicine* 4, 340–351 (2003).

[378] Cowan, D.T., *et al.* A randomized, double-blind, placebo-controlled, cross-over pilot study to assess the effects of long-term opioid drug consumption and subsequent abstinence in chronic noncancer pain patients receiving controlled-release morphine. *Pain Medicine* 6, 113–121 (2005).

[379] Davies, A., *et al.* Consistency of efficacy, patient acceptability, and nasal tolerability of fentanyl pectin nasal spray compared with immediate-release morphine sulfate in breakthrough cancer pain. *Journal of Pain and Symptom Management* 41, 358–366 (2011).

[380] Deyo, R.A., *et al.* Prescription opioids for back pain and use of medications for erectile dysfunction. *Spine* 38, 909–915 (2013).

[381] Dunn, K.M., *et al.* Opioid prescriptions for chronic pain and overdose: A cohort study. *Annals of Internal Medicine* 152, 85–92 (2010).

[382] Fleming, M.F., Balousek, S.L., Klessig, C.L., Mundt, M.P. & Brown, D.D. Substance use disorders in a primary care sample receiving daily opioid therapy. *Journal of Pain* 8, 573–582 (2007).

[383] Gomes, T., Mamdani, M.M., Dhalla, I.A., Paterson, J.M. & Juurlink, D.N. Opioid dose and drug-related mortality in patients with nonmalignant pain. *Archives of Internal Medicine* 171, 686–691 (2011).

[384] Gomes, T., *et al.* Opioid dose and risk of road trauma in Canada: A population-based study. *JAMA Internal Medicine* 173, 196–201 (2013).

[385] Hartung, D.M., *et al.* Rates of adverse events of long-acting opioids in a state Medicaid program. *Annals of Pharmacotherapy* 41, 921–928 (2007).

[386] Hojsted, J., Nielsen, P.R., Guldstrand, S.K., Frich, L. & Sjogren, P. Classification and identification of opioid addiction in chronic pain patients. *European Journal of Pain* 14, 1014–1020 (2010).

[387] Krebs, E.E., *et al.* Comparative mortality among Department of Veterans Affairs patients prescribed methadone or long-acting morphine for chronic pain. *Pain* 152, 1789–1795 (2011).

[388] Li, L., Setoguchi, S., Cabral, H. & Jick, S. Opioid use for noncancer pain and risk of myocardial infarction amongst adults. *Journal of Internal Medicine* 273, 511–526 (2013).

[389] Li, L., Setoguchi, S., Cabral, H. & Jick, S. Opioid use for noncancer pain and risk of fracture in adults: A nested case-control study using the general practice research database. *American Journal of Epidemiology* 178, 559–569 (2013).

[390] Mitra, F., Chowdhury, S., Shelley, M. & Williams, G. A feasibility study of transdermal buprenorphine versus transdermal fentanyl in the long-term management of persistent non-cancer pain. *Pain Medicine* 14, 75–83 (2013).

[391] Moore, T.M., Jones, T., Browder, J.H., Daffron, S. & Passik, S.D. A comparison of common screening methods for predicting aberrant drug-related behavior among patients receiving opioids for chronic pain management. *Pain Medicine* 10, 1426–1433 (2009).

[392] Naliboff, B.D., *et al.* A randomized trial of 2 prescription strategies for opioid treatment of chronic nonmalignant pain. *Journal of Pain* 12, 288–296 (2011).

[393] Portenoy, R.K., Messina, J., Xie, F. & Peppin, J. Fentanyl buccal tablet (FBT) for relief of breakthrough pain in opioid-treated patients with chronic low back pain: A randomized, placebo-controlled study. *Current Medical Research and Opinion* 23, 222–232 (2007).

394 Ralphs, J.A., Williams, A.C.D., Richardson, P.H., Pither, C.E. & Nicholas, M.K. Opiate reduction in chronic pain patients: A comparison of patient-controlled reduction and staff-controlled cocktail methods. *Pain* 56, 279–288 (1994).

395 Saffier, K., Colombo, C., Brown, D., Mundt, M.P. & Fleming, M.F. Addiction Severity Index in a chronic pain sample receiving opioid therapy. *Journal of Substance Abuse Treatment* 33, 303–311 (2007).

396 Salzman, R.T., *et al.* Can a controlled-release oral dose form of oxycodone be used as readily as an immediate-release form for the purpose of titrating to stable pain control? *Journal of Pain and Symptom Management* 18, 271–279 (1999).

397 Saunders, K.W., *et al.* Relationship of opioid use and dosage levels to fractures in older chronic pain patients. *Journal of General Internal Medicine* 25, 310–315 (2010).

398 Simpson, D.M., Messina, J., Xie, F. & Hale, M. Fentanyl buccal tablet for the relief of breakthrough pain in opioid-tolerant adult patients with chronic neuropathic pain: A multicenter, randomized, double-blind, placebo-controlled study. *Clinical Therapeutics* 29, 588–601 (2007).

399 Tennant, F.S. & Rawson, R.A. Outpatient treatment of prescription opioid dependence: Comparison of two methods. *Archives of Internal Medicine* 142, 1845–1847 (1982).

400 Wasan, A.D., *et al.* Does report of craving opioid medication predict aberrant drug behavior among chronic pain patients? *Clinical Journal of Pain* 25, 193–198 (2009).

401 Webster, L.R. & Webster, R.M. Predicting aberrant behaviors in opioid-treated patients: Preliminary validation of the opioid risk tool. *Pain Medicine* 6, 432–442 (2005).

402 Webster, L.R., Slevin, K.A., Narayana, A., Earl, C.Q. & Yang, R.H. Fentanyl buccal tablet compared with immediate-release oxycodone for the management of breakthrough pain in opioid-tolerant patients with chronic cancer and noncancer pain: A randomized, double-blind, crossover study followed by a 12-week open-label phase to evaluate patient outcomes. *Pain Medicine* 14, 1332–1345 (2013).

403 Wild, J.E., *et al.* Long-term safety and tolerability of Tapentadol extended release for the management of chronic low back pain or osteoarthritis pain. *Pain Practice* 10, 416–427 (2010).

404 Tayeb, B.O., Barreiro, A.E., Bradshaw, Y.S., Chui, K.K.H. & Carr, D.B. Durations of opioid, nonopioid drug, and behavioral clinical trials for chronic pain: Adequate or inadequate? *Pain Medicine* 17, 2036–2046 (2016).

405 Els, C., *et al.* High-dose opioids for chronic non-cancer pain: An overview of Cochrane Reviews. *Cochrane Database of Systematic Reviews* (2017).

406 Carr, D.B. Evidence-based pain medicine: Inconvenient truths. *Pain Medicine* 18, 2049–2050 (2017).

[407] Els, C., *et al.* Adverse events associated with medium- and long-term use of opioids for chronic non-cancer pain: An overview of Cochrane Reviews. *Cochrane Database of Systematic Reviews* (2017).

[408] Ramiro, S., *et al.* Combination therapy for pain management in inflammatory arthritis (rheumatoid arthritis, ankylosing spondylitis, psoriatic arthritis, other spondyloarthritis). *Cochrane Database of Systematic Reviews* (2011).

[409] Ramiro, S., *et al.* Combination therapy for pain management in inflammatory arthritis: A Cochrane systematic review. *Journal of Rheumatology* 39, 47–55 (2012).

[410] Lunde, C.E. & Sieberg, C.B. Walking the tightrope: A proposed model of chronic pain and stress. *Frontiers in Neuroscience* 14 (2020).

[411] Solomon, D.H., *et al.* The comparative safety of analgesics in older adults with arthritis. *Archives of Internal Medicine* 170, 1968–1976 (2010).

[412] Miller, M., Sturmer, T., Azrael, D., Levin, R. & Solomon, D.H. Opioid analgesics and the risk of fractures in older adults with arthritis. *Journal of the American Geriatrics Society* 59, 430–438 (2011).

[413] Coluzzi, F., Pergolizzi, J., Raffa, R.B. & Mattia, C. The unsolved case of "bone-impairing analgesics": The endocrine effects of opioids on bone metabolism. *Therapeutics and Clinical Risk Management* 11, 515–523 (2015).

[414] Fraser, L.A., *et al.* Oral opioids for chronic non-cancer pain: Higher prevalence of hypogonadism in men than in women. *Experimental and Clinical Endocrinology & Diabetes* 117, 38–43 (2009).

[415] Gruss, I., Firemark, A., Mayhew, M., McMullen, C.K. & Debar, L.L. Taking opioids in times of crisis: Institutional oversight, chronic pain and suffering in an integrated healthcare delivery system in the US. *International Journal of Drug Policy* 74, 62–68 (2019).

[416] Andraka-Christou, B., Rager, J.B., Brown-Podgorski, B., Silverman, R.D. & Watson, D.P. Pain clinic definitions in the medical literature and US state laws: An integrative systematic review and comparison. *Substance Abuse Treatment Prevention and Policy* 13, Art. No. 17 (2018).

[417] Schatman, M.E. The American chronic pain crisis and the media: About time to get it right? *Journal of Pain Research* 8, 885–887 (2015).

[418] Meldrum, M.L. Brief history of multidisciplinary management of chronic pain, 1900–2000. In: Schatman ME, Campbell A, editors. *Chronic Pain Management: Guidelines for Multidisciplinary Program Development.* 1–13 (2007).

[419] Schmidt, C. Experts worry about chilling effect of federal regulations on treating pain. *Journal of the National Cancer Institute* 97, 554–555 (2005).

[420] Fischer, W. Pain drug crackdown hits "nobodies" the hardest. *Inter Press Service News Agency.* May 24, 2006.

[421] Coyne, C.J. & Hall, A.R. Four decades and counting: The continued failure of the war on drugs. *Policy Analysis CATO Institute* 811 (2017).

[422] Netherland, J. & Hansen, H.B. The war on drugs that wasn't: Wasted whiteness, "dirty doctors," and race in media coverage of prescription opioid misuse. *Culture Medicine and Psychiatry* 40, 664–686 (2016).

423 Shultz, G.P. & Aspe, P. The failed war on drugs. *The New York Times.* December 31, 2017.

424 Socias, M.E. & Wood, E. Epidemic of deaths from fentanyl overdose: Another serious side effect of the war on drugs. *BMJ-British Medical Journal* 358, Art. No. j4355 (2017).

425 James, J.R., *et al.* Mortality after discontinuation of primary care-based chronic opioid therapy for pain: A retrospective cohort study. *Journal of General Internal Medicine* 34, 2749–2755 (2019).

426 Beall, P. How the Post calculated the shift from oxycodone to heroin. *West Palm Beach Post.* July 13, 2018.

427 Beall, P. Proving the unprovable: How the Post got the story. *West Palm Beach Post.* July 13, 2018.

428 Davis, C.S. & Carr, D.H. Self-regulating profession? Administrative discipline of "pill mill" physicians in Florida. *Substance Abuse* 38, 265–268 (2017).

429 Beall, P. Methadone clinics: Florida hinders help for heroin addiction. *West Palm Beach Post.* July 10, 2018.

430 Beall, P. How bad is the heroin crisis? Bad numbers mean no one even knows. *West Palm Beach Post.* July 30, 2018.

431 Beall, P. Oxy to heroin: Four people who made the deadly switch. *West Palm Beach Post.* July 11, 2018.

432 Passik, S.D. Nonmedical prescription opioid use for the self-treatment of pain in young adults: A national shame. *Journal of Addiction Medicine* 11, 248–249 (2017).

433 Fishbain, D.A., Goldberg, M., Rosomoff, R.S. & Rosomoff, H. Completed suicide in chronic pain. *Clinical Journal of Pain* 7, 29–36 (1991).

434 Kikuchi, N., *et al.* Pain and risk of completed suicide in Japanese men: A population-based cohort study in Japan (Ohsaki cohort study). *Journal of Pain and Symptom Management* 37, 316–324 (2009).

435 Rose, M.E. Are prescription opioids driving the opioid crisis? Assumptions vs facts. *Pain Medicine* 19, 793–807 (2018).

436 Sullum, J. Opioid-related deaths keep rising as pain pill prescriptions fall. *Reason.* November 29, 2018.

437 Case, A. & Deaton, A. Deaths of Despair and the Future of Capitalism. Kindle Edition (2020).

438 Eisinger, J. & Bandler, J. Walmart was almost charged criminally over opioids. Trump appointees killed the indictment. *ProPublica.* March 25, 2020.

439 Hiassen, C. Florida's "pill mill" clinics multiply, drug overdoses climb. *The Miami Herald.* April. 5, 2009.

440 Hiassen, C. Feds raid three South Florida pain clinics over illegal painkiller suspicions. *The Miami Herald.* March 4, 2010.

441 Hiassen, C. Inside Broward County's pill mills. *The Miami Herald.* April 5, 2009.

442 Rigg, K.K., March, S.J. & Iniciardi, J.A. Prescription drug abuse and diversion: Role of the pain clinic. *Journal of Drug Issues* 40, 681–701 (2010).

[443] Facher, L. Report: DEA did too little to constrain opioid supply even as crisis escalated. *Stat.* October 1, 2019.

[444] Beall, P. How Florida spread oxy across America. *West Palm Beach Post.* July 6, 2018.

[445] Sullum, J. Opioid omission mistakenly blames pain treatment for drug deaths. *Reason.* November 2, 2017.

[446] McMillan, B. Intractable Pain Act unanimously repealed. *Herald-Citizen.* March 21, 2015.

[447] Skerrett, P. For some chronic pain patients "without opioids, life would be torture." *STAT.* July 15, 2016.

[448] DHHS (Department of Health and Human Services). Report on pain management best practices: Updates, gaps, inconsistencies, and recommendations. https://www.hhs.gov/ash/advisory-committees/pain/reports/index.html. September 9, 2019.

[449] Yasinski, E. The other opioids epidemic. *ASH Clinical News.* October 1, 2019.

[450] Chapman II, R.W. How not to run a pain clinic: Attorney takes us on an inspection. *MedPage Today.* April 30, 2019.

[451] Greene, J. Opioid laws hit physicians, patients in unintended ways. *Modern Healthcare.* July 30, 2018.

[452] Rosner, B., Neicun, J., Yang, J.C. & Roman-Urrestarazu, A. Opioid prescription patterns in Germany and the global opioid epidemic: Systematic review of available evidence. *PLOS One* 14, Art. No. e0221153 (2019).

[453] UN. Narcotic Drugs—Estimated World Requirement for 2020. United Nations International Narcotics Control Board (2019).

[454] McCall, B. Differences in opioid use and abuse between the UK and US. *Medscape.* February 11, 2020.

[455] Luthra, S. How Germany averted an opioid crisis. *Kaiser Health News.* November 11, 2019.

[456] Stoicea, N., *et al.* Current perspectives on the opioid crisis in the US healthcare system: A comprehensive literature review. *Medicine* 98, Art. No. e15425 (2019).

[457] Jung, B. & Reidenberg, M.M. Physicians being deceived. *Pain Medicine* 8, 433–437 (2007).

[458] Griffin, O.H. & Spillane, J.F. Pharmaceutical regulation failures and changes: Lessons learned from OxyContin abuse and diversion. *Journal of Drug Issues* 43, 164–175 (2013).

[459] Beall, P. Rudi Giuliani, the DEA and the free flow of oxy. *West Palm Beach Post.* July 3, 2018.

[460] Brighthaupt, S.C., Stone, E.M., Rutkow, L. & McGinty, E.E. Effect of pill mill laws on opioid overdose deaths in Ohio & Tennessee: A mixed-methods case study. *Preventive Medicine* 126, Art. No. 105736 (2019).

[461] Ljungvall, H., Rhodin, A., Wagner, S., Zetterberg, H. & Asenlof, P. "My life is under control with these medications": An interpretative phenomenological

analysis of managing chronic pain with opioids. *BMC Musculoskeletal Disorders* 21, Art. No. 61 (2020).

[462] Board, E. DEA database could have exposed overprescription of opioids much earlier. *The San Diego Union-Tribune.* August 19, 2019.

[463] Mercadante, S. Potential strategies to combat the opioid crisis. *Expert Opinion on Drug Safety* 18, 211–217 (2019).

[464] Tauben. Interview with David Tauben: University of Washington, Chief of the Division of Pain Medicine. *Pain Management* 7, 233–238 (2017).

[465] Benjamin, D.M. Prosecution of physicians for prescribing opioids to patients. *Clinical Pharmacology & Therapeutics* 81, 797–798 (2007).

[466] Ariens, S. Who is the DEA listening to? *National Pain Report.* April 1, 2018.

[467] Reidenberg, M.M. & Willis, O. Prosecution of physicians for prescribing opioids to patients. *Clinical Pharmacology & Therapeutics* 81, 903–906 (2007).

[468] Kertesz, S.G. & Nicholson, K.M. No more "shortcuts" in prescribing opioids for chronic pain. Millions of Americans need nuanced care. *STAT.* April 26, 2019.

[469] Lawhern, R.A. Stop persecuting doctors for legitimately prescribing opioids for chronic pain. *STAT.* June 28, 2019.

[470] Stark, M. Dozens denied pain drugs after DEA raid. *The Billings Gazette.* May 3, 2005.

[471] Pergolizzi, J.V., Rosenblatt, M. & LeQuang, J.A. Three years down the road: The aftermath of the CDC Guideline for prescribing opioids for chronic pain. *Advances in Therapy* 36, 1235–1240 (2019).

[472] Prevention. Opioid Prescribing Estimates Workgroup. Atlanta: Centers for Disease Control and Prevention Observations presented to the National Center for Injury Prevention and Control's Board of Scientific Counselors. Available at https://www.cdc.gov/injury/pdfs/bsc/NCIPC_BSC_OpioidPrescribing EstimatesWorkgroupReport_December-12_2018-508.pdf. December 12, 2018.

[473] Kertesz, S.G., Satel, S.L. & Gordon, A.J. Opioid prescription control: When the corrective goes too far. *Health Affairs.* Available at https://www.healthaffairs.org/action/showDoPubSecure?doi=10.1377%2Fhblog 20180117.832392&format=full&. January 19, 2018.

[474] CDC. https://www.cdc.gov/media/releases/2019/s0424-advises-misapplication-guideline-prescribing-opioids.html (2019).

[475] Rosenfeld, M.L. State pain laws: A case for intractable pain centers part III. *Practical Pain Management* 5. December 2011.

[476] Perrone, J., Weiner, S.G. & Nelson, L.S. Stewarding recovery from the opioid crisis through health system initiatives. *Western Journal of Emergency Medicine* 20, 198–202 (2019).

[477] Kennedy, L.C., *et al.* "Those conversations in my experience don't go well": A qualitative study of primary care provider experiences tapering long-term opioid medications. *Pain Medicine* 19, 2201–2211 (2018).

[478] Oliva, E.M., *et al.* Associations between stopping prescriptions for opioids, length of opioid treatment, and overdose or suicide deaths in US veterans: Observational evaluation. *BMJ-British Medical Journal* 368 (2020).

[479] Levine, A. How the VA Fueled the national opioid crisis and is killing thousands of veterans. *Newsweek.* October 12, 2017.

[480] Driscoll, M.A., *et al.* Patient experiences navigating chronic pain management in an integrated health care system: A qualitative investigation of women and men. *Pain Medicine* 19, S19–S29 (2018).

[481] Breuer, B., Pappagallo, M., Tai, J.Y. & Portenoy, R.K. US board-certified pain physician practices: Uniformity and census data of their locations. *Journal of Pain* 8, 244–250 (2007).

[482] Haroon, E., Miller, A.H. & Sanacora, G. Inflammation, glutamate, and glia: A trio of trouble in mood disorders. *Neuropsychopharmacology* 42, 193–215 (2017).

[483] Thomas, M.A. Pain management—the challenge. *Pain Management* 5, 15–21 (2003).

[484] Fishbain, D.A., Lewis, J.E., Jinrun Gao, J., Cole, B. & Rosomoff, R.S. Alleged medical abandonment in chronic opioid analgesic therapy: Case report. *Pain Medicine* 10, 722–729 (2009).

[485] Cowles, C. The war on us. *St. Paul, Minnesota, Fidalgo Press* (2019).

[486] Dowell, D., Haegerich, T. & Chou, R. No shortcuts to safer opioid prescribing. *New England Journal of Medicine* 380, 2285–2287 (2019).

[487] IQVIA. Medicine use and spending in the U.S. *Institute for Human Data Science, Parsippany: IQVIA.* May 9, 2019.

[488] CDC. National Center for Health Statistics / National Death Index. *Center for Disease Control and Prevention.* https://www.cdc.gov/nchs/ndi/index.htm (2020).

[489] Beletsky, L. & Goulka, J. The federal agency that fuels the opioid crisis. *The New York Times.* September 17, 2018.

[490] Dupont, R.L. & Greene, M.H. Dynamics of a heroin addiction epidemic. *Science* 181, 716–722 (1973).

[491] Jalal, H., *et al.* Changing dynamics of the drug overdose epidemic in the United States from 1979 through 2016. *Science* 361, 1218–1225 (2018).

[492] Paulozzi, L.J., Budnitz, D.S. & Xi, Y.L. Increasing deaths from opioid analgesics in the United States. *Pharmacoepidemiology and Drug Safety* 15, 618–627 (2006).

[493] Modarai, F., *et al.* Relationship of opioid prescription sales and overdoses, North Carolina. *Drug and Alcohol Dependence* 132, 81–86 (2013).

[494] Hedegaard, H., Miniño, A.M. & Warner, M. Drug overdose deaths in the United States, 1999–2018. *NCHS Data Brief No. 166* 356(2020).

[495] Iniciardi, J.A. & Cicero, T.J. Black beauties, gorilla pills, footballs and hillbilly heroin: Some reflections on drug abuse and diversion over the past 40 years. *Journal of Drug Issues* 39, 101–114 (2009).

[496] Rudd, R.A., *et al.* Increases in heroin overdose deaths—28 states, 2010 to 2012. *MMWR-Morbidity and Mortality Weekly Report* 63, 849–854 (2014).

[497] Rudd, R.A., Seth, P., David, F. & Scholl, L. Increases in drug and opioid-involved overdose deaths—United States, 2010–2015. *MMWR-Morbidity and Mortality Weekly Report* 65, 1445–1452 (2016).

[498] Piper, B.J., Shah, D.T., Simoyan, O.M., McCall, K.L. & Nichols, S.D. Trends in medical use of opioids in the US, 2006–2016. *American Journal of Preventive Medicine* 54, 652–660 (2018).

[499] Jaffe, J.H. & O'Keeffe, C. From morphine clinics to buprenorphine: Regulating opioid agonist treatment of addiction in the United States. *Drug and Alcohol Dependence* 70, S3–S11 (2003).

[500] Fareed, A., Vayalapalli, S., Byrd-Sellers, J., Casarella, J. & Drexler, K. Safety and efficacy of long-term buprenorphine maintenance treatment. *Addictive Disorders & Their Treatment* 10, 123–130 (2011).

[501] Wolff, R.F., *et al.* Systematic review of efficacy and safety of buprenorphine versus fentanyl or morphine in patients with chronic moderate to severe pain. *Current Medical Research and Opinion* 28, 833–845 (2012).

[502] Louie, D.L., Assefa, M.T. & McGovern, M.P. Attitudes of primary care physicians toward prescribing buprenorphine: A narrative review. *BMC Family Practice* 20, Art. No. 157 (2019).

[503] Beall, P. El Chapo saw heroin coming, changed his business model. *West Palm Beach Post.* July 13, 2018.

[504] Beall, P. The history of heroin: From King Tut to cough remedy. *West Palm Beach Post.* June 28, 2018.

[505] Beall, P. Purdue Pharma plants the seeds of the opioid epidemic in a tiny Virginia town and others. *West Palm Beach Post* Jan 31 2019(2018).

[506] Kennedy-Hendricks, A., *et al.* Opioid overdose deaths and Florida's crackdown on pill mills. *American Journal of Public Health* 106, 291–297 (2016).

[507] Cicero, T.J., Ellis, M.S. & Surratt, H.L. Effect of abuse-deterrent formulation of OxyContin. *New England Journal of Medicine* 367, 187–189 (2012).

[508] Johnson, H., Paulozzi, L., Porucznik, C., Mack, K. & Herter, B. Decline in drug overdose deaths after state policy changes—Florida, 2010–2012. *MMWR-Morbidity and Mortality Weekly Report* 63, 569–574 (2014).

[509] Frieden, T.R. & Houry, D. Reducing the risks of relief: The CDC Opioid-Prescribing Guideline. *New England Journal of Medicine* 374, 1501–1504 (2016).

[510] Cicero, T.J., Ellis, M.S. & Kasper, Z.A. Increased use of heroin as an initiating opioid of abuse. *Addictive Behaviors* 74, 63–66 (2017).

[511] Ringwalt, C., Roberts, A.W., Gugelmann, H. & Skinner, A.C. Racial disparities across provider specialties in opioid prescriptions dispensed to Medicaid beneficiaries with chronic noncancer pain. *Pain Medicine* 16, 633–640 (2015).

[512] Pouget, E.R., Fong, C. & Rosenblum, A. Racial/ethnic differences in prevalence trends for heroin use and non-medical use of prescription opioids among

entrants to opioid treatment programs, 2005–2016. *Substance Use & Misuse* 53, 290–300 (2018).

513 Cicero, T.J., Ellis, M.S., Surratt, H.L. & Kurtz, S.P. The changing face of heroin use in the United States: A retrospective analysis of the past 50 years. *JAMA Psychiatry* 71, 821–826 (2014).

514 Strickler, G.K., Kreiner, P.W., Halpin, J.F., Doyle, E. & Paulozzi, L.J. Opioid prescribing behaviors: Prescription behavior surveillance system, 11 states, 2010–2016. *MMWR Surveillance Summaries* 69, 1–14 (2020).

515 Morizio, K.M., Baum, R.A., Dugan, A., Martin, J.E. & Bailey, A.M. Characterization and management of patients with heroin versus nonheroin opioid overdoses: Experience at an academic medical center. *Pharmacotherapy* 37, 781–790 (2017).

516 Lennihan, M. & Wilbur, D.Q. 12 million pills and 700 deaths: How a few pill mills helped fan the U.S. opioid inferno. *The Los Angeles Times/Associated Press.* June 14, 2019.

517 Ryan, H., Girion, L. & Glover, S. More than 1 million OxyContin pills ended up in the hands of criminals and addicts. What the drugmaker knew. *The Los Angeles Times.* July 10, 2016.

518 City News Service, N.P. The San Diego physician wrote fake prescriptions for dead or jailed patients, with medication then illegally distributed, prosecutors said. *Patch / La Mesa and Mount Helix, CA.* January 21, 2020.

519 Flynt, N. Ex-doctor sentenced to 11 years for fraud, operating pill mill. *Organized Crime and Corruption Reporting Project.* November 19, 2019.

520 Horwitz, S., Higham, S., Miroff, N. & Zezima, K. The flow of fentanyl: In the mail, over the border. *The New York Times.* August 23, 2019.

521 Zoorob, M. Fentanyl shock: The changing geography of overdose in the United States. *International Journal of Drug Policy* 70, 40–46 (2019).

522 Irving, D. Fentanyl: The most dangerous illegal drug in America. *Rand Review.* January 13, 2020.

523 Fishman, S.M., *et al.* Scope and nature of pain- and analgesia-related content of the United States medical licensing examination (USMLE). *Pain Medicine* 19, 449–459 (2018).

524 Hill, C.S. Government regulatory influences on opioid prescribing and their impact on the treatment of pain of nonmalignant origin. *Journal of Pain and Symptom Management* 11, 287–298 (1996).

525 Frank, J.W., *et al.* Patients' perspectives on tapering of chronic opioid therapy: A qualitative study. *Pain Medicine* 17, 1838–1847 (2016).

526 Facher, L. Tapered to zero: In radical move, Oregon's Medicaid program weighs cutting off chronic pain patients from opioids. *STAT.* August 15, 2018.

527 Llorente, E. As doctors taper or end opioid prescriptions, many patients driven to despair, suicide. *Fox News.* December 10, 2018.

528 Okie, S. Calif. jury finds doctor negligent in managing pain. *The Washington Post.* June 15, 2001.

[529] DEA. Director of the Pain and Policy Studies Group at the University of Wisconsin's Comprehensive Cancer Center. *A Joint State from 21 Health Organizations and the DEA.* https://www.deadiversion.usdoj.gov/pubs/advisories/painrelief.pdf (2002).

[530] Schulte, K. Giuliani's consulting firm helped halt Purdue opioid investigation in Florida. *Kaiser Health News.* September 5, 2018.

[531] Cicero, T.J., *et al.* Multiple determinants of specific modes of prescription opioids diversion. *Journal of Drug Issues* 41, 283–304 (2011).

[532] Iniciardi, J.A., Surratt, H.L., Kurtz, S.P. & Cicero, T.J. Mechanisms of prescription drug diversion among drug-involved club- and street-based populations. *Pain Medicine* 8, 171–183 (2007).

[533] Iniciardi, J.A. & Goode, J.L. OxyContin and prescription drug abuse. *Consumer Research* 7, 17–21 (2003).

[534] Cicero, T.J., *et al.* The development of a comprehensive risk-management program for prescription opioid analgesics: Researched abuse, diversion and addiction-related surveillance (RADARS (R)). *Pain Medicine* 8, 157–170 (2007).

[535] Iniciardi, J.A., *et al.* Prescription drugs purchased through the internet: Who are the end users? *Drug and Alcohol Dependence* 110, 21–29 (2010).

[536] Zezima, K. & Bernstein, L. "Hammer on the abusers": Mass. attorney general alleges Purdue Pharma tried to shift blame for opioid addiction. *The Washington Post* January 15, 2019.

[537] Keefe, P. The family that built an empire of pain. *The New Yorker.* October 23, 2017.

[538] Leung, M. To manage chronic pain, use the whole toolkit, not just opioids. *STAT.* June 5, 2016.

[539] McGreal, C. Rudy Giuliani won deal for OxyContin maker to continue sales of drug behind opioid deaths. *The Guardian* May 22, 2018.

[540] Hiassen, C. Money talked and opioids walked. *Apalachicola and Carrabelle Times.* August 6, 2019.

[541] Ahmad, R., Alaei, S. & Omidian, H. Safety and performance of current abuse-deterrent formulations. *Expert Opinion on Drug Metabolism & Toxicology* 14, 1255–1271 (2018).

[542] Mackey, T., Kalyanam, J., Klugman, J., Kuzmenko, E. & Gupta, R. Solution to detect, classify, and report illicit online marketing and sales of controlled substances via Twitter: Using machine learning and web forensics to combat digital opioid access. *Journal of Medical Internet Research* 20, Art. No. e10029 (2018).

[543] Peacock, A., *et al.* Post-marketing studies of pharmaceutical opioid abuse-deterrent formulations: A framework for research design and reporting. *Addiction* 114, 389–399 (2019).

[544] Augusta. OxyContin abuse: Maine's newest epidemic. Maine Office of Substance Abuse, Augusta, Maine. January 2002.

[545] Meier, B. & Lipton, E. Under attack, drug maker turned to Giuliani for help. *New York Times*. December 28, 2007.

[546] Jones, G.H., Bruera, E., Abdi, S. & Kantarjian, H.M. The opioid epidemic in the United States: Overview, origins, and potential solutions. *Obstetrical & Gynecological Survey* 74, 278–279 (2019).

[547] Kuehn, B.M. FDA tightens indications for using long-acting and extended-release opioids to treat chronic pain. *JAMA-Journal of the American Medical Association* 310, 1547–1548 (2013).

[548] Severtson, S.G., *et al.* Sustained reduction of diversion and abuse after introduction of an abuse deterrent formulation of extended release oxycodone. *Drug and Alcohol Dependence* 168, 219–229 (2016).

[549] Joseph, A. "A blizzard of prescriptions": Documents reveal new details about Purdue's marketing of OxyContin. *STAT.* January 15, 2019.

[550] Armstrong, D. Divulged private emails show Purdue Pharma's deception about the strength of OxyContin. *Pacific Standard.* February 26, 2019.

[551] Joseph, A. Purdue appeals order to unseal OxyContin records to Kentucky Supreme Court. *STAT.* January 14, 2019.

[552] Armstrong, D. Secret trove reveals bold "crusade" to make OxyContin a blockbuster. *STAT.* September 22, 2016.

[553] Armstrong, D. Purdue's Sackler embraced plan to conceal OxyContin's strength from doctors, sealed deposition shows. *ProPublica.* February 21, 2019.

[554] Lin, D.H., Lucas, E., Murimi, I.B., Kolodny, A. & Alexander, G.C. Financial conflicts of interest and the Centers for Disease Control and Prevention's 2016 guideline for prescribing opioids for chronic pain. *JAMA Internal Medicine* 177, 427–428 (2017).

[555] Kolodny, A. & Frieden, T.R. Ten steps the federal government should take now to reverse the opioid addiction epidemic. *JAMA-Journal of the American Medical Association* 318, 1537–1538 (2017).

[556] DrugWonks.com. CDC and opioids. Conflict? What conflict? *DrugWonks. com.* October 14, 2015.

[557] Minhee, C. & Calandrillo, S. The cure for America's opioid crisis? End the war on drugs. *Harvard Journal of Law and Public Policy* 42, 547–623 (2019).

[558] Incarceration Rate in the United States, 1960–2012. *The Brookings Institution* (2012).

[559] Whittaker, B. Ex-DEA agent: Opioid crisis fueled by drug industry and Congress. *60 Minutes.* October 17, 2017.

[560] Paulozzi, L.J., *et al.* A history of being prescribed controlled substances and risk of drug overdose death. *Pain Medicine* 13, 87–95 (2012).

[561] Hall, A.J., *et al.* Patterns of abuse among unintentional pharmaceutical overdose fatalities. *JAMA-Journal of the American Medical Association* 300, 2613–2620 (2008).

[562] Sagonowsky, E. Senators question whether Giuliani's influence scored Purdue Pharma leniency from feds. *Fierce Biotech.* August 27, 2018.

[563] Jung, B. & Reidenberg, M.M. The risk of action by the drug enforcement administration against physicians prescribing opioids for pain. *Pain Medicine* 7, 353–357 (2006).

[564] Foxhall, K. DEA enforcement versus pain practice. *Practical Pain Management* 5. June 29, 2016.

[565] Lawhern, R.A. An open letter to the governor of California about Trini Yaeger. *National Pain Report.* December 20, 2019.

[566] Adcock, C. The kingpin. *Frontier.* January 22, 2018.

[567] Denzel, S. Richard Paey. *National Registry of Exonerations* (2007).

[568] Taguchi, E., Lefferman, J., McNiff, E., Sergi, S. & Effron, L. Insys founder John Kapoor sentenced for role in fraud, bribery scheme that contributed to opioid crisis. *ABC News.* January 23, 2020.

[569] Emanuel, G. & Thomas, K. Top executives of Insys, an opioid company, are found guilty of racketeering. *New York Times.* May 2, 2019.

[570] Raymond, N. Judge partly vacates convictions of opioid maker Insys' founder, executives. *Reuters.* November 26, 2019.

[571] Compton, W.M., Boyle, M. & Wargo, E. Prescription opioid abuse: Problems and responses. *Preventive Medicine* 80, 5–9 (2015).

[572] Powell, D., R. L. Pacula & Taylor, E.A. How increasing medical access to opioids contributes to the opioid epidemic. *Rand Corporation Report.* September (2016).

[573] Wiese, A.D., *et al.* Long-acting opioid use and the risk of serious infections: A retrospective cohort study. *Clinical Infectious Diseases* 68, 1862–1869 (2019).

[574] Gallagher, R. Opioid-related harms: Simplistic solutions to the crisis ineffective and cause collateral damage. *Health Services Insights* 11(2018).

[575] Parks, T. Address patient shame, stigma when treating opioid misuse. *American Medical Association* website. November 2, 2016.

[576] Brinkley-Rubinstein, L., *et al.* Risk of fentanyl-involved overdose among those with past year incarceration: Findings from a recent outbreak in 2014 and 2015. *Drug and Alcohol Dependence* 185, 189–191 (2018).

[577] Szott, K. "Heroin is the devil": Addiction, religion, and needle exchange in the rural United States. *Critical Public Health* 30, 68–78 (2020).

[578] Jones, C.M. Syringe services programs: An examination of legal, policy, and funding barriers in the midst of the evolving opioid crisis in the US. *International Journal of Drug Policy* 70, 22–32 (2019).

[579] Proctor, S.L., Birch, A. & Herschman, P.L. Medication treatment with methadone or buprenorphine: Differential reasons for premature discharge. *Journal of Addiction Medicine* 13, 113–118 (2019).

[580] McLean, K. & Kavanaugh, P.R. "They're making it so hard for people to get help:" Motivations for non-prescribed buprenorphine use in a time of treatment expansion. *International Journal of Drug Policy* 71, 118–124 (2019).

[581] Merrill, J. Policy progress for physician treatment of opiate addiction. *Journal of General Internal Medicine* 17, 361–368 (2002).

582 Ries, R. & Saxon, A.J. Most people with opioid addictions don't get the right treatment: Medication-assisted therapy. *STAT.* September 21, 2017.

583 Payne, B.E., *et al.* Effect of lowering initiation thresholds in a primary care-based buprenorphine treatment program. *Drug and Alcohol Dependence* 200, 71–77 (2019).

584 Skerrett, P. Hey, doctors: Why aren't you stepping up to treat people with opioid addiction? *STAT.* July 5, 2018.

585 Daniulaityte, R., *et al.* Patterns of non-prescribed buprenorphine and other opioid use among individuals with opioid use disorder: A latent class analysis. *Drug and Alcohol Dependence* 204, Art. No. 107574 (2019).

586 Gudin, J. & Fudin, J. A narrative pharmacological review of buprenorphine: A unique opioid for the treatment of chronic pain. *Pain and Therapy* 9, 41–54 (2020).

587 Plosker, G.L. Buprenorphine 5, 10 and 20 mu g/h transdermal patch: A review of its use in the management of chronic non-malignant pain. *Drugs* 71, 2491–2509 (2011).

588 Chou, R., Ballantyne, J. & Lembke, A. Buprenorphine for long-term chronic pain management: Still looking for the evidence. *Annals of Internal Medicine* 172, 294 (2020).

589 Chavoustie, S., *et al.* Buprenorphine implants in medical treatment of opioid addiction. *Expert Review of Clinical Pharmacology* 10, 799–807 (2017).

590 Rinker, B. 32 churches and no methadone clinic: Struggling with addiction in an opioid "treatment desert." *STAT.* August 10, 2017.

591 Barglow, P. Commentary: The opioid overdose epidemic: Evidence-based interventions. *American Journal on Addictions* 27, 605–607 (2018).

592 Fiscella, K. & Wakeman, S.E. Deregulating buprenorphine prescribing for opioid use disorder will save lives. *STAT.* March 12, 2019.

593 Jones, C.M., Campopiano, M., Baldwin, G. & McCance-Katz, E. National and state treatment need and capacity for opioid agonist medication-assisted treatment. *American Journal of Public Health* 105, E55–E63 (2015).

594 Hadland, S.E., *et al.* Trends in receipt of buprenorphine and naltrexone for opioid use disorder among adolescents and young adults, 2001–2014. *JAMA Pediatrics* 171, 747–755 (2017).

595 Zhu, H. & Wu, L.T. National trends and characteristics of inpatient detoxification for drug use disorders in the United States. *BMC Public Health* 18, Art. No. 1073 (2018).

596 Hser, Y.I., Hoffman, V., Grella, C.E. & Anglin, M.D. A 33-year follow-up of narcotics addicts. *Archives of General Psychiatry* 58, 503–508 (2001).

597 Johnson, E.M., *et al.* Unintentional prescription opioid-related overdose deaths: Description of decedents by next of kin or best contact, Utah, 2008–2009. *Journal of General Internal Medicine* 28, 522–529 (2013).

598 Chen, L.H., Hedegaard, H. & Warner, M. Drug-poisoning deaths involving opioid analgesics: United States, 1999–2011. *NCHS Data Brief No. 166* (2014).

[599] Huhn, A.S., Strain, E.C., Tompkins, D.A. & Dunn, K.E. A hidden aspect of the US opioid crisis: Rise in first-time treatment admissions for older adults with opioid use disorder. *Drug and Alcohol Dependence* 193, 142–147 (2018).

[600] Manchikanti, L., *et al.* Opioid epidemic in the United States. *Pain Physician* 15, ES9–ES38 (2012).

[601] SAMHSA. Results from the 2012 National Survey on Drug Use and Health: Summary of National Findings. NSDUH Ser. H-46, DHHS Publ. No. SMA 13-4795. Rockville, MD. Substance Abuse and Mental Health Services Administration (2013).

[602] Dart, R.C., *et al.* Trends in opioid analgesic abuse and mortality in the United States. *New England Journal of Medicine* 372, 241–248 (2015).

[603] Fugelstad, A., Thiblin, I., Johansson, L.A., Agren, G. & Sidorchuk, A. Opioid-related deaths and previous care for drug use and pain relief in Sweden. *Drug and Alcohol Dependence* 201, 253–259 (2019).

[604] Adewumi, A.D., Hollingworth, S.A., Maravilla, J.C., Connor, J.P. & Alati, R. Prescribed dose of opioids and overdose: A systematic review and meta-analysis of unintentional prescription opioid overdose. *CNS Drugs* 32, 101–116 (2018).

[605] Bohnert, A.S.B., *et al.* Association between opioid prescribing patterns and opioid overdose-related deaths. *JAMA-Journal of the American Medical Association* 305, 1315–1321 (2011).

[606] Jones, C.M., Mack, K.A. & Paulozzi, L.J. Pharmaceutical overdose deaths, United States, 2010. *JAMA-Journal of the American Medical Association* 309, 657–659 (2013).

[607] Jeffery, M.M., *et al.* Rates of physician coprescribing of opioids and benzodiazepines after the release of the Centers for Disease Control and Prevention Guidelines in 2016. *JAMA Network Open* 2, Art. No. e198325 (2019).

[608] Nuckols, T.K., *et al.* Opioid prescribing: A systematic review and critical appraisal of guidelines for chronic pain. *Annals of Internal Medicine* 160, 38–+ (2014).

[609] Fadulu, L. A simple reason so many older Americans are overdosing on opioids. *The Atlantic.* August 11, 2018.

[610] Zedler, B., *et al.* Development of a risk index for serious prescription opioid-induced respiratory depression or overdose in Veterans' Health Administration patients. *Pain Medicine* 16, 1566–1579 (2015).

[611] Fischer, B., Jones, W., Tyndall, M. & Kurdyak, P. Correlations between opioid mortality increases related to illicit/synthetic opioids and reductions of medical opioid dispensing-exploratory analyses from Canada. *BMC Public Health* 20, Art. No. 143 (2020).

[612] Ilgen, M. Pain, opioids, and suicide mortality in the United States *Annals of Internal Medicine* 169, 498–499 (2018).

[613] Petrosky, E., *et al.* Chronic pain among suicide decedents, 2003 to 2014: Findings from the national violent death reporting system. *Annals of Internal Medicine* 169, 448–455 (2018).

[614] Zarroli, J. "Deaths of Despair" examines the steady erosion of U.S. working-class life. *National Public Radio.* March 18, 2020.

[615] Webster, L.R. Pain and suicide: The other side of the opioid story. *Pain Medicine* 15, 345–346 (2014).

[616] Berezow, A. Andrew Kolodny says chronic pain patients are PR pawns for big pharma. *American Council on Science and Health.* April 8 (2019).

[617] Jones, C.M. Trends and key correlates of prescription opioid injection misuse in the United States. *Addictive Behaviors* 78, 145–152 (2018).

[618] Graham, G.G., Davies, M.J., Day, R.O., Mohamudally, A. & Scott, K.F. The modern pharmacology of paracetamol: Therapeutic actions, mechanism of action, metabolism, toxicity and recent pharmacological findings. *Inflammopharmacology* 21, 201–232 (2013).

[619] Krueger, C. Ask the expert: Do NSAIDs cause more deaths than opioids? *Practical Pain Management.* November–December (2013).

[620] Kaufman, D.W., *et al.* The risk of acute major upper gastrointestinal bleeding among users of aspirin and ibuprofen at various levels of alcohol consumption. *American Journal of Gastroenterology* 94, 3189–3196 (1999).

[621] Blot, W.J., *et al.* Outcome of upper gastro-intestinal bleeding and use of ibuprofen versus paracetamol. *Pharmacy World & Science* 26, 319–323 (2004).

[622] McCrae, J.C., Morrison, E.E., MacIntyre, I.M., Dear, J.W. & Webb, D.J. Long-term adverse effects of paracetamol: A review. *British Journal of Clinical Pharmacology* 84, 2218–2230 (2018).

[623] Singh, G. & Triadafilopoulos, G. Epidemiology of NSAID induced gastrointestinal complications. *Journal of Rheumatology* 26, 18–24 (1999).

[624] Cryer, B. NSAID-associated deaths: The rise and fall of NSAID-associated GI mortality. *American Journal of Gastroenterology* 100, 1694–1695 (2005).

[625] Tarone, R.E., Blot, W.J. & McLaughlin, J.K. Nonselective nonaspirin nonsteroidal anti-inflammatory drugs and gastrointestinal bleeding: relative and absolute risk estimates from recent epidemiologic studies. *American Journal of Therapeutics* 11, 17–25 (2004).

[626] Saragiotto, B.T., *et al.* Paracetamol for low back pain. *Cochrane Database of Systematic Reviews* (2016).

[627] Radner, H., *et al.* Pain management for inflammatory arthritis (rheumatoid arthritis, psoriatic arthritis, ankylosing spondylitis and other spondylarthritis) and gastrointestinal or liver comorbidity. *Cochrane Database of Systematic Reviews* (2012).

[628] Whittle, S.L., Richards, B.L., Husni, E. & Buchbinder, R. Opioid therapy for treating rheumatoid arthritis pain. *Cochrane Database of Systematic Reviews* (2011).

[629] Huskisson, E.C. Simple analgesics for arthritis. *BMJ-British Medical Journal* 4, 196–200 (1974).

630 Stein, C. & Baerwald, C. Opioids for the treatment of arthritis pain. *Expert Opinion on Pharmacotherapy* 15, 193–202 (2014).

631 Schofferman, J. Long-term use of opioid analgesics for the treatment of chronic pain of non-malignant origin. *Journal of Pain and Symptom Management* 8, 279–288 (1993).

632 Kern, D.M., *et al.* Treatment patterns of newly diagnosed rheumatoid arthritis patients from a commercially insured population. *Rheumatology and Therapy* 5, 355–369 (2018).

633 Hamilton, G.M., *et al.* A population-based comparative effectiveness study of peripheral nerve blocks for hip fracture surgery. *Anesthesiology* 131, 1025–1035 (2019).

634 Kratz, T., *et al.* Impact of regional femoral nerve block during general anesthesia for hip arthroplasty on blood pressure, heart rate and pain control: A randomized controlled study. *Technology and Health Care* 23, 313–322 (2015).

635 Samanta, S., Samanta, S., Chatterjee, D. & Gupta, V. Anesthesia and psoriatic arthropathy: Challenges and literature review. *Anaesthesia Pain & Intensive Care* 19, 402–404 (2015).

636 Zhao, J.L. & Davis, S.P. An integrative review of multimodal pain management on patient recovery after total hip and knee arthroplasty. *International Journal of Nursing Studies* 98, 94–106 (2019).

637 Parris, W.C.V., Janicki, P.K., Johnson, B., Livengood, J. & Mathews, L. Persistent pain associated with long-term intrathecal morphine administration. *Southern Medical Journal* 89, 417–419 (1996).

638 Hansen, H., *et al.* A systematic evaluation of the therapeutic effectiveness of sacroiliac joint interventions. *Pain Physician* 15, E247–E278 (2012).

639 Sato, K.L., Johanek, L.M., Sanada, L.S. & Sluka, K.A. Spinal cord stimulation reduces mechanical hyperalgesia and glial cell activation in animals with neuropathic pain. *Anesthesia and Analgesia* 118, 464–472 (2014).

640 Crow, J.M. Biomedicine: Move over, morphine. *Nature* 535, S4–S6 (2016).

641 Kapural, L., *et al.* Novel 10-kHz high-frequency therapy (HF10 therapy) is superior to traditional low-frequency spinal cord stimulation for the treatment of chronic back and leg pain. *Anesthesiology* 123, 851–860 (2015).

642 Verrills, P., Sinclair, C. & Barnard, A. A review of spinal cord stimulation systems for chronic pain. *Journal of Pain Research* 9, 481–492 (2016).

643 Dineen, K.K. & DuBois, J.M. Between a rock and a hard place: Can physicians prescribe opioids to treat pain adequately while avoiding legal sanction? *American Journal of Law and Medicine* 42, 7–52 (2016).

644 Sorge, J., Werry, C. & Pichlmayr, I. Strong opioids for treatment of chronic pain: A meta-analysis. *Schmerz* 11, 400–410 (1997).

645 Derby, S., Chin, J. & Portenoy, R.K. Systemic opioid therapy for chronic cancer pain: Practical guidelines for converting drugs and routes of administration. *CNS Drugs* 9, 99–109 (1998).

[646] Atkinson, T.J., Fudin, J., Pandula, A. & Mirza, M. Medication pain management in the elderly: Unique and underutilized analgesic treatment options. *Clinical Therapeutics* 35, 1669–1689 (2013).

[647] Arendt-Nielsen, L., *et al.* A double-blind, placebo-controlled study on the effect of buprenorphine and fentanyl on descending pain modulation: A human experimental study. *Clinical Journal of Pain* 28, 623–627 (2012).

[648] Pickworth, W.B., Johnson, R.E., Holicky, B.A. & Cone, E.J. Subjective and psychological effects of intravenous buprenorphine in humans. *Clinical Pharmacology & Therapeutics* 53, 570–576 (1993).

[649] Comer, S.D., Sullivan, M.A., Whittington, R.A., Vosburg, S.K. & Kowalczyk, W.J. Abuse liability of prescription opioids compared to heroin in morphine-maintained heroin abusers. *Neuropsychopharmacology* 33, 1179–1191 (2008).

[650] Williams, J.T., *et al.* Regulation of mu-opioid Receptors: Desensitization, phosphorylation, internalization, and tolerance. *Pharmacological Reviews* 65, 223–254 (2013).

[651] Mao, J., Gold, M.S. & Backonj, M. Combination drug therapy for chronic pain: A call for more clinical studies. *Journal of Pain* 12, 157–166 (2011).

[652] Bravo, L., Mico, J.A. & Berrocoso, E. Discovery and development of tramadol for the treatment of pain. *Expert Opinion on Drug Discovery* 12, 1281–1291 (2017).

[653] Vosburg, S.K., *et al.* Assessment of Tapentadol API abuse liability with the researched abuse, diversion and addiction-related surveillance system. *Journal of Pain* 19, 439–453 (2018).

[654] Morgan, C.L., Jenkins-Jones, S., Currie, C. & Baxter, G. Outcomes associated with treatment of chronic pain with tapentadol compared with morphine and oxycodone: A UK primary care observational study. *Advances in Therapy* 36, 1412–1425 (2019).

[655] Knotkova, H., Fine, P.G. & Portenoy, R.K. Opioid rotation: The science and the limitations of the equianalgesic dose table. *Journal of Pain and Symptom Management* 38, 426–439 (2009).

[656] Fine, P.G. & Portenoy, R.K. Establishing "best practices" for opioid rotation: Conclusions of an expert panel. *Journal of Pain and Symptom Management* 38, 418–425 (2009).

[657] Freye, E. & Latasch, L. Development of opioid tolerance: Molecular mechanisms and clinical consequences. *Anasthesiologie Intensivmedizin Notfallmedizin Schmerztherapie* 38, 14–26 (2003).

[658] Raith, K. & Hochhaus, G. Drugs used in the treatment of opioid tolerance and physical dependence: A review. *International Journal of Clinical Pharmacology and Therapeutics* 42, 191–203 (2004).

[659] Slatkin, N.E. Opioid switching and rotation in primary care: Implementation and clinical utility. *Current Medical Research and Opinion* 25, 2133–2150 (2009).

[660] Vorobeychik, Y., Chen, L., Bush, M.C. & Mao, J.R. Improved opioid analgesic effect following opioid dose reduction. *Pain Medicine* 9, 724–727 (2008).

[661] Kleinmann, B. & Wolter, T. Managing chronic non-malignant pain in the elderly: Intrathecal therapy. *Drugs & Aging* 36, 789–797 (2019).

[662] Choquette, D., *et al.* Transdermal fentanyl improves pain control and functionality in patients with osteoarthritis: an open-label Canadian trial. *Clinical Rheumatology* 27, 587–595 (2008).

[663] Pavelka, K., Le Loet, X., Bjorneboe, O., Herrero-Beaumont, G. & Richarz, U. Benefits of transdermal fentanyl in patients with rheumatoid arthritis or with osteoarthritis of the knee or hip: An open-label study to assess pain control. *Current Medical Research and Opinion* 20, 1967–1977 (2004).

[664] Tennant, F. & Herman, L. The use of transdermal & transmucosal fentanyl in abstinent heroin addicts with severe chronic pain. *Journal of Addictive Diseases* 21, 140 (2002).

[665] Woodroffe, M.A. & Hays, H. Fentanyl transdermal system: Pain management at home. *Canadian Family Physician* 43, 268–272 (1997).

[666] Adler, J.A. & Mallick-Searle, T. An overview of abuse-deterrent opioids and recommendations for practical patient care. *Journal of Multidisciplinary Healthcare* 11, 323–332 (2018).

[667] Tennant, F. Why oral opioids may not be effective in a subset of chronic pain patients. *Postgraduate Medicine* 128, 18–22 (2016).

[668] Anderson, V.C., Cooke, B. & Burchiel, K.J. Intrathecal hydromorphone for chronic nonmalignant pain: A retrospective study. *Pain Medicine* 2, 287–297 (2001).

[669] Krames, E.S. Intraspinal opioid therapy for chronic nonmalignant pain: Current practice and clinical guidelines. *Journal of Pain and Symptom Management* 11, 333–352 (1996).

[670] Jain, S., Malinowski, M., Chopra, P., Varshney, V. & Deer, T.R. Intrathecal drug delivery for pain management: Recent advances and future developments. *Expert Opinion on Drug Delivery* 16, 815–822 (2019).

[671] Zhou, K., Sheng, S. & Wang, G.G. Management of patients with pain and severe side effects while on intrathecal morphine therapy: A case study. *Scandinavian Journal of Pain* 17, 37–40 (2017).

[672] Leibrock, L.G., Thorell, W.E., Tomes, D.J. & Keber, T.L. Long-term efficacy of continuous intrathecal opioid treatment for malignant and nonmalignant pain. *Neurosurgery Quarterly* 12, 122–131 (2002).

[673] Deer, T.R., Pope, J.E., Hanes, M.C. & McDowell, G.C. Intrathecal therapy for chronic pain: A review of morphine and ziconotide as firstline options. *Pain Medicine* 20, 784–798 (2019).

[674] Schweitzer, E. & Fitzgerald, R. Drug-based pain management Its role in a multimodal therapeutic concept. *Manuelle Medizin* 58, 22–26 (2020).

[675] Farghaly, H.S. M., Elbadr, M.M., Ahmed, M.A. & Abdelhaffez, A.S. Effect of single and repeated administration of amitriptyline on neuropathic pain model in rats: Focus on glutamatergic and upstream nitrergic systems. *Life Sciences* 233, Art. No. 116752 (2019).

676 Stepanenko, Y.D., *et al.* Dual action of amitriptyline on NMDA receptors: enhancement of Ca-dependent desensitization and trapping channel block. *Scientific Reports* 9, Art. No. 19454 (2019).

677 Nilges, M. R., Bondy, Z.B., Grace, J.A. & Winsauer, P.J. Opioid-Enhancing Antinociceptive Effects of Delta-9-Tetrahydrocannabinol and Amitriptyline in Rhesus Macaques. *Experimental and Clinical Psychopharmacology* 28, 355–364 (2020).

678 Kane, C.M., *et al.* Opioids combined with antidepressants or antiepileptic drugs for cancer pain: Systematic review and meta-analysis. *Palliative Medicine* 32, 276–286 (2018).

679 Brzezinski, K. Opioid induced hyperalgesia-case report. *Medycyna Paliatywna-Palliative Medicine* 4, 33–36 (2012).

680 Qin, Z.L., *et al.* Analysis of the analgesic effects of tricyclic antidepressants on neuropathic pain, diabetic neuropathic pain, and fibromyalgia in rat models. *Saudi Journal of Biological Sciences* 27, 2485–2490 (2020).

681 Chakrabarty, S., *et al.* Pregabalin and Amitriptyline as Monotherapy or as Low-Dose Combination in Patients of Neuropathic Pain: A Randomized, Controlled Trial to Evaluate Efficacy and Safety in an Eastern India Teaching Hospital. *Annals of Indian Academy of Neurology* 22, 437–441 (2019).

682 Frech, F., Qian, C.L., Gore, M. & Zhang, Q.Y. Cost Implications of Early Treatment Initiation Among Patients with Newly Diagnosed Fibromyalgia. *American Journal of Pharmacy Benefits* 9, 200–+ (2017).

683 Hutchinson, M.R., *et al.* Exploring the Neuroimmunopharmacology of Opioids: An Integrative Review of Mechanisms of Central Immune Signaling and Their Implications for Opioid Analgesia. *Pharmacological Reviews* 63, 772–810 (2011).

684 Akbari, E., Mirzaei, E., Rezaee, L., Zarrabian, S. & Haghparast, A. The effect of amitriptyline administration on pain-related behaviors in morphine-dependent rats: Hypoalgesia or hyperalgesia? *Neuroscience Letters* 683, 185–189 (2018).

685 Aguado, D., Abreu, M., Benito, J., Garcia-Fernandez, J. & de Segura, I.A.G. Amitriptyline, minocycline and maropitant reduce the sevoflurane minimum alveolar concentration and potentiate remifentanil but do not prevent acute opioid tolerance and hyperalgesia in the rat A randomised laboratory study. *European Journal of Anaesthesiology* 32, 248–254 (2015).

686 Portenoy, R.K. Managing cancer pain poorly responsive to systemic opioid therapy. *Oncology-New York* 13, 25–29 (1999).

687 Kennedy, M.C., Pallotti, P., Dickinson, R. & Harley, C. "If you can't see a dilemma in this situation you should probably regard it as a warning": A metasynthesis and theoretical modelling of general practitioners' opioid prescription experiences in primary care. *British Journal of Pain* 13, 159–176 (2019).

688 Swegle, J.M. & Logemann, C. Management of common opioid-induced adverse effects. *American Family Physician* 74, 1347–1354 (2006).

[689] Labianca, R., *et al.* Adverse effects associated with non-opioid and opioid treatment in patients with chronic pain. *Clinical Drug Investigation* 32, 53–63 (2012).

[690] Schug, S.A., Merry, A.F. & Acland, R.H. Treatment principles for the use of opioids in pain of nonmalignant origin. *Drugs* 42, 228–239 (1991).

[691] Tehrani, M., Aguiar, M. & Katz, J.D. Narcotics in Rheumatology. *Health Services Insights* 6, 39–45 (2013).

[692] King, S., Forbes, K., Hanks, G.W., Ferro, C.J. & Chambers, E.J. A systematic review of the use of opioid medication for those with moderate to severe cancer pain and renal impairment: A European Palliative Care Research Collaborative opioid guidelines project. *Palliative Medicine* 25, 525–552 (2011).

[693] Zhang, Y.T., Zheng, Q.S., Pan, J. & Zheng, R.L. Oxidative damage of biomolecules in mouse liver induced by morphine and protected by antioxidants. *Basic & Clinical Pharmacology & Toxicology* 95, 53–58 (2004).

[694] Streicher, J.M. & Bilsky, E.J. Peripherally acting mu-opioid receptor antagonists for the treatment of opioid-related side effects: Mechanism of action and clinical implications. *Journal of Pharmacy Practice* 31, 658–669 (2018).

[695] Roy, S., Liu, H.C. & Loh, H.H. mu-Opioid receptor-knockout mice: The role of mu-opioid receptor in gastrointestinal transit. *Molecular Brain Research* 56, 281–283 (1998).

[696] Dhingra, L., *et al.* A qualitative study to explore psychological distress and illness burden associated with opioid-induced constipation in cancer patients with advanced disease. *Palliative Medicine* 27, 447–456 (2013).

[697] Imam, M.Z., Kuo, A., Ghassabian, S. & Smith, M.T. Progress in understanding mechanisms of opioid-induced gastrointestinal adverse effects and respiratory depression. *Neuropharmacology* 131, 238–255 (2018).

[698] Bohn, L.M., *et al.* Enhanced morphine analgesia in mice lacking beta-arrestin 2. *Science* 286, 2495–2498 (1999).

[699] Sommers, T., *et al.* Emergency department burden of constipation in the United States from 2006 to 2011. *Am J Gastroenterol.* 110, 572–579 (2015).

[700] Bader, S., Weber, M. & Becker, G. Is the pharmacological treatment of constipation in palliative care evidence based? A systematic literature review. *Schmerz* 26, 568–572 (2012).

[701] Brock, C., *et al.* Opioid-induced bowel dysfunction pathophysiology and management. *Drugs* 72, 1847–1865 (2012).

[702] Garcia-Carrasco, M., *et al.* Functional gastrointestinal disorders in women with systemic lupus erythematosus: A case-control study. *Neurogastroenterology and Motility* 31, Art. No. e13693 (2019).

[703] Urits, I., *et al.* Advances in the understanding and management of chronic pain in multiple sclerosis: A comprehensive review. *Current Pain and Headache Reports* 23 Art. No. 59 (2019).

[704] Maddocks, I., Somogyi, A., Abbott, F., Hayball, P. & Parker, D. Attenuation of morphine-induced delirium in palliative care by substitution with infusion of oxycodone. *Journal of Pain and Symptom Management* 12, 182–189 (1996).

[705] Dale, R., Edwards, J. & Ballantyne, J. Opioid risk assessment in palliative medicine. *Journal of Community and Supportive Oncology* 14, 94–100 (2016).

[706] Galski, T., Williams, J.B. & Ehle, H.T. Effects of opioids on driving ability. *Journal of Pain and Symptom Management* 19, 200–208 (2000).

[707] Paqueron, X., *et al.* Is morphine-induced sedation synonymous with analgesia during intravenous morphine titration? *British Journal of Anaesthesia* 89, 697–701 (2002).

[708] Ganesh, A. & Maxwell, L.G. Pathophysiology and management of opioid-induced pruritus. *Drugs* 67, 2323–2333 (2007).

[709] Coluzzi, F., Billeci, D., Maggi, M. & Corona, G. Testosterone deficiency in non-cancer opioid-treated patients. *Journal of Endocrinological Investigation* 41, 1377–1388 (2018).

[710] Abs, R., *et al.* Endocrine consequences of long-term intrathecal administration of opioids. *Journal of Clinical Endocrinology & Metabolism* 85, 2215–2222 (2000).

[711] Sibille, K.T., McBeth, J., Smith, D. & Wilkie, R. Allostatic load and pain severity in older adults: Results from the English Longitudinal Study of Ageing. *Experimental Gerontology* 88, 51–58 (2017).

[712] Caporali, R., *et al.* Comorbid conditions in the AMICA study patients: Effects on the quality of life and drug prescriptions by general practitioners and specialists. *Seminars in Arthritis and Rheumatism* 35, 31–37 (2005).

[713] Chawla, P.S. & Koshar, N.S. Effect of pain and nonsteroidal analgesics on blood pressure. *Wisconsin Medical Journal: Official Publication of the State Medical Society of Wisconsin* 98, 22–25 (1999).

[714] Snowden, S. & Nelson, R. The effects of nonsteroidal anti-inflammatory drugs on blood pressure in hypertensive patients. *Cardiology in Review* 19, 184–191 (2011).

[715] Biondi, D.M., Xiang, J., Etropolski, M. & Moskovitz, B. Evaluation of blood pressure and heart rate in patients with hypertension who received tapentadol extended release for chronic pain: A post hoc, pooled data analysis. *Clinical Drug Investigation* 34, 565–576 (2014).

[716] Hardo, P.G., Wasti, S.A. & Tennant, A. Night pain in arthritis: Patients at risk from prescribed night sedation. *Annals of the Rheumatic Diseases* 51, 972–973 (1992).

[717] Kusnecov, A.W. & Rabin, B.S. Stressor-induced alterations of immune function: Mechanisms and issues. *International Archives of Allergy and Immunology* 105, 107–121 (1994).

[718] Bair, M.J. & Sanderson, T.R. Coanalgesics for chronic pain therapy: A narrative review. *Postgraduate Medicine* 123, 140–150 (2011).

[719] van den Bussche, H., *et al.* Which chronic diseases and disease combinations are specific to multimorbidity in the elderly? Results of a claims data based cross-sectional study in Germany. *BMC Public Health* 11, Art. No. 101 (2011).

[720] Masotti, A., *et al.* Circulating microRNA profiles as liquid biopsies for the characterization and diagnosis of fibromyalgia syndrome. *Molecular Neurobiology* 54, 7129–7136 (2017).

[721] Cerda-Olmedo, G., Mena-Duran, A.V., Monsalve, V. & Oltra, E. Identification of a microRNA signature for the diagnosis of fibromyalgia. *PLOS One* 10, Art. No. e0121903 (2015).

[722] Dayer, C.F., *et al.* Differences in the miRNA signatures of chronic musculoskeletal pain patients from neuropathic or nociceptive origins. *PLOS One* 14, Art. No. e0219311 (2019).

[723] Fan, Y.S., *et al.* Serum miRNAs are potential biomarkers for the detection of disc degeneration, among which miR-26a-5p suppresses Smad1 to regulate disc homeostasis. *Journal of Cellular and Molecular Medicine* 23, 6679–6689 (2019).

[724] Martirosyan, N.L., *et al.* The role of microRNA markers in the diagnosis, treatment, and outcome prediction of spinal cord injury. *Frontiers in Surgery* 3 (2016).

[725] Douglas, S.R., *et al.* Analgesic response to intravenous ketamine is linked to a circulating microRNA signature in female patients with complex regional pain syndrome. *Journal of Pain* 16, 814–824 (2015).

[726] Budd, E., Nalesso, G. & Mobasheri, A. Extracellular genomic biomarkers of osteoarthritis. *Expert Review of Molecular Diagnostics* 18, 55–74 (2018).

[727] Dragic, L.L., Wegrzyn, E.L., Schatman, M.E. & Fudin, J. Pharmacogenetic guidance: Individualized medicine promotes enhanced pain outcomes. *Journal of Pain Research* 11, 37–40 (2018).

[728] Fudin, J. Opioid allergy, pseudo-allergy, or adverse effect? *Pharmacy Times.* March 6, 2018 (2018).

[729] Fisher, M.M., Harle, D.G. & Baldo, B.A. Anaphalactoid reactions to narcotic analgesics. *Clinical Reviews in Allergy* 9, 309–318 (1991).

[730] Saljoughian, M. Opioids: Allergy vs. Pseudoallergy. *US Pharm.* 7, HS-5-HS-9 (2006).

[731] Harle, D.G., Baldo, B.A., Coroneos, N.J. & Fisher, M.M. Anaphylaxis following administration of papaveretum: Case report—implication of IgE antibodies that react with morphine and codeine and identification of an allergenic determinant. *Anesthesiology* 71, 489–494 (1989).

[732] Nasser, S.M.S. & Ewan, P.W. Opiate-sensitivity: Dlinical characteristics and the role of skin prick testing. *Clinical and Experimental Allergy* 31, 1014–1020 (2001).

[733] Anselme, A., Metz-Favre, C. & de Blay, F. Narcotic allergy. *Revue Francaise D Allergologie* 51, 548–552 (2011).

[734] Li, P.H., Ue, K.L., Wagner, A., Rutkowski, R. & Rutkowski, K. Opioid hypersensitivity: Predictors of allergy and role of drug provocation testing. *Journal of Allergy and Clinical Immunology-in Practice* 5, 1601–1606 (2017).

[735] Swerts, S., *et al.* Allergy to illicit drugs and narcotics. *Clinical and Experimental Allergy* 44, 307–318 (2014).

[736] Tripp, D.M. & Brown, G.R. Pharmacist assessment of drug allergies. *American Journal of Hospital Pharmacy* 50, 95–98 (1993).

[737] Klyne, D.M., Moseley, G.L., Sterling, M., Barbe, M.F. & Hodges, P.W. Are signs of central sensitization in acute low back pain a precursor to poor outcome? *Journal of Pain* 20, 994–1009 (2019).

[738] Waxman, A.R., Arout, C., Caldwell, M., Dahan, A. & Kest, B. Acute and chronic fentanyl administration causes hyperalgesia independently of opioid receptor activity in mice. *Neuroscience Letters* 462, 68–72 (2009).

[739] Schug, S.A. Opioid-induced hyperalgesia: What to do when it occurs? *Annals of Palliative Medicine* 1, 6–7 (2012).

[740] Chu, L.F., *et al.* Analgesic tolerance without demonstrable opioid-induced hyperalgesia: A double-blinded, randomized, placebo-controlled trial of sustained-release morphine for treatment of chronic nonradicular low-back pain. *Pain* 153, 1583–1592 (2012).

[741] Mercado-Reyes, J., Almanza, A., Segura-Chama, P., Pellicer, F. & Mercado, F. D2-like receptor agonist synergizes the mu-opioid agonist spinal antinociception in nociceptive, inflammatory and neuropathic models of pain in the rat. *European Journal of Pharmacology* 853, 56–64 (2019).

[742] Martinez-Navarro, M., Maldonado, R. & Banos, J.E. Why mu-opioid agonists have less analgesic efficacy in neuropathic pain? *European Journal of Pain* 23, 435–454 (2019).

[743] Roeckel, L.A., *et al.* Morphine-induced hyperalgesia involves mu opioid receptors and the metabolite morphine-3-glucuronide. *Scientific Reports* 7, Art. No. 10406 (2017).

[744] Hogan, D., Baker, A.L., Moron, J.A. & Carlton, S.M. Systemic morphine treatment induces changes in firing patterns and responses of nociceptive afferent fibers in mouse glabrous skin. *Pain* 154, 2297–2309 (2013).

[745] Ferrini, F., *et al.* Morphine hyperalgesia gated through microglia-mediated disruption of neuronal Cl-homeostasis. *Nature Neuroscience* 16, 183–192 (2013).

[746] Tappe, A., *et al.* Synaptic scaffolding protein Homer1a protects against chronic inflammatory pain. *Nature Medicine* 12, 677–681 (2006).

[747] Juni, A., Klein, G. & Kest, B. Morphine hyperalgesia in mice is unrelated to opioid activity, analgesia, or tolerance: Evidence for multiple diverse hyperalgesic systems. *Brain Research* 1070, 35–44 (2006).

[748] Celerier, E., Gonzalez, J.R., Maldonado, R., Cabanero, D. & Puig, M.M. Opioid-induced hyperalgesia in a murine model of postoperative pain: Role of nitric oxide generated from the inducible nitric oxide synthase. *Anesthesiology* 104, 546–555 (2006).

[749] Bryant, C.D., Eitan, S., Sinchak, K., Fanselow, M.S. & Evans, C.J. NMDA receptor antagonism disrupts the development of morphine analgesic tolerance

in male, but not female C57BL/6J mice. *American Journal of Physiology-Regulatory Integrative and Comparative Physiology* 291, R315–R326 (2006).

750 Li, X.Q., Angst, M.S. & Clark, J.D. A murine model of opioid-induced hyperalgesia. *Molecular Brain Research* 86, 56–62 (2001).

751 Qiu, C.Y., Sora, I., Ren, K., Uhl, G. & Dubner, R. Enhanced delta-opioid receptor-mediated antinociception in mu-opioid receptor-deficient mice. *European Journal of Pharmacology* 387, 163–169 (2000).

752 Mayer, D.J., Mao, J.R., Holt, J. & Price, D.D. Cellular mechanisms of neuropathic pain, morphine tolerance, and their interactions. *Proceedings of the National Academy of Sciences of the United States of America* 96, 7731–7736 (1999).

753 Niesters, M., Aarts, L., Sarton, E. & Dahan, A. Influence of ketamine and morphine on descending pain modulation in chronic pain patients: A randomized placebo-controlled cross-over proof-of-concept study. *British Journal of Anaesthesia* 110, 1010–1016 (2013).

754 Gaskell, H., Moore, R.A., Derry, S. & Stannard, C. Oxycodone for neuropathic pain and fibromyalgia in adults. *Cochrane Database of Systematic Reviews* (2014).

755 Gaskell, H., Derry, S., Stannard, C. & Moore, R.A. Oxycodone for neuropathic pain in adults. *Cochrane Database of Systematic Reviews* (2016).

756 Maeda, M., Tsuruoka, M., Hayashi, B., Nagasawa, I. & Inoue, T. Descending pathways from activated locus coeruleus/subcoeruleus following unilateral hindpaw inflammation in the rat. *Brain Research Bulletin* 78, 170–174 (2009).

757 Caraci, F., *et al.* Rescue of noradrenergic system as a novel pharmacological strategy in the treatment of chronic pain: Focus on microglia activation. *Frontiers in Pharmacology* 10 (2019).

758 Parada, C.A., Vivancos, G.G., Tambeli, C.H., Cunha, F.D. & Ferreira, S.H. Activation of presynaptic NMDA receptors coupled to NaV1.8-resistant sodium channel C-fibers causes retrograde mechanical nociceptor sensitization. *Proceedings of the National Academy of Sciences of the United States of America* 100, 2923–2928 (2003).

759 Weber, C. NMDA receptor antagonists in pain therapy. *Anasthesiologie Intensivmedizin Notfallmedizin Schmerztherapie* 33, 475–483 (1998).

760 Angst, M.S., Koppert, W., Pahl, I., Clark, D.J. & Schmelz, M. Short-term infusion of the mu-opioid agonist remifentanil in humans causes hyperalgesia during withdrawal. *Pain* 106, 49–57 (2003).

761 Son, S. & Ko, S. Does intraoperative remifentanil infusion really make more postoperative pain? *Korean Journal of Anesthesiology* 61, 187–189 (2011).

762 Li, Y.Z., *et al.* Inhibition of glycogen synthase kinase-3 beta prevents remifentanil-induced hyperalgesia via regulating the expression and function of spinal N-methyl-D-aspartate receptors in vivo and vitro. *PLOS One* 8, Art. No. e77790 (2013).

[763] Roeckel, L.A., Le Coz, G.M., Gaveriaux-Ruff, C. & Simonin, F. Opioid-induced hyperalgesia: Cellular and molecular mechanisms. *Neuroscience* 338, 160–182 (2016).

[764] Boettger, M.K., Weber, K., Gajda, M., Brauer, R. & Schaible, H.G. Spinally applied ketamine or morphine attenuate peripheral inflammation and hyperalgesia in acute and chronic phases of experimental arthritis. *Brain Behavior and Immunity* 24, 474–485 (2010).

[765] Angst, M.S. & Clark, J.D. Opioid-induced hyperalgesia: A qualitative systematic review. *Anesthesiology* 104, 570–587 (2006).

[766] Sandkuhler, J. Models and mechanisms of hyperalgesia and allodynia. *Physiological Reviews* 89, 707–758 (2009).

[767] Colvin, L.A., Bull, F. & Hales, T.G. Perioperative opioid analgesia—when is enough too much? A review of opioid-induced tolerance and hyperalgesia. *Lancet* 393, 1558–1568 (2019).

[768] Fletcher, D. & Martinez, V. Opioid-induced hyperalgesia in patients after surgery: A systematic review and a meta-analysis. *British Journal of Anaesthesia* 112, 991–1004 (2014).

[769] Kars, M.S., *et al.* Fentanyl versus remifentanil-based TIVA for pediatric scoliosis repair: Does it matter? *Regional Anesthesia and Pain Medicine* 44, 627–631 (2019).

[770] Guo, W., *et al.* Long lasting pain hypersensitivity following ligation of the tendon of the masseter muscle in rats: A model of myogenic orofacial pain. *Molecular Pain* 6, Art. No. 40 (2010).

[771] Lee, L.H., Irwin, M.G. & Lui, S.K. Intraoperative remifentanil infusion does not increase postoperative opioid consumption compared with 70% nitrous oxide. *Anesthesiology* 102, 398–402 (2005).

[772] Cortinez, L.I., Brandes, V., Munoz, H.R., Guerrero, M.E. & Mur, M. No clinical evidence of acute opioid tolerance after remifentanil-based anaesthesia. *British Journal of Anaesthesia* 87, 866–869 (2001).

[773] Hansen, E.G., Duedahl, T.H., Romsing, J., Hilsted, K.L. & Dahl, J.B. Intra-operative remifentanil might influence pain levels in the immediate post-operative period after major abdominal surgery. *Acta Anaesthesiologica Scandinavica* 49, 1464–1470 (2005).

[774] Compton, P., Canamar, C.P., Hillhouse, M. & Ling, W. Hyperalgesia in heroin dependent patients and the effects of opioid substitution therapy. *Journal of Pain* 13, 401–409 (2012).

[775] Lee, M., Silverman, S., Hansen, H., Patel, V. & Manchikanti, L. A comprehensive review of opioid-induced hyperalgesia. *Pain Physician* 14, 145–161 (2011).

[776] Chu, L.F., Angst, M.S. & Clark, D. Opioid-induced hyperalgesia in humans: Molecular mechanisms and clinical considerations. *Clinical Journal of Pain* 24, 479–496 (2008).

[777] Chu, L.F., Dairmont, J., Zamora, A.K., Young, C.A. & Angst, M.S. The endogenous opioid systemi is not involved in modulation of opioid-induced hyperalgesia. *Journal of Pain* 12, 108–115 (2011).

[778] Fishbain, D.A., Cole, B., Lewis, J.E., Gao, J. & Rosomoff, R.S. Do opioids induce hyperalgesia in humans? An evidence-based structured review. *Database of Abstracts of Reviews of Effects (DARE): Quality-assessed Reviews* 10, 829–839 (2009).

[779] Higgins, C., Smith, B.H. & Matthews, K. Evidence of opioid-induced hyperalgesia in clinical populations after chronic opioid exposure: a systematic review and meta-analysis. *British Journal of Anaesthesia* 122, E114–E126 (2019).

[780] Mercadante, S., Ferrera, P., Arcuri, E. & Casuccio, A. Opioid-induced hyperalgesia after rapid titration with intravenous morphine: Switching and re-titration to intravenous methadone. *Annals of Palliative Medicine* 1, 10–13 (2012).

[781] Hooten, W.M., Mantilla, C.B., Sandroni, P. & Townsend, C.O. Associations between heat pain perception and opioid dose among patients with chronic pain undergoing opioid tapering. *Pain Medicine* 11, 1587–1598 (2010).

[782] Ruscheweyh, R., Stumpenhorst, F., Knecht, S. & Marziniak, M. Comparison of the cold pressor test and contact thermode-delivered cold stimuli for the assessment of cold pain sensitivity. *Journal of Pain* 11, 728–736 (2010).

[783] Cook, C.D. & Nickerson, M.D. Nociceptive sensitivity and opioid antinociception and antihyperalgesia in Freund's adjuvant-induced arthritic male and female rats. *Journal of Pharmacology and Experimental Therapeutics* 313, 449–459 (2005).

[784] Hay, J.L., *et al.* Hyperalgesia in opioid-managed chronic pain and opioid-dependent patients. *Journal of Pain from 11th World Congress on Pain* 10, 316–322 (2009).

[785] Doverty, M., *et al.* Methadone maintenance patients are cross-tolerant to the antinociceptive effects of morphine. *Pain* 93, 155–163 (2001).

[786] Compton, P., Charuvastra, V.C. & Ling, W. Pain intolerance in opioid-maintained former opiate addicts: Effect of long-acting maintenance agent. *Drug and Alcohol Dependence* 63, 139–146 (2001).

[787] Dyer, K.R., *et al.* Steady-state pharmacokinetics and pharmacodynamics in methadone maintenance patients: Comparison of those who do and do not experience withdrawal and concentration-effect relationships. *Clinical Pharmacology & Therapeutics* 65, 685–694 (1999).

[788] Ballantyne, J.C. Assessing the prevalence of opioid misuse, abuse, and addiction in chronic pain. *Pain* 156, 567–568 (2015).

[789] Santo, T., *et al.* Correlates of indicators of potential extra-medical opioid use in people prescribed opioids for chronic non-cancer pain. *Drug and Alcohol Review* 39, 128–134 (2020).

[790] Wachholtz, A., Gonzalez, G. & Ziedonis, D. Psycho-physiological response to pain among individuals with comorbid pain and opioid use disorder: Implications for patients with prolonged abstinence. *American Journal of Drug and Alcohol Abuse* 45, 495–505 (2019).

[791] Volkow, N.D., Jones, E.B., Einstein, E.B. & Wargo, E.M. Prevention and treatment of opioid misuse and addiction: A review. *JAMA Psychiatry* 76, 208–216 (2019).

[792] Chabal, C., Erjavec, M.K., Jacobson, L., Mariano, A. & Chaney, E. Prescription opiate abuse in chronic pain patients: Clinical criteria, incidence, and predictors. *Clinical Journal of Pain* 13, 150–155 (1997).

[793] Weaver, M. & Schnoll, S. Abuse liability in opioid therapy for pain treatment in patients with an addiction history. *Clinical Journal of Pain* 18, S61–S69 (2002).

[794] Gilam, G., *et al.* Negative affect-related factors have the strongest association with prescription opioid misuse in a cross-sectional cohort of patients with chronic pain. *Pain Medicine* 21, E127–E138 (2020).

[795] Fishman, S.M. Commentary in response to Paulozzi et al.: Prescription drug abuse and safe pain management. *Pharmacoepidemiology and Drug Safety* 15, 628–631 (2006).

[796] Solomon, R.L. The opponent process theory of acquired motivation: The costs of pleasure and the benefits of pain. *American Psychologist* 35, 691–712 (1980).

[797] Solomon, R.L. & Corbit, J.D. Opponent-process theory of motivation 1: Temporal dynamics of affect. *Psychological Review* 81, 119–145 (1974).

[798] Koob, G.F. & Le Moal, M. Addiction and the brain antireward system. *Annual Review of Psychology* 59, 29–53 (2008).

[799] Koob, G.F. & Le Moal, M. Drug addiction, dysregulation of reward, and allostasis. *Neuropsychopharmacology* 24, 97–129 (2001).

[800] Koob, G.F. Neurobiology of opioid addiction: Opponent process, hyperkatifeia, and negative reinforcement. *Biological Psychiatry* 87, 44–53 (2020).

[801] Borsook, D., Youssef, A.M., Simons, L., Elman, I. & Eccleston, C. When pain gets stuck: The evolution of pain chronification and treatment resistance. *Pain* 159, 2421–2436 (2018).

[802] Leknes, S., Brooks, J.C.W., Wiech, K. & Tracey, I. Pain relief as an opponent process: A psychophysical investigation. *European Journal of Neuroscience* 28, 794–801 (2008).

[803] Small, D.M., Zatorre, R.J., Dagher, A., Evans, A.C. & Jones-Gotman, M. Changes in brain activity related to eating chocolate: From pleasure to aversion. *Brain* 124, 1720–1733 (2001).

[804] Kringelbach, M.L., O'Doherty, J., Rolls, E.T. & Andrews, C. Activation of the human orbitofrontal cortex to a liquid food stimulus is correlated with its subjective pleasantness. *Cerebral Cortex* 13, 1064–1071 (2003).

[805] Cabanac, M. Sensory pleasure. *Quarterly Review of Biology* 54, 1–29 (1979).

[806] Raheemullah, A., Andruska, N., Saeed, M. & Kumar, P. Improving residency education on chronic pain and opioid use disorder: Evaluation of CDC Guideline-based education. *Substance Use & Misuse* 55, 684–690 (2019).

[807] Turk, D.C., Brody, M.C. & Okifuji, E.A. Physicians attitudes and practices regarding the long-term prescribing of opioids for noncancer pain. *Pain* 59, 201–208 (1994).

[808] Huang, Z.R., *et al.* Clinical consumption of opioid analgesics in China: A retrospective analysis of the national and regional data 2006–2016. *Journal of Pain and Symptom Management* 59, 829–835 (2020).

[809] Lewy, J. The army disease: Drug addiction and the civil war. *War in History* 21, 102–119 (2014).

[810] Courtwright, D.T. Dark Paradise: A History of Opiate Addiction in America. Cambridge, MA, Harvard University Press (2001).

[811] Kandall, S.R. Women and addiction in the United States—1850 to 1920. *Substance and Shadow: A History of Women and Addiction in the United States—1850 to the Present.* Cambridge, MA; Harvard University Press (1996).

[812] Supreme & Court. Linder v. United States. *US 5* 268 (1925).

[813] McNamara, J.D. The drug war: The American junkie. *Hoover Digest* No. 2. Spring issue (2004).

[814] Jenerette, C.M. & Brewer, C. Health-related stigma in young adults with sickle cell disease. *Journal of the National Medical Association* 102, 1050–1055 (2010).

[815] Bulgin, D., Tanabe, P. & Jenerette, C. Stigma of sickle cell disease: A systematic review. *Issues in Mental Health Nursing* 39, 675–686 (2018).

[816] Sinha, C.B., Bakshi, N., Ross, D. & Krishnamurti, L. Management of chronic pain in adults living with sickle cell disease in the era of the opioid epidemic A qualitative study. *JAMA Network Open* 2, Art. No. e194410 (2019).

[817] Gallegos, A. CDC clarifies opioid prescribing guidelines in cancer, sickle cell disease. *Hematology News.* April 15 (2019).

[818] Wyatt, R. Pain and ethnicity. *American Medical Association Journal of Ethics* 15, 449–454 (2013).

[819] Furlan, A.D., Sandoval, J.A., Mailis-Gagnon, A. & Tunks, E. Opioids for chronic noncancer pain: A meta-analysis of effectiveness and side effects. *Canadian Medical Association Journal* 174, 1589–1594 (2006).

[820] Busse, J.W., *et al.* Opioids for chronic non-cancer pain: A protocol for a systematic review of randomized controlled trials. *Systematic Reviews* 2 (2013).

[821] Kahan, M., Mailis-Gagnon, A. & Tunks, E. Canadian guideline for safe and effective use of opioids for chronic non-cancer pain: Implications for pain physicians. *Pain Research & Management* 16, 157–158 (2011).

[822] Kahan, M. & Srivastava, A. Canadian guideline for safe and effective use of opioids for chronic non-cancer pain: A primer for addiction medicine physicians. *Canadian Journal of Addiction* 1, 14–24 (2010).

[823] Kalso, E., *et al.* Recommendations for using opioids in chronic non-cancer pain. *European Journal of Pain* 7, 381–386 (2003).

[824] Gallagher, H. & Galvin, D. Opioids for chronic non-cancer pain. *BJA Education* 18, 337–341 (2018).

[825] Asthana, R., *et al.* Framing of the opioid problem in cancer pain management in Canada. *Current Oncology* 26, E410–E413 (2019).

[826] Hauser, W., Schubert, T., Scherbaum, N. & Tolle, T. Guideline-recommended vs high-dose long-term opioid therapy for chronic noncancer pain is associated with better health outcomes: Data from a representative sample of the German population. *Pain* 159, 85–91 (2018).

[827] Moisset, X., *et al.* Use of strong opioids in chronic non-cancer pain in adults: Evidence-based recommendations from the French society for the study and treatment of pain. *Presse Medicale* 45, 447–462 (2016).

[828] Bannwarth, B., Bertin, P. & Queneau, P. Strong opioids for chronic non-cancer pain. *Presse Medicale* 30, 947–950 (2001).

[829] Khazan, O. How France cut heroin overdoses by 79 percent in 4 years. *The Atlantic.* April 16 (2018).

[830] Clay, R.A. How Portugal is solving its opioid problem *American Psychological Association* 49, 20 (2018).

[831] Ferreira, S. Portugal's radical drugs policy is working. Why hasn't the world copied it? *The Guardian.* December 5, 2017 (2017).

[832] Sumitani, M., *et al.* Executive summary of the clinical guidelines of pharmacotherapy for neuropathic pain: Second edition by the Japanese society of pain clinicians. *Journal of Anesthesia* 32, 463–478 (2018).

[833] Shindo, Y., Iwasaki, S. & Yamakage, M. Efficacy and practicality of opioid therapy in Japanese chronic noncancer pain patients. *Pain Management Nursing* 20, 222–231 (2019).

[834] Kim, E.D., *et al.* Guidelines for prescribing opioids for chronic non-cancer pain in Korea. *Korean Journal of Pain* 30, 18–33 (2017).

[835] Allan, L., *et al.* Randomised crossover trial of transdermal fentanyl and sustained release oral morphine for treating chronic non-cancer pain. *British Medical Journal* 322, 1154–1158 (2001).

[836] Rowbotham, M.C., Reisnerkeller, L.A. & Fields, H.L. Both intravenous lidocaine and morphine reduce the pain of postherpetic neuralgia. *Neurology* 41, 1024–1028 (1991).

[837] Dellemijn, P.L.I. & Vanneste, J.A.L. Randomised double-blind active-placebo-controlled crossover trial of intravenous fentanyl in neuropathic pain. *Lancet* 349, 753–758 (1997).

[838] Gostick, N., Allen, J. & Cranfield, R. A comparison of the efficacy and adverse effects of controlled-release dihydrocodeine and immediate-release dihydrocodeine in the treatment of pain in osteoarthritis and chronic back pain. In Twycross RG, ed. *Proceedings of The Edinburgh Symposium on Pain Control and Medical Education*, 137–143 (1989).

[839] Harke, H., Gretenkort, P., Ladleif, H.U., Rahman, S. & Harke, O. The response of neuropathic pain and pain in complex regional pain syndrome I

to carbamazepine and sustained-release morphine in patients pretreated with spinal cord stimulation: A double-blinded randomized study. *Anesthesia and Analgesia* 92, 488–495 (2001).

840 Eriksen, J., Sjogren, P., Bruera, E., Ekholm, O. & Rasmussen, N.K. Critical issues on opioids in chronic non-cancer pain: An epidemiological study. *Pain* 125, 172–179 (2006).

841 Wiffen, P.J., Derry, S., Naessens, K. & Bell, R.F. Oral tapentadol for cancer pain. *Cochrane Database of Systematic Reviews* (2015).

842 Imanaka, K., *et al.* Efficacy and safety of oral tapentadol extended release in Japanese and Korean patients with moderate to severe, chronic malignant tumor-related pain. *Current Medical Research and Opinion* 29, 1399–1409 (2013).

843 Devulder, J., Richarz, U. & Nataraja, S.H. Impact of long-term use of opioids on quality of life in patients with chronic, non-malignant pain. *Current Medical Research and Opinion* 21, 1555–1568 (2005).

844 Milligan, K., *et al.* Evaluation of long-term efficacy and safety of transdermal fentanyl in the treatment of chronic noncancer pain. *Journal of Pain* 2, 197–204 (2001).

845 Strumpf, M., Dertwinkel, R., Wiebalck, A., Bading, B. & Zenz, M. Role of opioid analgesics in the treatment of chronic non-cancer pain. *CNS Drugs* 14, 147–155 (2000).

846 Strumpf, M., Willweber-Strumpf, A., Herberg, K.W. & Zenz, M. Safety-relevant performance of patients on chronic opioid therapy. *Schmerz* 19, 426–433 (2005).

847 Strumpf, M., Linstedt, U., Wiebalck, A. & Zenz, M. Treatment of low back pain: Significance, principles and danger. *Schmerz* 15, 453–460 (2001).

848 Sommer, C., Klose, P., Welsch, P., Petzke, F. & Hauser, W. Opioids for chronic non-cancer neuropathic pain: An updated systematic review and meta-analysis of efficacy, tolerability and safety in randomized placebo-controlled studies of at least 4 weeks' duration. *European Journal of Pain* 24, 3–18 (2019).

849 George, J.M., Menon, M., Gupta, P. & Tan, M.G.E. Use of strong opioids for chronic non-cancer pain: a retrospective analysis at a pain centre in Singapore. *Singapore Medical Journal* 54, 506–510 (2013).

850 Welsch, P., Petzke, F., Klose, P. & Hauser, W. Opioids for chronic osteoarthritis pain: An updated systematic review and meta-analysis of efficacy, tolerability and safety in randomized placebo-controlled studies of at least 4 weeks double-blind duration. *European Journal of Pain* 24, 685–703 (2020).

851 Hermans, L., *et al.* Influence of morphine and naloxone on pain modulation in rheumatoid arthritis, chronic fatigue syndrome/fibromyalgia, and controls: A double-blind, randomized, placebo-controlled, cross-over study. *Pain Practice* 18, 418–430 (2018).

[852] Le Loet, X., Pavelka, K. & Richarz, U. Transdermal fentanyl for the treatment of pain caused by osteoarthritis of the knee or hip: An open, multicentre study. *BMC Musculoskeletal Disorders* 6, Art. No. 31 (2005).

[853] Roux, P., *et al.* Buprenorphine/naloxone as a promising therapeutic option for opioid abusing patients with chronic pain: Reduction of pain, opioid withdrawal symptoms, and abuse liability of oral oxycodone. *Pain* 154, 1442–1448 (2013).

[854] Laird, B.J.A., et al. Cancer pain and its relationship to systemic inflammation: An exploratory study. *Pain* 152, 460–463 (2011).

[855] Chatham, M.S., Ashley, E.S.D., Svengsouk, J.S. & Juba, K.M. Dose Ratios between High Dose Oral Morphine or Equivalents and Oral Methadone. *Journal of Palliative Medicine* 16, 947–950 (2013).

ABOUT THE AUTHOR

⥬

Stefan Franzen is a professor of chemistry at North Carolina State, specializing in physical and biophysical chemistry. He received a BS in chemistry at the University of California in Berkeley in 1982 and a PhD in physical chemistry at Stanford University in 1992. He served in the US Peace Corps in Kenya from 1982 to 1985. His primary research areas at North Carolina State are the structure and function of multifunctional enzymes, infrared plasmonic materials from conducting metal oxides, and plant virus biotechnology. He has published more than two hundred peer-reviewed research journal articles. He became an expert in biomedical research based on research on plant viruses as drug-delivery agents in collaboration with groups from Duke University and University of North Carolina Medical Schools. In the field of education, he had taught physical chemistry to premedical students for many years. He initiated several major study-abroad programs in both Poznan, Poland; and Hangzhou, China; where has conducted research and published with research groups. He is fluent in Swedish, Dutch, German, French, Spanish, Polish, Chinese, Portuguese, Italian, Swahili, and Russian. Dr. Franzen's interest in pain management and research is based on personal experience. Although he himself is not a pain patient, he has witnessed the workings of pain clinics and the attitudes of medical professionals from firsthand experience. He gives a unique perspective on the issues of pain and addiction. His goal is to provide a comprehensive view of the issues that affect pain patients when they seek medical care.

CPSIA information can be obtained
at www.ICGtesting.com
Printed in the USA
BVHW080628110921
616280BV00001B/4